International Handbook of
Medical Education

International Handbook of Medical Education

A Guide for Students

Edited by
Ibrahim Al Alwan
Mohi Eldin Magzoub
Margaret Elzubeir

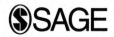

Los Angeles • London • New Delhi • Singapore • Washington DC

SAGE Publications Ltd
1 Oliver's Yard
55 City Road
London EC1Y 1SP

SAGE Publications Inc.
2455 Teller Road
Thousand Oaks, California 91320

SAGE Publications India Pvt Ltd
B 1/I 1 Mohan Cooperative Industrial Area
Mathura Road
New Delhi 110 044

SAGE Publications Asia-Pacific Pte Ltd
3 Church Street
10-04 Samsung Hub
Singapore 049483

Library of Congress Control Number: 2011942341

British Library Cataloguing in Publication data

A catalogue record for this book is available from the British Library

ISBN 978-1-4462-4721-1 (pbk)

Typeset by Cenveo Publisher Services
Printed and bound by CPI Group (UK) Ltd, Croydon,
CR0 4YY (for Antony Rowe)
Printed on paper from sustainable resources

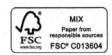

Contents

Foreword

World events, dwindling educational opportunities for Saudi students abroad and an ever-increasing population in demand of high quality healthcare, were contributing factors that led to the establishment of King Saud bin Abdulaziz University of Health Sciences in Riyadh, Saudi Arabia, in 2005.

The university staff is unique in that it is made up of international experts from the four corners of the world. Another unique characteristic of our university is that our academic programs comprise curricula that have been adopted from prestigious universities in the United States, Australia and Europe, as well as locally developed curricula profiting from both Saudi and international expertise in medical education. This blend of experts and expertly developed curricula has proved to be a very successful model for us and, I believe, one that makes us uniquely qualified to write an international handbook for students in medical education.

As University President, I face the dilemmas encountered by other institutes of higher education worldwide. That is, how to make the most of our resources while balancing the advantage of smaller classroom sizes with the demands for increased enrolment to meet the healthcare needs of our country. The answer for many of us was found in an innovative student-centered and, in some cases, student-directed learning environment that is well structured and adequately assessed to ensure excellent outcomes. However, for such a model to be successful, we realized that our students must possess the study skills necessary to be capable, independent, life-long learners. In recognizing this need, we reached out to other international experts in medical education, only to find that very little student-focused information was available. This shortfall became the driving force behind our university's quest to develop a handbook to guide students, not only in Saudi Arabia but internationally as well, through the conundrums of medical education.

I trust that this handbook will become an invaluable resource for students, and hope that it is only the first of editions to come, as we adapt and update our knowledge to meet the ever-changing and ever-challenging innovations in medical education.

Bandar Al Knawy
President
King Saud bin Abdulaziz University for Health Sciences

Editors and Contributors

Editors

Dr Ibrahim Al Alwan, MRCP (UK), FAAP, FRCPC, is Dean of the College of Medicine and Associate Professor of Pediatrics at King Saud bin Abdulaziz University for Health Sciences (KSAU-HS). Dr Al Alwan also serves as a Consultant, Pediatrician, and Pediatric Endocrinologist at the National Guard Health Affairs. In March 2011, he was also appointed President of the Association for Medical Education in the Eastern Mediterranean Region (AMEEMR).

Professor Margaret Elzubeir, BA (Hons), PhD, has been contributing to innovations in health professions education in the UK and the Middle East for over twenty years. She undertook her undergraduate and postgraduate education in Education and Educational Psychology at the University of Wales, College of Cardiff, UK. Professor Elzubeir was a Senior Lecturer and Director of Small Group Learning at Peninsula College of Medicine & Dentistry in UK prior to joining King Saud bin Abdulaziz University for Health Sciences, responsible for the Curriculum Development Unit of the Department of Medical Education and Coordinator of two Blocks in the Masters in Medical Education Program.

Professor Mohi Eldin Mohamed Ali Magzoub, MBBS, MSc, PhD, MFPHM, is Chairman of the Department of Medical Education, College of Medicine, King Saud bin Abdulaziz University for Health Sciences (KSAU-HS). His teaching and research interests include a wide range of topics in Medical Education and Community Medicine: Problem-Based Learning, Community-Based Medicine, and Epidemiology and Health System Management.

Contributors

Dr Zulkifli Ahmad is Professor of Public Health at the School of Medical Sciences, Universiti Sains Malaysia. He obtained his Bachelor of Medicine and Surgery degree from the University of Malaya, and Masters in Public Health from University of Sydney, Australia, and his PhD from the University of Malaya. Dr Zulkifli's research interests are in child health issues, tobacco control, and community-based education.

Dr Nadia Al Attas, Pediatrician and Medical Educationalist at the College of Medicine, King Saud bin Abdulaziz University for Health Sciences (KSAU-HS).

She is involved in student assessment, educational project development, and faculty enhancement activities. Her current focus is on simulation-based education.

Dr Hanan Al Kadri, Assistant Professor, is Associate Dean, Female Medical Student Branch, College of Medicine, King Saud bin Abdulaziz University for Health Sciences, Riyadh, Saudi Arabia, and Consultant, Obstetrics and Gynaecology, at the National Guard Health Affairs. Her major interests/working fields are high-risk pregnancy, pediatrics, gynaecology, and medical education (student assessment).

Mohamed S. Al Moamary is Assistant Vice President, Educational Affairs, King Saud bin Abdulaziz University for Health Sciences (KSAU-HS), and an Associate Professor and Consultant Pulmonologist at King Abdulaziz Medical City, Riyadh, Saudi Arabia. He was the founding Associate Dean, Clinical Affairs, College of Medicine, KSAU-HS, from 2006 to 2011. He has led the initiative to integrate patient safety in the medical curriculum and introduced an innovative framework for medical interns' competencies. He is the primary author of the Saudi Initiative for Asthma, and has published many scientific papers in pulmonary medicine and medical education. Dr Al Moamary is the founding editor-in-chief of the *Annals of Thoracic Medicine*.

Dr Ahmed Al Rumayyan is Associate Dean, Academic and Student Affairs, College of Medicine, KSAU-HS, Riyadh, Saudi Arabia. He is a graduate of King Saud University, Riyadh (1983–1989), obtaining his MBBS in 1990. He completed his Pediatric Residency Training (1993–1996) at the Children's Hospital, University of Manitoba, Canada, and his Pediatric Neurology Fellowship Training (1997–1999) at the Children's Hospital, University of British Columbia, Canada. Dr Al Rumayyan was certified by the American Board of Pediatrics (1996) and the Royal College of Physicians and Surgeons of Canada in Pediatrics (1997). He was also certified by the Royal College of Physicians and Surgeons of Canada in Neurology (2001). Following his return to Saudi Arabia, Dr Al Rumayyan was appointed Consultant, Pediatric Neurologist, and later Head of the Division of Pediatric Neurology, where he served from 2002 to 2010. Dr Al Rumayyan was appointed Deputy Director of the Ambulatory Care Center, KAMC-Riyadh, from 2006. In addition to his clinical and administrative appointments, Dr Al Rumayyan was an Honorary Clinical Assistant Professor at the College of Medicine, King Saud University, Riyadh, from 2003 to 2005. He joined the College of Medicine, KSAU-HS, Riyadh, as an Assistant Professor of Pediatrics in December 2005. He obtained his Masters Degree in Medical Education from KSAU-HS in June 2010. Dr Al Rumayyan is an active member on several KAMC committees, has presented a number of research studies, published several articles, and has attended many different national and international conferences and symposiums.

Dr Tariq Al Tokhais, MBBS, Registrar, Plastic Surgery, King Khalid University, Riyadh, Saudi Arabia, and at present a Fellow Resident, Pediatric Surgery, King Fahad National Guard Hospital, Riyadh.

Dr Abdullah Mohammed Al Zahem, BDS, MME, works as a program director in National Guard Health Affairs and King Saud bin Abdulaziz University for Health Sciences, with responsibility for all dental training programs and the postgraduate AEGD residency program, in addition to his practice in the Orofacial Pain Clinic as consultant. He has done research in the field of dentistry related to stress, dental education, and orofacial pain. He lectured nationally and internationally with innovative instructional methods including problem-based learning. He focuses on stress management for dental students and its relation with curricula construction.

Dr Zubair Amin is a practicing pediatrician and medical educator. He is Associate Professor in Pediatrics and Assistant Dean for Education at the Yong Loo Lin School of Medicine, National University of Singapore. Dr Amin has a Masters in Health Profession Education (MHPE) from the University of Illinois, Chicago, USA. His interests in medical education are in faculty development, assessment, and international medical education. He is one of the editors of *Medical Education Online* and *Anatomical Science Educators*.

Andleeb Arshad has worked as a Medical Educationist in universities in Saudi Arabia and Pakistan. He is also a Medical Education Consultant for the Ministry of Health, Saudi Arabia. He has enjoyed supervisory roles in Faculty Enhancement, e-Learning, and Program Evaluation. He has been involved in setting up three Masters in Medical Education programs internationally. He has an excellent academic track record, with an Overall Merit in the postgraduate degree. He received his MBBS from Sind Medical College, Pakistan, and his MA in Education from University of Leeds, United Kingdom. He has written about, and made numerous presentations, on innovations in Teaching and Learning.

Hanan Balkhy, MD, MMed, FAAP, CIC, is Assistant Professor of Pediatric Infectious Diseases, College of Medicine, King Saud bin Abdulaziz University, for Health Sciences (KSAU-HS), and Deputy Executive Director, Infection Prevention and Control, National Guard Health Affairs. Dr Balkhy also holds the position of Head, Research Promotion and Education Section, King Abdullah International Medical Research Center, KSAU-HS.

Professor John Bligh, BSc, MBChB, MMEd, MA, MD, FRCGP, Hon FAcadMEd, is Dean of Medical Education, Cardiff University School of Medicine, UK. He has wide international experience of curriculum design and reform, and was formerly International Fellow for Saudi Arabia for the Royal College of General Practitioners. He led the Expert Advisory Panel on assessment and selection for the Tooke Inquiry into Modernising Medical Careers, and was editor-in-chief of *Medical Education* between 1998 and 2005. He is the author or co-author of over 150 published papers, and his most recent book, co-authored with Alan Bleakley and Julie Browne, is *Medical Education for the Future: Identity, Power and Location*.

Geke A. Blok is Head of Medical Education and Science at the Reinier de Graaf Teaching Hospital in Delft, the Netherlands. Formerly, she worked at the University of Maastricht. She is interested in several aspects of professional learning, learning on the job, and student-centered learning. Her current work and research aims at professional development, assessment of professional competence, design of powerful (professional) learning environments, and expertise development in professional education. She has ample experience with the development of curricula and educational programmes, training with simulation patients, faculty/ clinical teacher development and assessment of competence of faculty/clinical teachers. She is also a clinical psychologist and a registered psychotherapist.

Julie Browne, BA, FAcadMEd, is External Relations Manager at the School of Postgraduate Medical and Dental Education, Cardiff University: The Wales Deanery, UK. Her professional background is in publishing, and she was formerly Managing Editor of *Medical Education* and *The Clinical Teacher*. She coordinated the work of the Expert Advisory Panel on assessment for the Tooke Inquiry into Modernising Medical Careers. She was Executive Officer of the Academy of Medical Educators from 2007 to 2010. Her published work focuses primarily on medical education publishing, ethics, and practices.

Dr Susan Case is Director of Testing, National Conference of Bar Examiners, since 2001. Prior to this, she was Senior Evaluation Officer, National Board of Medical Examiners, from 1976 to 2001 (25 years). Her education list includes the University of Connecticut (1966–1968); Wheaton College (MA) (1964–1966); and Northfield Mt. Hermon.

Nayef Dajim, BSc (PT), MBBS, is Resident, Orthopaedics Surgery Department, King Fahad Medical City, Riyadh, Saudi Arabia. He graduated from King Saud bin Abdulaziz University for Health Sciences with Bachelor of Medicine and Surgery in July 2009 and finished his Compulsory Internship (September 2009–August 2010) at the same university. He also holds the degree of Bachelor of Physical Therapy and Rehabilitation Sciences from King Saud University (September 2000–July 2005). Dr Dajim is an active member of the IFMSA, Riyadh Chapter.

Diana H. J. M. Dolmans, PhD, is an educational psychologist. She works as an associate professor at the Department of Educational Development and Research, Maastricht University, Faculty of Health Medicine and Life Sciences, the Netherlands. Her research interests are in problem-based learning.

Robert J. Duvivier is an MD/PhD student from Maastricht University, the Netherlands. His research focuses on clinical skills. He has been involved in medical education issues on the local, national, and international levels. He was recently elected Liaison Officer on Medical Education issues to the executive board of the International Federation of Medical Students' Associations (IFMSA), representing medical students on the executive board of the AMEE and executive council of the WFME. He has also worked with WHO in its Reference Group on Medical Education as expert consultant.

Hana M. A. Fakhoury is an assistant professor at the Department of Basic Sciences, College of Medicine, King Saud bin Abdulaziz University for Health Sciences. In 1992, Dr Fakhoury obtained her Bachelor of Science degree in Biology from the American University of Beirut, and completed her Doctor of Philosophy degree in Biochemistry and Molecular Biology at the Victoria University of Manchester, UK, in 1998. She worked at the same university for five years, which qualified her for the title of Senior Postdoctoral Fellow. Dr Fakhoury is an active researcher with several publications in medical journals, including *The Lancet*.

Rania Ghazi Zaini, PhD, is Associate Dean of E-Learning and Distance Learning, and Assistant Professor of Medical Education at the Umm Al-Qua University, Makkah, Saudi Arabia.

Willem de Grave, PhD, received his doctorate from Maastricht University in 1998 and is now an Educational Psychologist at the Department of Educational Development and Research, Faculty of Health, Medicine and Life Sciences, Maastricht University. His major interests are in the areas of PBL and Faculty Development. His research work is focused on PBL (cognitive processes in tutorial groups, the Role of the Tutor). He has served as an Educational Consultant in PBL in higher education and has produced several video tapes about PBL.

Ali H. Hajeer is Chairman, Department of Basic Medical Sciences, College of Medicine at King Saud bin Abdulaziz University for Health Sciences.

Emily Hall, MD, is a resident in Obstetrics and Gynecology at New York Methodist Hospital and a graduate of Columbia University's College of Physicians and Surgeons. Her research interests include medical education, team training, and patient safety. Prior to medical school, Dr Hall spent six years as a writer and a senior analyst at Morningstar in Chicago. Emily serves as educational consultant on projects where her experiences as a medical student, writer, and scholar converge. This includes consulting with faculty implementing team-based learning for the first time.

Professor Bashir Hamad, MBBS, MD, DTPH, DCMT, Dip Ed (medical), is the founding Dean of Faculty of Medicine, University of Gezira, Sudan (1979–1984) and Faculty of Medicine and Health Sciences, United Arab Emirates University (1986–1989). Known for innovative, community-oriented, and problem-solving approaches, Professor Hamad was the Regional Advisor in health personnel education in EMRO (1984) and a Consultant on Education Development at WHO/EMRO (1990). He was also a member of the Executive Committee of the World Federation for Medical Education (WFME) and an adjunct professor of health professions at the Department of Medical Education at the Medical Center, University of Illinois, Chicago. His research work and publications are mainly in student health, tropical medicine, and health professions education.

Professor Hossam Hamdy, an international authority on medical education, is currently serving as Vice Chancellor for the Medical and Health Sciences Colleges, and Dean for the College of Medicine, University of Sharjah, UAE. Prior to this, he served as a Senior Consultant in Pediatric Surgery at Qassimi Hospital in UAE. He graduated with honors from the Faculty of Medicine, Alexandria University, Egypt, in 1967. He completed his Fellowship in Medical Education at Boston University, USA, and earned his PhD in Medical Education from the University of Groningen, the Netherlands. He is a Fellow of the Royal College of Surgeons (Edinburgh) and American College of Surgeons. He has also served as Director of Medical Education for the Ministry of Health in Bahrain, and as Dean for the College of Medicine and Medical Sciences in the Arabian Gulf University.

Professor John Hamilton has worked extensively in Africa and has been centrally involved in innovative schools in McMaster (Canada), Ilorin (Nigeria), Durham (England), and was Dean in Newcastle, Australia. He graduated in 1960, and was Chair of the Australian Medical Council accreditation committee, and the Australian Quality of Health Care study. He was Chair of the WHO Diarrheal Disease Control programme and Consultant in Medical Education. He is now Professor Emeritus at Newcastle and assists medical schools in many countries. In 2006, he was appointed an Officer of the Order of the British Empire (OBE) by Her Majesty the Queen for services to international medical education.

Peter H. Harasym, PhD, Med, Bed, BSc, is Associate Dean of International Affairs and CFD, College of Medicine, I-Shou University, and Professor of Healthcare Administration, College of Medicine, I-Shou University. Professor Harasym is a recipient of Medical Educational Consultant (1988–2010) award from the WHO. Prior to his appointment at the I-Shou University, he was Professor, Department of Community Health Sciences, Faculty of Medicine, University of Calgary, Alberta.

Professor Ronald M. Harden, OBE, MD, FRCP (GLAS), FRCPC, FRCSEd, is the General Secretary, Association of Medical Education in Europe, and editor of *Medical Teacher*. He has held posts as Professor of Medical Education, Director of the Centre for Medical Education, and Teaching Dean, University of Dundee, UK. He also has an appointment as Professor of Medical Education at Al-Imam University, Riyadh, Saudi Arabia. He is a leading authority in medical education and has published more than 400 papers on the subject. He has received numerous awards for his contribution to medical education, including the Karolinska Prize for Research in Medical Education.

Professor Clarke Hazlett is Professor Emeritus Faculty of Medicine at the University of Alberta (Edmonton), Canada, where he is Chair of Community Medicine and Public Health Sciences. He continues to be an Adjunct Professor at the Chinese University of Hong Kong (China) after his retirement as Professor of Medical Education for 16 years (1993–2008). Professor Hazlett established the IDEAL Consortium at the Chinese University of Hong Kong and is presently serving as the consortium's Secretary-General. During his academic career, he has run over 120 faculty development workshops, across 22 countries, on topics such as EBM, teaching enhancement, presentation skills, life-long learning, grant writing, preparing publications, and assessment.

Rogayah Jaafar is Professor of Medical Education at the School of Medical Sciences, Universiti Sains Malaysia, and was the founding Head of the Department of Medical Education during its inception in 1986. She obtained her Bachelor of Medicine and Surgery degree from the University of Cairo, Egypt, Master of Health Professional Education from the University of New South Wales, Australia, and her postgraduate fellowship certificate in Health Leadership Development from the University of Chicago, USA. Dr Rogayah's research interests include curriculum development, problem-based learning, community-based medical education, partnership and leadership development, and women's health issues.

Rachelle Kamp holds an MSc degree in Cognitive Neurosciences and an MSc degree in Educational Sciences. Since November 2008, she is a PhD candidate at the department of Educational Development and Research at Maastricht University, the Netherlands. Her PhD deals with problem-based learning and focuses on peer ratings about students' contributions to the tutorial group and their relationship with students' test scores.

Rana Faisal Kattan is a pediatrician (Saudi and Arab Board certified). She took her Masters Degree in Medical Education from King Saud bin Abdulaziz University for Health Sciences (KSAU-HS), Riyadh. She is currently working in King Abdulaziz Medical City as an Associate Consultant in General Pediatrics and Chief of Clinical Services. She is an active member of the Pediatric Residency educational committee and has contributed as a clinical supervisor to the Pediatric Block (College of Medicine, KSAU-HS). She is involved in research programs and as a mentor in research summer school, and has co-directed a course about scientific writing conducted in Riyadh and Jeddah, Saudi Arabia.

Silvia Mamede is a scientific researcher at Erasmus University Rotterdam, Institute of Psychology and Department of Internal Medicine. She graduated as a physician at the Federal University of Ceará, Brazil, holds a Master's degree from the Instituto Superiore di Sanitá, Italy (1999), and a PhD from the Erasmus University Rotterdam (2006), with studies on the reflective practice in medicine conducted under the supervision of Professor Henk G. Schmidt. From 1995 to 2003, she was the Dean of the School of Public Health in Ceará, Brazil, one of the first institutions to adopt problem-based learning for health profession's higher education in the country.

Fadi Munshi, MD, MSc, PhD (c), is a graduate student in medical education at the University of Calgary, and is a Medical Educator at King Fahad Medical City, Saudi Arabia. He was a graduate student at Maastricht University (2006–2008); a Neurology Resident at King Fahad Medical City (2003–2006); and graduated as a Medical Student from Umm Al-Qura University, Saudi Arabia (1996–2002).

Dr Samuel Scott Obenshain, Emeritus Professor of Pediatrics and Family and Community Medicine, University of New Mexico School of Medicine. He joined the faculty as an Assistant Professor and Director of Ambulatory Pediatrics in 1970. He was appointed Assistant Dean and later Associate Dean of Undergraduate Medical Education in 1973, a position he held for over 30 years. He retired from the University in 2003 and assumed the position of Executive Dean of Ross University School of Medicine in Dominica for one-and-a-half-years.

Melinda Perlo, MA, recently concluded her masters in Educational Psychology at Teachers College, Columbia University, and served as an educational specialist in the Center for Education Research and Evaluation at Columbia University Medical Center. Prior to moving to New York, she worked at the David Geffen School of Medicine at UCLA.

Jamie Read is currently in the second year of his postgraduation from the Peninsula Medical School in South West England, UK. His current post is in both general medicine and medical education, which involves the teaching and training of medical students, nursing staff and junior doctors in the South West Peninsula. He is also involved with the Academy of Medical Educators and Chairs one of the working groups focused on supporting careers in medical education. His career aims are to pursue a profession in an acute medical specialty while maintaining a strong link to medical education.

Boyd Richards is Assistant Vice President for Education Research and Evaluation at the Columbia University. Since earning a PhD from Indiana University in Instructional Systems Technology, Dr Richards has focused his administrative, service, and research activities on educational scholarship and promotions, teaching academies, clinical performance examinations, problem-based learning curricula, team-based learning interventions, and programs for improving faculty teaching, all within medical education. He also serves on the editorial board for MedEdPortal and Teaching and Learning in Medicine, and as consulting editor for *Academic Medicine*. He formerly served as editor of the Performance Improvement Quarterly.

Dr Chris Roberts, MBChB, DRCOG, MRCGP, ILTHE, M.Med.Sci, PhD, is Associate Professor in Medical Education, Associate Dean (Educational Development), and Director of the Office of Postgraduate Medical Education at the University of Sydney. Prior to these appointments, he was Associate Dean (Learning and Teaching) and Director of the Centre for Professional Health Education and Research, University of Sydney. He is involved in a number of collaborative projects themed around assessment and clinical education.

Henk G. Schmidt holds professorial positions at Maastricht University and Erasmus University, the Netherlands. Presently, he is Rector Magnificus of Erasmus University. His research interests are learning and memory, and have publications on problem-based learning, long-term memory, and the development of expertise in medicine. He received numerous awards for his work in medical education, among them honorary degree of the Université de Sherbrooke in Canada and the Distinguished Career Award of the American Educational Research Association. In 2004, the Karolinska Institutet, Stockholm, Sweden, announced him to be the first winner of its international medical education research prize.

Dr Francis Michael Seefeldt, PhD, MFA, MA, has a long background in both international consultation and US domestic evaluation of community-based health and service programs, having worked with community-centered programs throughout the USA. His primary expertise is program evaluation, and he has taught and conducted research at the University of Illinois, College of Medicine, since 1979. At present, he is involved in educational psychology, faculty and curriculum evaluation, and humanities in medicine at the Department of Medical Education, College of Medicine, King Saud bin Abdulaziz University for Health Sciences (KSAU-HS) through its Masters in Medical Education Program.

Dr Hani Tamim received his BS in Biology from the American University of Beirut (1994), his Master of Public Health degree from Emory University (1995), and a Doctor of Philosophy degree in Epidemiology and Biostatistics from McGill University of Montreal – Faculty of Medicine. After that, Dr Tamim joined the College of Medicine at King Saud bin Abdulaziz University for Health Sciences, Riyadh, Saudi Arabia, as an Assistant Professor of Epidemiology and Biostatistics (2005–2009), and later as Associate Professor (2009–2011). Dr Tamim's research interests include cancer, pharmacoepidemiology, critical care, research methodology, and statistics. He has authored more than 70 publications in national and international peer-reviewed journals.

Floris van Blankenstein holds an MSc degree in Psychology and a PhD from Maastricht University, the Netherlands. His PhD was on problem-based learning and dealt with research on the working ingredient behind problem-based learning, being elaboration. He obtained his PhD degree in 2011. Currently, he is employed at the Inholland University of Applied Sciences in the Netherlands.

Jan van Dalen, PhD, is Coordinator of Communication Skills, Training, and Assessment, Skills Laboratory, Maastricht University, the Netherlands. His main activities are production of teaching materials and evaluation instruments, teaching of trainers, and research into the development of students' communication skills and coordinates faculty development programme of the skillslab staff. He is also Associate Secretary General of the Network TUFH; Associate Editor of *Education for Health*; and Programme Director, Master of Health Professions Education programme.

Professor Henk T. Van der Molen is Professor of Psychology and Chair and Educational Director of the Institute of Psychology, Faculty of Social Sciences, at Erasmus University Rotterdam since 2005. He is also Professor of Psychology at the

Open University of the Netherlands since 1992 and has been Professor of Psychology in Methods of Psychological Practice at the University of Groningen (1997–2002). He got his MA and his PhD (cum laude) at the Rijksuniversiteit Groningen (1980–1985). His research interests are: development and evaluation of skill acquisition programs in different areas, clinical and personality psychology, problem-based learning, and assessment of skills acquisition.

Professor Cess van der Vleuten is Chair, Department of Educational Development and Research, Faculty of Health, Medicine and Life Sciences, Maastricht University. Professor Vleuten has been trained as a personality psychologist and psychometrician, and has a PhD in Educational Sciences from Maastricht University (1989). He was also appointed as Scientific Director of the School of Health Professions Education. His area of expertise lies in evaluation and assessment. He has published widely on these topics, and holds several academic awards for his work, including several career awards.

Professor Merrilyn Walton, BA, BSW, MSW, PhD, is Professor of Medical Education (Patient Safety), Sydney School of Public Health, Faculty of Medicine, University of Sydney. Prior to this, she was Associate Professor of Medical Education, Office of Postgraduate Medical Education, Faculty of Medicine, University of Sydney, from 2006 to 2010. Professor Walton is also a member of the Australian Health Ethics Committee, National Health and Medical Research Council, since 2009.

Professor James Ware is Director of Medical Education and Postgraduate Studies, Department of Medical Education and Postgraduate Studies for the Saudi Commission for Health Specialties, Riyadh, Saudi Arabia. Prior to this appointment, he was Director of Medical Education, Centre of Medical Education, Faculty of Medicine, Centre of Health Sciences, Safat, Kuwait.

Dr Mohammed Zamakhshary, MD, FRCSc, FAAP, graduated from the College of Medicine, King Abdulaziz University, in 1999, and finished his residency training program at the Division of General Surgery in Dalhousie University, Halifax, Nova Scotia. He also completed his Masters in Medical Education through a joint program between Mount St. Vincent and Dalhousie universities, in addition to completing his Masters in Clinical Epidemiology and Public Health. Dr Zamakhshary holds the position of Assistant Professor of Surgery, Department of Medical Education, in the College of Medicine, King Saud bin Abdulaziz University for Health Sciences (KSAU-HS), and the Department of Epidemiology and Biostatistics in the College of Public Health and Health Informatics, KSAU-HS. Additionally, he is directly responsible for the Clinical Investigator Program at the King Abdullah International Medical Research Center. His main research interests are surgical outcomes, access to care, and population-based childhood research.

Preface

Medical education has grown expeditiously in the last decade in both content and process. This development was triggered by innovations in educational approaches, namely: problem-based learning (PBL) and community-based education (CBE). It has lead to medical schools establishing departments for medical education and developing special introductory courses for undergraduate curricula. As a result, an enormous amount of literature in the form of books, articles, and other forms, is now available for teachers and medical educators, but there is still nothing available for students.

The King Saud bin Abdulaziz University for Health Sciences (KSAU-HS) is proud to take the lead in publishing this handbook with the student as the main focus. The aim is to provide students with a tool to guide them on the *"road to success"* during their academic lives and beyond. This handbook—The International Handbook of Medical Education: A Guide for Students—will provide students access to basic medical education knowledge and skills, presented in a simple and interactive format. The handbook is designed to help students improve their study skills, such as reading, writing, searching and research, and provide them with essential information on assessment skills, such as answering MCQs, preparing for OSCE, and the like.

The book is divided into nine sections: Foundation, Study Skills, Learning in the Classroom, Learning in the Skills Lab, Learning in the Hospital, Learning in the Community, Getting the Most of Assessment and Evaluation, Student Support, and International Student Education.

In keeping with our mission and, in this instance, extending it to include an international audience, King Saud bin Abdulaziz University for Health Sciences, presents this handbook as a guide for students to develop the knowledge, skills and attitudes that will advance their careers and, ultimately, enhance the health of the population and contribute to the advancement of medicine.

Editors

Ibrahim Al Alwan, MRCP (UK) FAAP, FRCPC, is the Dean of the College of Medicine, KSAU-HS and President of the Association of Medical Education in the Eastern Mediterranean Region (AMEEMR). Dr. Alwan as an Associate Professor of Pediatrics has been teaching and participating in all academic activities at the KSAU-HS.

Dr. Alwan has been active in research works with several presentations and publications and is also a member of various committees in the University and the

National Guard Health Affairs where he serves as a Consultant, Pediatrician and Pediatric Endocrinologist.

Professor Mohi Eldin Mohammed Ali Magzoub, MBBS, MSC, PhD, MFPHM, Chairman, Department of Medical Education, College of Medicine, KSAU-HS. Prof. Magzoub was instrumental in establishing the Department of Medical Education and the inception of the Masters in Medical Education Program. He acted as a Consultant in medical education for many medical schools worldwide and his research interest includes a wide range of topics in medical education and community medicine. He has published more than 40 peer reviewed articles and books in medical education.

Professor Magzoub is the newly appointed Secretary General of the Association of Medical Education in the Eastern Mediterranean Region (AMEEMR).

Professor Margaret Elzubeir, B.A. (Hons.), PhD has been contributing to innovations in the health professions education in the UK and the Middle East for over twenty years. She is responsible for the Curriculum Development Unit of the Department of Medical Education, College of Medicine, KSAU-HS and a Coordinator of two Blocks in the Masters in Medical Education Program.

Professor Elzubeir has over 25 peer reviewed publications, conference presentations and has served as invited speaker at medical schools in the Middle East. Her professional interests include application of adult learning and psychological principles.

Acknowledgements

We would like to express our gratitude to all those who helped us complete the *International Handbook of Medical Education: A Guide for Students*.

To Prof. Youssef Al Eissa, Vice President, Educational Affairs, King Saud bin Abdulaziz University for Health Sciences (KSAU-HS), our sincerest appreciation for giving us his encouragement and support from the very first instance of conceptualizing this Handbook. To Ms. Susan El Masri, Senior Coordinator, Academic Affairs, College of Medicine, KSAU-HS for her stimulating and motivating assistance, our deepest thanks.

We would also like to extend our heartfelt appreciation to all the contributing authors for the extraordinary lengths they took to help make this Handbook a reality by providing their chapters. We value your collaboration; the medical education health profession has continued to grow with people like you.

Also outstanding during the preparation of this Handbook is the effort and long hours of work put in by our administrative staff: Ms. Jennifer Perry and Ms. Lilian Rivera Carandang; we are very pleased and proud to have you both in this endeavor.

Many thanks to Ms. Tessa Picknett, Ms. Delia Alfonso Martinez, and Ms. Alana Clogan at SAGE Publications for helping us achieve the challenge of putting out our first international handbook into such a remarkable edition.

I

FOUNDATION

Chapter 1

Applying Adult Learning

Margaret Elzubeir

Objectives

- To define learning, learning principles, and strategies.
- To differentiate between Andragogy and Pedagogy while understanding that all human beings have innate tendencies to emerge as adult learners as they mature.
- To list and explain eight adult learning principles.
- To apply knowledge of adult learning principles in an educational setting.

Introduction

Internationally, higher education institutions are revitalizing their undergraduate and postgraduate education programs through an increasing shift from a conventional teacher-centered pedagogy to a contemporary learner-centered focus. While this is very encouraging, it is noteworthy that the literature and practical applications of learner-centered approaches have focused primarily on teaching strategies and perspectives. It is, however, equally important for students to understand the principles underpinning the shift in emphasis and to consider practical implications for their responsibilities as learners.

This is, however, often overlooked, and consequently many students transitioning from high school or conventional undergraduate courses to a contemporary medical education environment sometimes feel ill-prepared for the change. Part of the problem may be a mismatch between individual conceptions of learning and conceptions of adult learning that underpin most of the university teaching methods in courses students opt for. It is therefore increasingly evident that students need to be assisted in developing an understanding of themselves as learners, their motives and approaches, and practical strategies that will enhance their learning. All are keys to a successful transition to lifelong learning.

This student handbook is designed to appeal to medical students who have an active interest in developing a deeper understanding of themselves as learners and of teaching and learning in medicine in the 21st century. In keeping with this general aim, this chapter describes principles and suggestions for implementation of adult learning practices and illustrates how, when combined, they can create powerful educational strategies that students (and teachers) can utilize to achieve more effective learning. The first section focuses on what we know about adult learners and on the eight principles of adult learning espoused by Knowles[1, 2] and others.[3-5] I then suggest some ways in which students can consciously enact or apply the principles.

Definitions of learning, learning principles, and strategies

Based on several decades of research, what we know about learning, learning principles, and strategies has changed a great deal. The following are some working definitions of these concepts which should provide a background:

1. **Learning**
   For the purposes of this chapter, learning is defined as a "long-term change in mental representations or association as a result of experience."[6] It is a means through which we acquire not only knowledge, but also values, attitudes, and emotional reactions. It is, however, important to note that most psychologists would also emphasize that learning cannot be said to have occurred unless there is a change in behavior and that learning is influenced by several variables including culture, intelligence, experience, and environment.

2. **Learning principles and theories**
   As a result of systematic research to understand the nature of learning, psychologists have been able to make generalizations about learning processes through formulation of both principles and theories of learning. Principles of learning identify certain factors that influence learning (i.e., how learning takes place) while learning theories provide explanations about the underlying mechanisms that are involved in learning (i.e., processes or why learning takes place). While principles of learning tend to be fairly stable over time, theories of learning continue to evolve.

3. **Learning strategies**
   As with "learning", there are multiple definitions for learning strategies that differ in sometimes subtle ways. However, in general they can be described as the tactics learners use or the various ways in which learners approach learning. More specifically, Weinstein and Mayer[7] define learning strategies as "behaviors and thoughts that a learner engages in during learning" which are "intended to influence the learner's encoding process" (p. 315). Hence, all individuals have preferred strategies for learning. For example, some prefer visual (written) information to auditory information (spoken) or experiential (learning by doing). McKeachie et al.[8] identified three main categories of learning strategies which, it would appear, successful learners employ. These are cognitive (i.e., to learn and understand information including

summarizing, paraphrasing, elaborating); meta-cognitive strategies which include planning, regulating, monitoring, and modifying cognitive learning processes. Finally, resource management strategies refer to strategies learners use to control resources such as time, effort, and support. The following sections will outline some main principles of adult learning and a combination of the above strategies that students can utilize to enhance successful learning.

4. **Andragogy and Pedagogy**
There are numerous books and articles devoted to adult learning.[15, 9-11] On the whole they support the idea that although many aspects of effective teaching and learning apply to all age groups, because adults have more life experiences and are more self-directed in their learning, teaching and learning as adults should be approached in a different way than teaching and learning as children.

Malcolm Knowles,[1, 2] who is considered the modern father of adult learning theory, used the term *andragogy* to describe the art and science of how adults learn, and distinguished adult learning from *pedagogy*; the study of how children learn. Initially the two concepts were seen as two distinct processes, but contemporary theory sees the two processes on a continuum. The quantity and quality of experiences learners have when they enter learning experiences and the amount of control that they have over the learning process and the learning environment are now considered the main determinants of location on the continnum.[12] Andragogic methods of learning and teaching are often associated with learner-centered methods whereas, in contrast, pedagogic methods are associated with teacher-centered methods. According to Knowles,[1, 2] traditional pedagogic methods alone are inappropriate for use with adults while andragogic methods are more appropriate. Since he first proposed the model, he has however modified it to include pre-adults (adolescents) as andragogic learners. He therefore now sees that adult learning is not a unique characteristic of adults and all human beings have innate tendencies to emerge as adult learners as they mature.

5. **Adult learning principles**
Knowles is considered a pioneer in the field of adult learning. He first described adult learning as a process of self-directed inquiry and identified six assumptions or principles of adult learning. Through the passage of time, these and other "principles" have been associated with adult learning. Table 1.1 provides an outline of a selection of these principles and suggestions of practical strategies that students can apply to enact them. Through an understanding of the principles, students should also be able to better evaluate what competent teaching and facilitation looks like.

Being an effective educator includes an understanding of how adults learn best. You will find most medical educators you encounter are aware of these principles and understand that acknowledging adults' prior knowledge and understanding

TABLE 1.1   Principles of adult learning and suggestions for students seeking to consciously activate the principles

Principle	Application to student learning strategies
Adults are autonomous and self-directed.	Self-directed learning is probably the most typical way in which adults choose to learn.[13] Take responsibility for your own learning. Diagnose your own learning needs. Generate your own task-oriented, measurable learning objectives for independent self-study; reflect on and evaluate the extent to which you have achieved objectives. However, do not overlook the importance of peer collaboration. Remember, collaborative learning can provide rich adult learning experiences. Use social networks, peers, and teachers as emotional and educational support mechanisms in your self-directed learning activities. Challenge, but do not overload, yourself. Use an effective time management system (i.e. study smart – pursue the right activities at the right time slots). Seek out alternative viewpoints. Critically evaluate resources such as journal articles, books, tutors, internet, and other learning resources efficiently. Where appropriate, make appointments to consult with content experts. Use all learning opportunities to broaden and deepen your understanding.
Adults bring a wealth of background knowledge and life experiences to learning contexts.	Experience lies at the heart of adult learning.[14] Draw on and share your prior knowledge and experiences as a starting point. These should be acknowledged and built on as far as possible by your teachers in all learning contexts. See your prior experiences and knowledge as representing valuable resources and draw on these when problem-solving, reflecting and applying knowledge. Associate what you learn with something you already know. Identify causal connections and apply to problems. Be confident in your own abilities but also question and address your own biases, assumptions, misconceptions or preconceived ideas developed in the past. Engage in deep processing. Make connections to prior knowledge and generate your own questions about information being learned.
Adults are goal-oriented.	You are more likely to retain and retrieve information if it is relevant to your future goals.[15] When regulating your study, determine what your overall goals are. In small-group learning share what you want to learn with peers and educators so they can ensure to the greatest extent possible that your goals are addressed. Prior to learning experiences ask yourself "what do I expect to learn?" and "how might I apply what I learned in the future?"; "how will this learning meet my own learning goals?" Your learning behaviors should be goal-directed rather than random. Categorize and organize new information.

Principle	Application to student learning strategies
	Brainstorm and clarify salient concepts. Use concept mapping[16] to make linkages and as a graphical means of organizing and representing knowledge. Keep your eye on your goals and verify their achievement, e.g. through vocalization of what you learn or through a visual representation such as concept maps.
Adults are relevancy-oriented and want to apply what they learn.	Adults have a desire to know why they should learn something in order to learn it effectively.[17] They are eager to apply new knowledge to solve problems and address real-life needs and situations immediately. Prior to learning experiences ask yourself "what do I expect to learn?"; "how will this learning be applied in my future professional role?" If not always provided by instructors seek out and construct your own learning objectives (especially in self-directed learning). Make connections to your own goals in order to see relevance and value. Make a personal commitment to apply what you have learned practically. Try to use and transfer learning in one context to other relevant contexts. Use different methods to integrate and make connections, e.g. concept mapping, diagrams, etc. Decide on how you will know you have learned something.
Adults are intrinsically (and extrinsically) motivated to learn.	Motivation is the natural human capacity to direct energy toward a goal.[18] Intrinsic motivators become increasingly more important than extrinsic ones. Find motivation to learn from within you and as a consequence of personal goals and external expectations, e.g. complying with fulfillment of your own expectations or recommendations of your instructors, preparing for service to the community, satisfying your inquiring mind. Tune out distractions. Take pride in your achievements. Just as you are able to assess your learning and adjust your strategies, you are also able to adjust your motivation. Strategies for regulation of motivation include goal-oriented self-talk, interest strategies, self-handicapping, and emotion regulation. Determine how your learning will benefit you practically. Challenge yourself to achieve more and better outcomes. Do not just attune your learning to assessment and teacher demands. Critical self-reflection and self-evaluation are principal methods of assessing progress. Through collaborative learning and sharing of resources you can often create greater energy for learning. Engage in meta-cognitive[19] processing, i.e. self awareness, self regulation and self monitoring of cognitive processes.

Continued

Principle	Application to student learning strategies
	Research tells us that good learners are those who are highly aware of their own thinking and memory and use this information to regulate learning. Regulate not only your learning but also your physical and social environment in order to motivate yourself. Construct supportive environments. Decide on how to deal with social or emotional impediments to learning. Record your critical reflections.
Adults learn best when they are active partici-pants in the learning process.	Engage in opportunities for problem solving, questioning, peer collaboration, sharing of experiences, and actively participate in group situations. Use opportunities for brainstorming, case-based learning and exercises that require you to practice a skill or apply knowledge. Practice skills frequently. Improve your integrative learning skills. Associate skills, observations and facts with what you already know to discover patterns and new relationships. Summarize what you learn frequently to increase retention and recall.
Adults learn more effectively when given timely and constructive feedback on their learning.	Adults need to know when they are learning correctly, so they can succeed.[20,21] Seek and use opportunities for feedback from instructors, peers, and patients. Reflect on your strengths and weaknesses and make a conscious effort to plan how you will use the information for personal development. Reflective practice[22,23] is an ideal to work towards throughout your professional career. It aids self knowledge, continuous renewal and development of your understanding.
Adults have different learning preferences/ styles.	Not all individuals learn in the same way. We all have different ways of processing and retaining information. Individual styles are influenced by experience, education, personality, intelligence, culture, and sensory and cognitive preferences. However, because there will be a variety of teaching and learning strategies encountered, it will be necessary to be versatile. Evaluate and understand your own learning preferences/styles while acknowledging that it is better to vary the methods by which you learn. Studies have shown that medical students prefer multiple learning styles.[24,25] Numerous learning style self assessment tools are available on the internet.[26, 27]

validates them as competent and capable learners. Your instructors will therefore begin by finding out what you already know about the topic, will encourage you to elaborate on your learning, and will generally trust you to seek and embrace responsibility for your own learning. In most cases, they will begin by helping you see the connections between prior learning and new information. For graduate-entry students this will be particularly important as they come with a wealth of prior knowledge and professional experience in social and applied health sciences. Your instructors may also encourage you to use concept mapping[24, 25] as a strategic method for articulating and organizing prior and current knowledge, stimulating meta-cognition and problem-solving.

Knowles also promoted the concept of self-directed learning. He felt that adults should create personal learning objectives that would allow them to set individual goals and to practice using new learning in practical ways. Self-regulated learning is the most lasting and pervasive.

Independent study can be facilitated by using resources at your disposal within and outside the learning institution. Personal tutors or facilitators can share your learning goals and intended agenda.

Take Home Messages

- Contemporary medical education curricula are designed bearing in mind adult learning principles.
- Although these principles are fairly straightforward and intuitive, they should be understood and applied by both students and teachers.
- Learning is about expanding new skills, developing new knowledge and perspectives and improving expertise. Development and change across the lifespan play a role in understanding how and why adults learn.
- Despite the numerous theories and models that describe or explain how adults learn, there is a general consensus about the central principles. In reviewing current models and theories, this chapter has identified eight key principles which include: autonomy and self direction, prior knowledge and experience, goal orientation; relevancy, intrinsic motivation, active participation in learning process, timely and constructive feedback, understanding of different learning styles.
- Adult learning principles have both individual and social components.
- Understanding principles of adult learning should enable students to better evaluate what competent teaching and facilitation should look like.
- Adult learners should consider how they may consciously activate adult learning.

References

1. Knowles MS. *The Modern Practice of Adult Education: From Pedagogy to Andragogy* (2nd edition). New York: Cambridge Books, 1980.
2. Knowles MS. Introduction: the art and science of helping adults learn. In: MS Knowles and associates. *Andragogy in Action: Applying Modern Principles of Adult Learning*. San Francisco: Jossey-Bass, 1984.
3. Marriam SB, Caffarella RS and Baumgartner LM. *Learning in Adulthood: A comprehensive guide* (3rd edition). San Francisco: Jossey Bass, 2007.
4. Brookfield S. *Understanding and Facilitating Adult Learning*. San Francisco: Jossey-Bass, 1986.
5. Boud D and Griffin V (eds). *Appreciating Adults Learning: from the Learner's Perspective*. London: Kogan Page, 1987.
6. Ormrod JE. *Human Learning* (5th edition). Ohio: Prentice Education, 2008.
7. Weinstein CE and Mayer RE. The teaching of learning strategies. In: MC Wittrock (ed.). *Handbook of Research on Teaching* (3rd edition), pp. 315–327. New York: Macmillan, 1986.
8. McKeachie WJ, Pintrich PR, Lin Y and Smith DA. *Teaching and Learning in the College Classroom: a review of the research literature*. University of Michigan, 1987.
9. Mezirow JA. A critical theory of adult learning and education. *Adult Educ,* (1), 1981; 32(1) (Fall): 3–24.
10. Jarvis P. *Towards a Comprehensive Theory of Human Learning*. London: Routledge, 2006
11. Tennant M. *Psychology and Adult ILarning* (3rd edition). London: Routledge, 2006.
12. Smith R. *Learning to Learn across the Lifespan*. San Francisco: Jossey-Bass, 1990.
13. Brockett RG and Hiemstra R. *Self Direction in Adult Learning: Perspectives on theory, research and practice*. New York: Routledge, 1991.
14. Kolb DA. *Experiential Learning*. Engelwood Cliffs, NJ: Prentice Hall, 1984.
15. Bash L. *Adult Learners in the Academy*. San Francisco: Jossey Bass, 1999.
16. Novak J. *Learning, Creating and Using Knowledge. Concept Maps as Facilitative tools in Schools and Corporations*. Mahwah, NJ: LEA, 1998.
17. Wlodkowski R. *Enhancing Adult Motivation to Learn: A comprehensive guide for teaching all adults* (3rd edition). San Francisco: Jossey Bass, 2008.
18. Wlodkowski R. Creating motivating learning environments. In: MW Galbraith, *Adult Learning Methods: A guide for effective instruction* (3rd edition). Malabar, FL: Krieger, 2004.
19. Flavell, J. H. Speculations about the nature and development of metacognition. In FE Weinert and RH Kluwe (eds), *Metacognition, Motivation and Understanding*, pp. 21–29. Hillside, NJ: Lawrence Erlbaum Associates, 1987.
20. Hewson MG and Little ML. Giving feedback in medical education: verification of recommended techniques. *J Gen Internal Med*, 1988; 13(2): 111–116.
21. van de Ridder JMM, Stiokking KM, McGaghie WC and ten Cate OTJ. What is feedback in clinical education? *Med Educ*, 2008; 42(2): 189–197.
22. Schon D. *The Reflective Practitioner: How Professionals Think in Action*. London: Arena, 1996.
23. Wald HS, Davis SW, Reis SP, Monroe AD and Borkan JM. Reflecting on reflections: enhancement of medical education curriculum with structured field notes and guided feedback. *Acad Med*, 2009; 84(7): 830–837.
24. Lujan HL and DiCarlo SE. First year medical students prefer multiple learning styles. *Adv in Physiol Edu*, 2006; 30: 13–16.

25. Curry L. Cognitive and learning styles in medical education. *Acad Med*, 1999; 74(4): 409–413.
26. Vark. A guide to learning styles. The Vark Questionnaire can be accessed at: http://www.vark-learn.com/english/page.asp?p=questionnaire
27. An online learning style inventory developed by Solomon BA and Felder RM can be accessed at: http://www.engr.ncsu.edu/learningstyles/ilsweb.html

Chapter 2

How is your Curriculum Designed?

What you should know about your curriculum

Ronald M. Harden

Objectives

By the end of this chapter, you will be able to answer the following questions:
- What is the aim of the training program?
- What learning outcomes are expected of you on the completion of your studies in medical school?
- What learning strategies have been incorporated in your curriculum?
- What learning opportunities are available to you?
- How is your achievement of the learning outcomes assessed?
- What is the educational environment in your school?

Introduction

An undergraduate curriculum was traditionally defined in terms of a series of courses and clinical attachments, and how these were time tabled within a 4-, 5-, or 6-year program of study. Each course was represented by a discipline or subject, knowledge of which was deemed necessary for a doctor. Subjects included basic medical sciences such as anatomy, biochemistry, physiology, paraclinical disciplines such as pathology or microbiology, and clinical specialties such as medicine, surgery or obstetrics and gynecology. Today the situation is very different. The curriculum is interpreted as much more than a syllabus or timetable. It is an overall learning experience and educational program which covers learning outcomes, how the program is planned and delivered to meet these, and how the learner's achievements are assessed.

In most schools, there has been a move away from a curriculum focused on subjects and disciplines to an integrated model or program, built most commonly around body systems and with closer integration of clinical and basic medical sciences. This chapter highlights the six questions you should ask regarding the curriculum in your medical school, and to which you should know the answers.

Let us digress for a moment before we consider the questions and your curriculum.

Imagine that arrangements have been made for you to spend a year in a country where you have had no previous experience. What would you want to know prior to your departure? You would certainly want information as to the purpose of your visit and what was expected of you on your return. What cities, towns, features or landmarks would you be expected to visit, and where would these be located in relation to each other? What were the options with regard to transport? What support, if any, could you expect to receive during the year and who would be available to advise you if you had a problem? Similar questions should be asked by you about your medical education journey. Your time in medical school should not be some sort of magical mystery tour with the destination, travel requirements and activities hidden en route. These should be transparent to you as a key player. You need to be familiar with the aims of the program, the expected learning outcomes, the educational strategies, the available learning opportunities, the assessment methods, and the education environment. We will explore each of these in more detail.

Question 1 – What is the aim of the training program?

The first question relates to the mission of the medical school. Is there a special emphasis, as noted in the mission statement, on the type of doctor produced? This may be a doctor with a particular interest and expertise in, for example, research, a community-minded physician, or a professional with an international focus and understanding. While there may be subtle differences in emphasis, most schools aim to produce graduates who are well trained, show potential and who are prepared to embark on the specialty training of their choice.

It has been increasingly recognized that the mission of a school should not be restricted to the production of doctors qualified to provide excellent care for individual patients. The school should have social responsibility and accountability for the population they serve and for international dimensions of medical care.[18] Is this vision reflected in the mission statement of your medical school?

Question 2 – What learning outcomes are expected of you on the completion of your studies at medical school?

The move to outcome-based education (OBE) has been described as the most significant development in medical education in the past decade. In OBE, the emphasis is on the product or the learning outcomes achieved, rather than on the process or methods used to achieve the goals. Fuller argued that "a good archer is known not by his arrows but by his aim."

A number of frameworks or models have been used to present the expected learning outcomes. Examples are: ACGME abilities, Brown abilities, Global Minimum Essential Requirements developed by the China Medical Board, CanMED competencies and 'The Scottish Doctor' learning outcomes. You can read more about the rationale for the move to outcome-based education in the AMEE Guide 14[1] and in the *Medical Teacher* themed issues of April 2002, September 2007, and August 2010.

The three-circle model[13] adopted in the Scottish Doctor learning outcomes is of particular interest. It presents a holistic approach with different outcome domains integrated, and highlights the doctor as a professional rather than a technician. The model includes:

- in the inner circle: technical competencies – clinical skills, practical procedures, patient management, communication skills, patient investigations, information handling, and health promotion;
- in the middle circle: how doctors should approach their practice – with scientific understanding, appropriate attitudes, ethics, and with appropriate decision-making strategies; and
- in the outer circle: the doctor as a professional – a member of a team working within the healthcare system, assessing their own competence, and keeping up-to-date with their practice.

Are these outcome domains addressed in your curriculum? Some learning outcomes that have been neglected in the past but now attract attention are: attitudes, professionalism, management skills, team work, patient safety, error management, and teaching skills. Do these feature in your curriculum?

Question 3 – What learning strategies have been incorporated in your curriculum?

The SPICES model for curriculum planning I described in 1984 is still valid today.[17] This identifies six key strategies in planning a curriculum and presents each as a continuum between two extremes.

- *Student-centered/teacher-centered*
  In a student-centered curriculum, what matters is the student and what the student learns. In a teacher-centered curriculum, the emphasis is on the teacher and what is taught. A typical teacher-centered approach is illustrated in this anecdote. An orthopedic surgeon complains to the professor of anatomy that students attending his clinic lack an understanding of the basic anatomy of the hand. The professor of anatomy responds that this was covered fully in his course, that two lectures were devoted to the subject and that there is clearly a problem with the students. In contrast, in a student-centered approach there would be an agreement as to the understanding of anatomy necessary and steps would be taken to ensure that the required

level of mastery was achieved by the students. A flexible approach would be adopted that would allow students to choose their method and pace of study.

In a student-centered approach, greater emphasis is placed on the teacher as a facilitator of the students' learning. For each course, study guides are provided to help the students to manage their own learning.[16] In the post-Flexner Carnegie review of medical education in the USA,[2] it is argued that "medical education should standardize learning outcomes and general competencies and then provide greater options for individualizing the learning experience for students and residents."

- *Problem-based/information gathering*
In a problem-based approach, a problem is used to drive the learning activities on a need-to-know basis. Students achieve the outcomes through tackling the problems presented. It is helpful to think of PBL as active learning, stimulated by and focused around a clinical, community or scientific problem.[4, 15]

In a more traditional curriculum, students are first presented with information on basic and clinical sciences and are expected to apply this knowledge later on to clinical problems with which they are faced. Integration of theory with practice is not easy. I remember one student in a final examination who gave me a textbook list of 50 or so causes of splenomegaly, but was unable to identify the three possible causes in the patient he was examining.

Problem-based learning became popular as a curriculum strategy, as it helped the student to relate theory to practice and provided a more authentic or work-related learning experience. Students found the approach motivating and interesting. When compared to the traditional curriculum, it has been likened to the difference between sex and artificial insemination. PBL is challenging and places more responsibility on you – the student. It is important that, in addition to thinking about the particular problem being studied, you generalize to other situations in medicine. In what other ways, for example, might the patient have presented and how could these features have been explained? What similarities and differences are there in related problems? Some schools are now less enthusiastic about a problem-based approach as initially described, and have adopted a task-based or presentation-centered variation, where the learning is centered around a set of 100 to 200 tasks commonly encountered by a doctor in medical practice.[5, 14]

- *Integrated/discipline-based*
In an integrated curriculum, the emphasis is on bringing together subjects from the same phase of the curriculum, such as medicine, surgery, obstetrics and gynecology, or physiology, anatomy and biochemistry (horizontal integration), or integrating the basic and clinical sciences from different phases of the curriculum (vertical integration).

One rationale for an integrated approach is that patients do not normally present with an identifiable medical or surgical problem. I recall asking a student in a final examination to take a history from and examine a woman who had presented with abdominal pain. The student asked whether I wanted a medical, surgical, or gynecological examination. They had been taught these separately and had not learned how to integrate them. Vertical integration and introducing clinical experience early in the course has a number of advantages and has been shown to influence career choice.[6]

- **Community-based/hospital-based**
  Teaching and learning in a community-based approach is centered in the community, e.g. in a health center. In a hospital-based approach, it is centered in a teaching hospital. Even if you intend to have your career in specialist hospital practice, experience in the community as a student can give you a valuable insight into medical practice that you will find useful later. It was demonstrated in Australia that students who spent a year based in a local community performed as well as or better than students studying in a hospital environment.

- **Elective/standard**
  The typical curriculum has two elements – a basic core studied by all students and an elective component, where the student can choose what they want to study either from a prescribed list or from a topic proposed by the student. The elective or student-selected course can address an aspect of the curriculum you want to study in more depth, perhaps because you are interested in a career in this area, or it can be a topic not normally covered, such as a foreign language. The proportion of time allocated to electives or student-selected courses varies from school to school. In medical schools in the UK, as recommended by the General Medical Council, this may be as high as 25%. The elective component provides you with an opportunity to further develop your independent learning and self-assessment skills in addition to mastering the topic covered.

- **Systematic (planned) apprenticeship (opportunistic)**
  In an opportunistic curriculum, what the student learned was dependent on what the teacher felt like teaching or on the availability of patients in the clinical setting. As described above, one of the most important developments in medical education has been the move to a more systematic approach with clearly defined learning outcomes. A map of the curriculum can be used to relate the learning outcomes to the curricular content, to the learning experiences or opportunities and to the assessment.[10]

Where on the SPICES dimension is your medical school and where would you like it to be? You might like to engage the teachers in your school in a discussion about this.

Question 4 – What learning opportunities are available to you?

Learning opportunities should be planned in the curriculum to allow you to achieve expected learning outcomes. We have seen, in recent years, the development of new, powerful learning tools and technologies including the internet and simulation.[7, 19, 20] As described by Prensky, you are the digital natives who came to medical school with thousands of hours of online experience whereas the teachers are often digital immigrants. In your medical studies you will find, as useful sources of information, search engines such as Google, Wikipedia and YouTube. A study from St Andrews University in the UK found more than 400 images available on YouTube relevant to a course in pathology. The challenge is to assess the quality or reliability of the information provided. In medical practice, you will not find it unusual for your patients to come and see you with a detailed knowledge of their condition obtained from the internet. Some more structured courses are also available online on a range of topics such as ELECTRO-CARDIOGRAPHY, pain control, and anatomy. You can also extend your clinical experience online using 'virtual patients' with whom you can interact.

Social networking through sites such as Facebook can also contribute to learning. You need to be cautioned, however, about ethical and personal considerations. What you put on your Facebook page may later be examined by potential employers in relation to a job for which you have applied. Students can collaborate usefully in the preparation of a medical school's code of conduct.

It is no longer necessary to try out a new skill or procedure for the first time on a real patient. A wide range of simulators is available on which you can practice skills. These range from rectal examination, venipuncture and wound suturing to more complicated procedures such as cardiopulmonary resuscitation or anesthesiology. The 'Harvey' cardiac manikin, for example, allows you to examine the radial pulse, blood pressure, jugular venous pulse and apex beat and to auscultate the heart in patients with a range of conditions. This is an invaluable experience that helps you not only to master the necessary clinical skills but also to gain an understanding of cardiopulmonary physiology and pathophysiology. Trained simulated patients are also widely used to assist students to acquire skills in history taking and physical examinations, including the more intimate examinations such as rectal and vaginal examinations.

Students should, as part of their medical studies, develop teaching skills. A significant development in medical education is the use of peer teaching, where more senior students, or students from the same year, contribute to the teaching program. This benefits both the tutor and the student. Ross and Cameron[21] provide a description of how this works in practice at the Edinburgh medical school.

Despite the introduction of these new technologies, lectures still have a role to play in the training program. There are no bad lectures, only bad lecturers. Lectures are not usually efficient as a method of transferring information, but can convey an enthusiasm or passion for the subject, a framework for the study of a topic and, importantly, can stimulate you to think and reflect.

Is appropriate use being made of new approaches to teaching and learning in your training? When you examine the learning outcomes expected of you, can you match the most appropriate learning experiences?

Question 5 – How is your achievement of the learning outcomes assessed?

It is useful to think of a further set of five questions when considering, as part of the curriculum, the assessment of your achievement of the learning outcomes.

- *What should be assessed?* The answer is obvious in outcome-based education – the learning outcomes expected at graduation and at each stage of training. In most schools, there is a move away from an emphasis on the recall of knowledge to an assessment of the application of knowledge and the skills expected of a doctor, including appropriate attitudes and professionalism.
- *How should it be assessed?* While written examinations, including multiple-choice questions, have a role to play, increasing emphasis is being placed on performance-based examinations. The Objective Structured Clinical Examination (OSCE) is now the gold standard. The competency of students is assessed at a series of 20 or so stations with a component of competence such as history taking, physical examination, practical skills, or problem solving assessed at each station. Students have reported that the OSCE, if properly conducted, is a fair and reliable assessment of their competence.

  A student portfolio is being increasingly used for assessment purposes. Portfolios are particularly useful in assessing learning outcomes such as professionalism and self-assessment skills. For a number of years, students at Dundee Medical School have been assessed in the final examination on the basis of a portfolio produced by them, in which they present evidence that they have achieved the expected learning outcomes in each of the domains as set out in the Scottish Doctor.[3]
- *Why assess?* The traditional purpose of assessment is to assess whether students have mastered the level of knowledge required of them, either to graduate or to pass on to the next stage of the program. There has been a move from the concept of 'assessment of learning' to the idea of 'assessment for learning', whereby the assessment is more closely integrated into the teaching and learning program. We will return to this idea in the final section – 'The curriculum of the future.' For the moment, the importance of feedback from the teacher to the student should be emphasized. It is important that you receive feedback as to your performance, not simply as a percentage mark, but with details of where there are gaps in your understanding of the subject or skills and how these can be remedied. One worrying finding, in a study from Aberdeen Medical School, was that students who had performed less satisfactorily in an examination were less likely to seek feedback on their performance. In general, however, feedback is valued by students. When I asked students on one occasion to identify what they perceived as their most useful learning experience in the previous six months, the one most commonly cited was "the feedback they were given as to their performance following an OSCE".

- **When to assess?** The classical answer to the question "when to assess?" is at the end of a course of study. With the use of portfolios, assessment is now becoming part of an ongoing process integrated with learning. It is also of interest to assess your competence in an area before you start a course.

   One interesting idea, now being implemented in some schools, is the concept of the progress test. This is a form of assessment where groups of students of different seniority (i.e. different classes in a curriculum) are given the same written test. The test is made comprehensive by sampling all relevant disciplines in a curriculum.[8]

- **Who should assess?** Currently, there is controversy as to whether the assessment of students should be the responsibility of the medical school or whether there should be a national or international examination. In some countries, such as the UK, the responsibility for assessment rests with the individual school and is monitored by the General Medical Council. In other countries, such as the USA, assessment is the responsibility of a national body – The National Board of Medical Examiners. I have argued, elsewhere, that while there are advantages of a national examination, these are outweighed by the disadvantages.[12]

When considering who should assess the student, the importance of self-assessment should not be ignored. Although self-assessment is notoriously unreliable, it is an ability that needs to be acquired by students by the time they qualify if they are to monitor their own performance as a doctor and keep themselves up-to-date. As a professional, you are expected to be an inquirer into your own competence.

Question 6 – What is the educational environment in your school?

Perhaps the most neglected factor, in consideration of the curriculum, is the educational environment or climate. This is because it is less tangible and not easily measured. The position has changed with the development of tools such as the Dundee Ready Education Environment Measure (DREEM), which has been accepted for use in a wide range of settings. The educational environment is important, as it has a profound effect on students' behavior and learning. Does it encourage, for example, scholasticism, propriety, social awareness, and cooperation between students? In your school, is there a measure of the educational environment and what type of environment is encouraged?

The curriculum of the future

I have presented, in this chapter, six questions that you should address regarding the curriculum in your school:

- What is the aim of the training program?
- What learning outcomes are expected at the completion of your studies?

- What learning strategies have been adopted in your curriculum?
- What learning opportunities are available to you?
- How is your achievement of learning outcomes assessed?
- What is the education environment in your school?

By answering these questions, you will be better equipped to plan and manage your own work program as a student. There is an important additional consideration. A greater knowledge and understanding of the curriculum will allow you to contribute to its further development. Students have an important role to play in this respect and often show considerable insight into problems or areas where change is advisable.

Looking to the future, what changes can be expected? Predicting the future is notoriously difficult, but two areas where we will see significant developments are adaptive learning and continuum of learning. With new learning technologies and an understanding of how we learn, it will be possible to tailor courses and the approaches to teaching to the needs of the individual student, based on an assessment of their progress. What will become fixed is the standard that students achieve and not the time scheduled in the curriculum. At present, all too often what is fixed is the time, and what is variable is the standard achieved. For example, a student may master the necessary cardiac auscultation skills, using Harvey, the cardiac simulator, in one hour, while others may require four hours or more.

For historical reasons, medical education has been organized, developed and funded in separate silos – undergraduate, postgraduate, and continuing medical education. Since 1932, or even earlier, the need for a more seamless continuum has been argued, but this has been difficult to achieve for historical, political and financial reasons. With current developments in medical education, new technologies and educational approaches, the time is now ripe to look again at creating a more seamless continuum of education. The losers will be those who remain inside their comfort zone and think only in terms of traditional medical education based on the three separate phases.

These and other visions for the future can be achieved. In medical education, we suffer primarily not from weaknesses in what we can do, but from illusions. We are haunted, not by reality, but by myths put in the place of reality.[11] As a student and a future doctor, you can help to ignite the transformation from vision to reality, and begin to shape its design and implementation. You are part of the solution.

References

1. AMEE Medical Education Guide No. 14 (1999) *Outcome-based Education*. Association for Medical Education in Europe, Dundee, UK.
2. Cooke, M., Irby, D.M. and O'Brien, B.C. (2010) *Educating Physicians: A call for Reform of Medical School and Residency*. Jossey-Bass, San Francisco, CA.

3. Davis, M.H., Friedman Ben-David, M., Harden, R.M., Howie, P., Ker, J., McGhee, C., Pippard, M.J. and Snadden, D. (2001) Portfolio assessment in medical students' final examinations, *Medical Teacher*, 23, pp. 357–366.
4. Davis, M.H. and Harden R.M. (1998) AMEE Medical Education Guide No. 15: Problem-based learning: a practical guide, *Medical Teacher*, 21(2), pp. 130–140.
5. Davis, M.H. and Harden, R.M. (2003) Planning and implementing an undergraduate medical curriculum: the lessons learned, *Medical Teacher*, 25(6), pp. 596–608.
6. Dornan, T., Littlewood, S., Margolis, S.A., Scherpbier A., Spencer, J. and Ypinazer, V. (2007) How can experience in clinical and community settings contribute to early medical education? A BEME systematic review. BEME Guide No. 6, *Medical Teacher*, 28(1), pp. 3–18.
7. Ellaway, R. and Masters, K. (2008) AMEE Guide 32: e-Learning in medical education. Part 1: Learning, teaching and assessment, *Medical Teacher*, 30(5), pp. 455–473.
8. Freeman, A. et al. (2010) Progress testing internationally, *Medical Teacher*, 32, pp. 451–455.
9. Harden, R.M. (1986) Ten questions to ask when planning a course or curriculum, *Medical Education*, 20, pp. 356–365.
10. Harden, R.M. (2001) Curriculum mapping: a tool for transparent and authentic teaching and learning. AMEE Medical Education Guide No. 21, *Medical Teacher*, 23(2), pp. 123–137.
11. Harden, R.M. (2002) Myths and e-learning, *Medical Teacher*, 24(5), pp. 469–472.
12. Harden, R.M. (2009) Five myths and the case against a European or national licensing examination, *Medical Teacher*, 31(3) pp. 217–220.
13. Harden, R.M., Crosby, J.R. and Davis, M.H. (1999) An introduction to outcome-based education, *Medical Teacher*, 21, pp. 7–14.
14. Harden, R.M., Crosby, J.R., Davis, M.H., Howie, P.W. and Struthers, A.D. (2002) Task-based learning: the answer to integration and problem-based learning in the clinical years, *Medical Education*, 34, pp. 391–397.
15. Harden, R.M. and Davis, M.H. (1998) The continuum of problem-based learning, *Medical Teacher*, 20(4), pp. 317–322.
16. Harden, R.M., Laidlaw, J.M. and Hesketh, E.A. (1999) AMEE Education Guide No. 16: Study guides – their use and preparation, *Medical Teacher*, 21(3), pp. 248–265.
17. Harden, R.M., Sowden, S. and Dunn, W.R. (1984) Educational strategies in curriculum development: the SPICES model, *Medical Education*, 18, pp. 284–297.
18. Hodges, B.D., Maniate, J.M., Martimianakis, M.A., Alsuwaidan, M. and Segouin, C. (2009) Cracks and crevices: Globalization discourse and medical education, *Medical Teacher*, 31, pp. 910–917.
19. Issenberg, S.B., McGaghie, W.C., Petrusa, E.R., Gordon, D.L. and Scalese, R.J. (2004) Features and uses of high-fidelity medical simulations that lead to effective learning: a BEME systematic review. BEME Guide 4. *Medical Teacher*, 27(1), pp. 10–28.
20. Masters, K. and Ellaway, R. (2008) AMEE Guide 32: e-Learning in medical education. Part 2: Technology, management and design, *Medical Teacher*, 30(5), pp. 474–489.
21. Ross, M.T. and Cameron, H.S. (2007) Peer assisted learning: A planning and implementation framework: AMEE Guide No. 30, *Medical Teacher*, 29, pp. 527–545.

Chapter 3

Current Trends in Medical Education

Rania Ghazi Zaini

Objectives

- To learn the "integration model" as a teaching strategy and integrated medical curricula.
- To learn problem-based learning as an instructional strategy and its underlying concepts and principles.
- To learn community perspectives in medical education and the difference between its two approaches: community-oriented medical education and community-based medical education.
- To learn about simulation learning.

Introduction

Changing patterns of healthcare delivery, ongoing scientific and specialty expansion, increased expectation of doctors' responsibilities by society and the shift in medical students and doctors themselves, propel change and innovation in medical education. Furthermore, new educational strategies, appropriate to adult learning and based on theory, will have emphasis in the new era.

In response to these changes, new trends in medical education have emerged and have compelled medical schools to restructure conventional curricula to ensure highly competent and qualified doctors. Harden and colleagues[27] illustrate an innovative medical curriculum as being one that seeks to decrease the amount of factual knowledge while providing opportunities for choice. It aims to have vertical and horizontal integration of disciplines, functions in hospital and community learning environments, seeks to define learning outcomes and emphasizes skills, attitudes, and knowledge. Innovative medical education has taken on a number of different concerns: the nature of the curriculum, teaching and instructional methods, assessment, and the management of the curriculum.

This chapter presents the most relevant themes in innovative medical education that have emerged since the early 1960s. It describes the integration model, problem-based learning (PBL), community prospective in the medical curriculum, and the drift towards outcome-based education (OBE). In addition, the recent international concerns regarding medical professionalism and simulation are discussed.

Integration model

An integration model is a teaching strategy in which content is drawn from several subject areas and disciplines and focuses on a particular theme or topic. The integrated curriculum attempts to fuse independent disciplines around one theme, either horizontally or vertically. In horizontal integration, the boundaries between parts of the course are removed, with integration across topics or subjects. In vertical integration, borders between sequential phases are lost, with fusion throughout the course.[30]

In the mid-twentieth century (the 1950s), the first horizontally and vertically integrated medical curriculum was adopted at Case Western Reserve University in Cleveland, Ohio. The curriculum was based on organ system instruction, coupled with an institutional commitment to correlate the basic sciences with clinical experience.[31, 35] There are various forms of integrated medical curricula. Harden's Integration Ladder[24] represents integration stages ranging from isolation (subject-based teaching) to a trans-disciplinary curriculum, which emphasized the flexibility of educational strategies.

An integrated approach has many advantages over subject-centered instruction, which benefits students and staff:

- Fuses distinct scientific and clinical disciplines, making learning more meaningful.
- Facilitates self- and active learning.
- Eliminates areas of redundancy and streamlines the content and length of courses, providing room for electives and self-learning.
- Unites the experience of medical education, bringing it closer to the work of the medical practitioner in a highly advanced integrated curriculum.
- Encourages cooperation between staff of different departments.
- Assists the endorsement of the core curriculum.[28, 35]

On the other hand, there are many potential obstacles to implementing an integrated medical curriculum. For example, unless there is careful planning and coordination of the integrative curriculum, many important topics may be overlooked. Also, medical teachers may find it difficult to teach integrated courses and there is therefore a need for effective staff development programs before implementation.

Integrated medical education has become the prime feature of recent medical education reform. There is an emphasis upon integrated medical education in national and international reports and accreditation standards.[4, 15–16, 18, 53–55]

Problem-based learning

Problem-based learning (PBL) is a learning instruction strategy in which students identify their learning needs and issues that are raised in relation to a particular (clinical) problem. This helps to develop an understanding about the underlying concepts and principles.

In PBL tutorials, students are divided into small groups and are represented with either a real or imaginary clinical situation. This is used as a springboard from which to explore various topics and identify learning needs. A member of the staff facilitates the PBL tutorial and ensures that students are equally participative, and that interaction focuses on relevant issues, but without instructions or dominating group discussions. Barrows[6] outlines the process of PBL in six steps:

- encountering the problem;
- problem-solving;
- identifying learning;
- needs interactive process involving self-study;
- applying newly gained knowledge to the problem; and
- summarizing what has been learned.

PBL is considered a paradigm shift in medical education instruction. It has become increasingly popular since first being developed by Howard Barrows at McMaster Medical School in Canada.[7] By the end of the 20th century, around 150 medical schools worldwide (some 10% of the total) have adopted PBL.[44] Nowadays, many medical schools use some form of PBL, ranging from a total PBL approach, such as the one used at McMaster University, to a hybrid approach, such as the one used at Sheffield University.[36] The PBL continuum is illustrated as 11 steps, ranging from "theoretical learning", which is facilitated by traditional lectures, to "task-based learning," as an ultimate step of PBL.[26] Within this continuum, PBL may be utilized as a supplemental tool to didactic lecture-based or other learning strategies.

PBL has many advantages – it corresponds with adult learning theories, encourages deep learning, and fits in well with integrated approaches in which students study various aspects of a problem. It also encourages student autonomy, building on their previous knowledge and identifying their learning needs.

On the other hand, many difficulties are associated with PBL curricula, in relation to design, implementation and staff and student responses. Students' orientation and staff development programs are essential in preparing students and teachers for the PBL curricula.

Community perspectives in medical education

A community perspective in medical education has been encouraged since the 1980s, especially with the establishment of the Network for Community-Oriented Educational Institutes for Health Sciences in 1997.[41] Many educational and logistical arguments encourage reducing the emphasis on hospital-based programs and favoring more emphasis on the community as a context for student learning. An international call has also recognized the need to re-orient medical education to meet the healthcare needs of individuals and communities.[9]

There are two approaches to a community perspective in medical education:

- Community-oriented medical education (COME) is defined as "relevant medical education and takes into consideration all aspects of its operations that prioritize health problems in the country in which it is conveyed"[21] COME emphasizes a health-oriented education, rather than the traditional disease-oriented education, and it aims to produce community-oriented doctors who are capable and willing to serve their communities and deal effectively with health problems at primary, secondary, and tertiary levels.

- Community-based medical education (CBME) is "a means of achieving educational relevance for community needs, and consequently, serves as a way of implementing a community oriented program."[33] CBME is about teaching medical students in the community rather than in the hospital.

The distinction between the two approaches is not very clear. Magzoub et al.[33] clarify this issue on the basis of objectives and learning activities. COME refers to the *objectives* of the school and their relevance to community health needs. Such objectives must be reflected in the content of the curriculum. On the other hand, CBME refers to *learning activities* that take place in a community setting which may, or may not, be relevant to community health needs.

By the new millennium, many medical schools had adopted community-oriented curricula with students spending 10% or more of their time in the community.[22] These community-based attachments are based on the schools' community, cultural resources, and vision. Gezira Medical School in Sudan is considered a distinguished model for a community-based, community-oriented program. The school has great involvement with its community. On a regular basis, it sends students for between one week and a month to attachments in rural areas.[32, 34]

Outcome-based education

According to William Spady,[43] the pioneer of outcome-based education (OBE), the term means "focusing and organizing everything in an educational system based around what is essential for students' success at the completion of their learning experience." Outcome-based education starts with a clear vision of what students are required to know, what they are able to do, and what values and attitudes are desirable by the end of the program or learning experience. Subsequently, course designers select and plan for the appropriate content and teaching and assessment methods. This process gives top priority to end-product "outcomes", which becomes the basis for curriculum instruction, assessment planning, and implementation. However, this does not consider the form of programs. The same outcomes could be delivered and measured by a variety of methods, suitable to the institution's resources.

Terry[51] identifies four main characteristics of outcome-based education:

- outcomes are clearly identified;
- achieving them determines progress;
- multiple instructional strategies and authentic assessment tools are used; and
- students are given time and assistance to reach their potentials.

Features of outcome-based education

1. *Curriculum design in outcome-based education*

   One of Spady's[43] principles of OBE is "designing back." Thus, the curriculum design follows a top-down approach. Once exit outcomes are defined, they are used to determine program, course, unit and lesson outcomes (see Figure 3.1). Furthermore, teaching in OBE requires the development of a clear vision regarding the essentials that students need to perform effectively, followed by designing and selecting teaching strategies that enable students to achieve these outcomes.

2. *Institutes and outcome-based education*

   A key feature of OBE is that the program is founded on defined, measurable learning outcomes, thereby increasing the accountability of programs. Learning outcomes are considered to provide a means of systematic and organizational accountability, as they are explicit, observable, and therefore assessable indicators of student achievement.

3. *Teachers and outcome-based education*

   OBE requires a fundamental change in the teacher's role, shifting the focus from teachers to students. Students and their achievements, weaknesses, and strengths become the focus of teachers and the curriculum planners. Teachers have to review the whole curriculum and display an in-depth understanding of their contribution to students' learning. They then plan and organize teaching to be consistent with the students' needs. In OBE, contemporary teachers have multiple roles – as information providers, role models, facilitators, assessors, and curriculum and resources planners.[23]

4. *Students and outcome-based education*

   The role of students or learners in the education process is a fundamental principle of OBE. They are challenged to be active learners rather than passive recipients and to be independent and motivated. OBE provides students/learners with an opportunity to be fully involved in their own educational experiences, since they know what the final outcomes are and what is expected of them along the way.

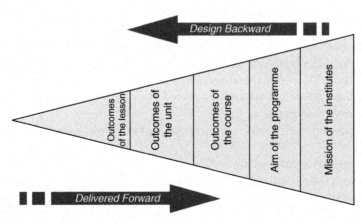

FIGURE 3.1   Designing-back approach in OBE

Moreover, OBE provides a balanced approach between autonomous learning and creative teaching. The curriculum explicitly and transparently encourages students' self-directed learning, as well as encouraging the faculty's liberty in selecting the content and methods of instruction.

Model of outcome-based education

There is an international move toward outcome-based education. Professional organizations have been concerned with medical programs and their outcomes and have developed competence-based or outcome-based frameworks.

In North America, the Association of American Medical Colleges (AAMC)[5] developed a consensus among leaders of the medical education community regarding the attributes required of physicians, which declares "Physicians must be altruistic ... knowledgeable ... skillful ... and dutiful." The Accreditation Council for Graduate Medical Education (ACGME)[2] developed six areas of competencies that all residents must demonstrate to qualify for independent practice. These comprise: patient care, medical knowledge, practice-based learning and improvement, interpersonal and communication skills, professionalism, and systems-based practice. In addition, the CanMEDS framework of the Royal College of Physicians and Surgeons of Canada (RCPSC)[40] defines the practicing specialist's key competencies and essential abilities that reflect societal needs (see Figure 3.2).

In the United Kingdom, as a response to the recommendation of the General Medical Council, "Tomorrow's Doctors",[15] the "*Scottish Doctor*" was developed as a consensus of the Scottish medical schools' views on essential "learning outcomes" for undergraduate medical education.[42] The Scottish Doctor highlighted 12 domains that relate to the doctor's competence and reflective practice, as illustrated in the three-circle outcome model[25] (see Table 3.1).

The Gulf Cooperation Council (GCC) Medical Colleges Deans' Committee[20] developed a consensus on the "learning outcomes" in the undergraduate medical programs for the medical schools in Arabian Gulf countries. The GCC's learning

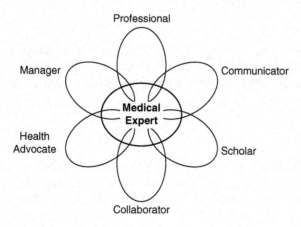

FIGURE 3.2 CanMEDS roles framework

TABLE 3.1 Scottish Doctor learning outcomes.

What the doctor is able to do:
'Doing the right thing'
Competence in clinical skills
Competence in practical procedures
Competence to investigate a patient
Competence in patient management
Competence in health promotion and disease prevention
Competence in communication
Competence in the handling and retrieval of information
How the doctor approaches practice
'Doing the thing right'
An understanding of basic and clinical sciences and underlying principles
Appropriate attitudes, ethical stance and legal responsibilities
Appropriate decision-making skills, clinical reasoning, and judgment
The doctor as professional
'The right person doing it'
An aptitude for personal development
Appropriate attitudes, ethical stance and legal responsibilities

outcomes expand on six fundamental themes of contemporary graduate and undergraduate medical education in six domains that are comparable to the ACGME Outcomes Project. They are as follows:

- patient care;
- medical knowledge;
- practice-based learning and improvement;
- interpersonal and communication skills;
- ethics and professionalism; and
- system-based practice.

In Saudi Arabia, the Medical Schools Deans' Committee has proposed a national framework of "Saudi MEDs" that highlight the desirable competencies of doctors and set the standard of expertise that trainees are required to achieve at each stage of their training.[57]

Simulation in learning

Simulation in medical education has developed and expanded over the last four decades. The innovative PBL curricula at McMaster and Maastricht have encouraged development and involvement of simulated patients, clinical skill centers and, more recently, high fidelity simulations.

- *Simulated patients*

Prior to embracing PBL as an educational model, Howard Barrows[6] developed the idea of the "simulated patient" to facilitate teaching and assessment during the clerkships in neurology. To Barrows, a simulated patient is a normal person who has been carefully trained to present the signs and symptoms of a real patient, in order to provide an opportunity for a student to learn or be evaluated on skills. Other names have been attached to this phenomenon – programmed patient, patient instructor, patient educator, and teaching associate.

The term "simulated patient" is sometimes used synonymously with the term "standardized patient", which was coined by Geoffrey Norman who used the term to refer to training the individual to present a standard, repeatable stimulus.[37] Standardized patients are now used in examinations by most professional bodies because high fidelity promises high validity of assessment. Yet the reliability of scores based on simulated patients depends on the scoring method and the degree of objectivity of the scoring system.[37]

In the 1970s, the utilization of simulated patients and simulators was expanded with the expansion of PBL, the foundation of Clinical Skill Centers and the development and growth of the Objective Structured Clinical Examination (OSCE). Nowadays, the role of the patients in medical education has been changed from passive participation to active partners with more involvement in the education and training of medical students.[45, 48, 56] Patients value their specific contribution to the education and training of medical students, which encourages their further involvement in the delivery of medical programs and the expansion of potential community-based teaching.[46]

- *Simulators*

Simulators are being designed to reproduce some aspects of clinical practice. This may vary from replicated aspects of a task to more complex, interactive environments such as operating theaters. Models and simulators range from simple static models to more interactive ones. The static models, such as those used for the insertion of intravenous lines, catheterization and endoscopy, permit students to practice single skills, but they do not respond to students' actions. The high level simulators, such as "SimMan" and "Harvey",[1, 19] provide sophisticated training and evaluation opportunities. SimMan was the first tested, computer-controlled patient simulator and a lifelike anesthetic training model developed by the University of Southern California School of Medicine in 1967.[1] Harvey is a full-sized mannequin who simulates 27 cardiac conditions and was first demonstrated in 1968 at the American Heart Association Scientific Sessions by Dr Michael Gordon of the University of Miami Medical School, under the title of a "Cardiology Patient Simulator".[19] Since SimMan, human patient simulators have advanced. The ultra-sophisticated simulators blink, speak and breathe, accurately mirroring human responses to such procedures as CPR, intravenous medication, intubation, ventilation, and catheterization.

Advanced simulators afford a technology base to train or evaluate students on single skills and procedures, as well as on whole scenarios that require teamwork, decision making, clinical reasoning, and individual skills and procedures.

Clinical skill centers

The perceived incompetence in clinical skills and procedures among medical graduates has led to a radical review in the approach to clinical teaching.[8] This has occurred at the same time as the call for medical graduates' competence in communication skills. Both of these factors have enforced the development of clinical skill units. In 1974, the first Skills Center was developed in Maastricht to facilitate the delivery of the PBL medical program that integrated the psychological and biomedical aspects of medical education.[10] The Maastricht skills lab has a wide remit and provides training for 150 procedures and communication skills.[52] Subsequently, Maastricht's successful experience has influenced other medical schools in developing clinical skill centers (CSCs), as well as adopting a PBL approach and utilizing simulated patients and simulators.

This trend has been developed in response to changes in healthcare policy and medical curricula, along with emphasis on quality assessment that confirms graduates' clinical and interpersonal competences. CSCs have become a fundamental element in the delivery and evaluation of medical programs for both undergraduates and postgraduates.

CSCs promise much potential:

- providing innovative ways of training in clinical skills by integrating theoretical knowledge and clinical practice;
- providing a clinically and emotionally safe environment for clinical skills training;
- enhancing assessment standards for student performance, affording the opportunity to tailor personalized training schemes; and
- enhancing the diagnosis of educational needs.

Dent[14] describes four core activities of CSCs:

- provision of various delivery methods;
- adoption of educational strategies;
- creation of self-assessment opportunities; and
- recognition of support mechanisms for both students and staff.

The potential scope of clinical skill centers is broad and encompasses not only clinical and communication skills but many others:[29,11]

- communication and history taking;
- professional attitudes and awareness of the ethical basis of health care;
- physical examination, procedural and clinical laboratory skills;
- diagnostic and therapeutic skills;

- resuscitation;
- critical thinking, reasoning, and problem-solving;
- teamwork, organization, and management;
- multi-professional practice; and
- information technology and medical informatics.

The development of CSCs must focus on the nature of the curriculum, the available resources (human and physical) and the scope of users (graduate/undergraduate). It must be flexible in its design and an integral part of the curriculum, with specific relevance and educational impact. Boulay and Medway[11] recognize the limitations of a skills center, because it can only provide simulated experiences which are adjunct to, but can never replace, real clinical experience. Thus, medical students must be encouraged to transfer their experience and competence with simulators to real patients.

Medical professionalism

The call for professional practice is not new. The concept of professionalism is well known, but is not easy to define. Accordingly, there is no consensus definition for professionalism. Cruess and Cruess[13] consider professionalism to be a physician's social responsibilities and a social contact between doctor and patient. The Royal College of Physicians[39] agrees that "medical professionalism signifies a set of values, behaviour and relationships that underpin the trust that the public has in doctors." Furthermore, a consensus of Physician's Charter among American and European professional bodies defines professionalism as "the basis of medicine's contract with society. It demands placing the interests of patients above those of the physician, setting and maintaining standards of competence and integrity, and providing expert advice to society on matters of health."[3] The charter specifies three fundamental principles: patient welfare, patient autonomy, and social justice. The following are ten professional responsibilities expected of physicians:

- commitment to professional competence;
- honesty with patients;
- patient confidentiality;
- maintaining appropriate relations with patients;
- improving the quality of care;
- improving access to care;
- distribution of finite resources;
- scientific knowledge; and
- maintaining trust.

Currently, professionalism and professional development have become a prominent topic in medical education. Many initiatives have been undertaken by educational and certifying bodies to accentuate the issue of medical professionalism in both graduates and undergraduates. The Accreditation Council for Graduate Medical Education[2] has adopted professionalism as one of the six core competencies that all residents must demonstrate to qualify for independent practice. The Association of American Medical Colleges (AAMC) considers professionalism a key outcome in its Medical Schools Objectives Project (MSOPI).[5] The CanMEDS roles[40] and the Scottish Doctor[42] also describe the knowledge, skills, and attitudes that define professionalism. The General Medical Council (GMC) statement of "Good Medical Practice"[17] defines professionalism and the professional standards that are expected of doctors in the UK.

Traditionally, medical schools were criticized for not enforcing professional behavior. Until recently, many medical schools had focused their assessment strategies on knowledge and skill and overlooked assessing professionalism during undergraduate studies. This may be related to vague understanding of the concept of professionalism and unclear teaching and assessment opportunities.[38] Professionalism used to be transmitted by role modeling, which is no longer considered appropriate or sufficient.[13]

Nowadays, the concept of professionalism is associated with some observed behavior that can be taught, fostered, and assessed in medical programs. Most medical schools have developed courses and learning opportunities that target professionalism. Much of the medical literature has discussed approaches to teaching and evaluating medical professionalism in undergraduate and graduate programs.[12-13, 47, 49-50] Stern and Papadakis[50] recommend a comprehensive program in teaching professionalism that includes three basic actions: setting expectations, providing experiences, and evaluating outcomes (see Table 3.2).

TABLE 3.2 Comprehensive program of teaching professionalism (from Stern and Papadakis).[50]

Setting expectations	
White-coat ceremonies Orientation sessions	Policies and procedures Codes and charters
Providing experiences	
Formal curriculum Problem-based learning Ethics courses Patient–doctor education International electives	Hidden curriculum Role models Parables The environment as teacher
Evaluation outcomes	

Assessment before entry into
    medical school
Assessment by faculty
Assessment by peers
	Assessment by patients (patient
	    satisfaction)
	Multi-perspective (360°) evaluation

Conclusion

As presented in this chapter, there is a universal drive for the development of medical education. Medical education worldwide has been exposed to the same drivers of change and has shared the paradigm of the future of medical education and practice. This has been reinforced with the international move toward establishing outcome-based education and global accreditation standards. It is obvious that medical schools in each country and region have to share this paradigm and commit to the international perspective of medical education.

References

1. Abrahamson, S., Denson, J.S. and Wolf, W.M. (1969) Effectiveness of a Simulator in Training Anesthesiology Residents. *Journal of Medical Education*, 44, 515–519.
2. Accreditation Council for Graduate Medical Education (1999) *General Competencies*. Chicago: Accreditation Council for Graduate Medical Education.
3. American Board of Internal Medicine (ABIM), Foundation American Board on Internal Medicine (ACP-ASIM), Foundation American College of Physical Medicine and American Society of Internal Medicine (2002) Medical Professionalism in the New Millennium: A Physician Charter. *Annual of Internal Medicine*, 136 (3), 243–246.
4. Association of American Medical Colleges (AAMC) (1984) Physicians for the Twenty-First Century: Report of the Project Panel on the General Professional Education of the Physician and College for Medicine. *Journal of Medical Education,* 59 (11), Supplement, Part 2:208.
5. Association of American Medical Colleges (AAMC) (1998) *Report I: Learning Objectives for Medical Student Education (MSOPI): Guidelines for Medical Schools.* Washington, DC: Association of American Medical Colleges.
6. Barrows, H.S. (1985) *How to Design a Problem-Based Curriculum for the Pre-Clinical Years,* New York, Springer.
7. Barrows, H.S. and Tamblyn, R.M. (1976) An Evaluation of Problem-Based Learning in Small Groups Utilizing a Simulated Patient. *Journal of Medical Education*, 51, 52–54.
8. Bligh, J. (1995) The Clinical Skills Unit. *Postgraduate Medical Journal*, 71, 730–732.
9. Boaden, N. and Bligh, J. (1999) *Community-based Medical Education: Towards a shared Agenda for Learning.* New York: Oxford University Press.
10. Bouhuijs, P.A.J., Schmidt, H.G., Snow, R.E. and Wijnen, W.H.F.W. (1978) The Rijksuniversiteit Limburg, Maastricht, the Netherlands: development of medical education. In F.M. Katz and T. Fülöp (Eds), *Personnel for Healthcare, Case Studies of Educational Programs.* Geneva: World Health Organization.
11. Boulay, C.D. and Medway, C. (1999) The Clinical Skills Resource: A Review of Current Practice. *Medical Education*, 33 (3), 185–191.
12. Cruess, R.L., McIlroy, J.H., Cruess, S.R., Ginsburg, S. and Stenert, Y. (2006) The Professionalism Mini-Evaluation Exercise: A Preliminary Investigation. *Academic Medicine*, 81, S74–S86.
13. Cruess, S.R. and Cruess, R.L. (1997) Professionalism Must be Taught. *British Medical Journal*, 315, 1674–1677.
14. Dent, J.A. (2001) Current Trends and Future Implications in the Developing Role of Clinical Skills Centers. *Medical Teacher*, 23, 483–489.

15. General Medical Council (GMC) (1993) *Tomorrow's Doctors. Recommendations on Undergraduate Medical Education.* London: The Education Committee of General Medical Council.

16. General Medical Council (GMC) (2002) *Tomorrow's Doctors. Recommendations on Undergraduate Medical Education,* 2nd Ed. London: The Education Committee of General Medical Council.

17. General Medical Council (GMC) (2006) *Good Medical Practice,* 3rd Ed. London: General Medical Council.

18. General Medical Council (GMC) (2009) *Tomorrow's Doctors. Recommendations on Undergraduate Medical Education,* 3rd Ed. London: The Education Committee of General Medical Council.

19. Gordon, M.S. (1974) Cardiology Patient Simulator: Development of an Automated Manikin to Teach Cardiovascular Disease. *American Journal of Cardiology,* 34, 350–355.

20. Gulf Countries Council's Medical College Deans' Committee (2005) *Medical Colleges Curriculum Outcomes: Competencies and Corresponding Curriculum Objectives.* Gulf Cooperation Council (unpublished document).

21. Hamad, B. (1991) Community-oriented Medical Education: What is it? *Medical Education,* 25 (1), 16–22.

22. Harden, R.M. (2001) Planning a Curriculum. In J. Dent and R.M. Harden (Eds.), *A Practical Guide for Medical Teachers.* Edinburgh and London: Churchill Livingstone and Harcourt.

23. Harden, R.M. and Crosby, J.R. (2000) The Good Teacher is more than a Lecturer: the Twelve Roles of the Teacher. *Medical Teacher,* 22, 334–347.

24. Harden, R.M. (2000) The Integration Ladder: A Tool for Curriculum Planning and Evaluation. *Medical Education,* 34, 551.

25. Harden, R.M., Crosby, J.R., Davis, M.H. and Friedman, M. (1999) AMEE Guide No. 14: Outcome-based Education: Part 5 – From Competency to Meta-Competence: A Model for the Specification of Learning Outcomes. *Medical Teacher,* 21, 546–552.

26. Harden, R.M. and Davias, M.H. (1998) The Continuum of Problem-based Learning. *Medical Teacher,* 20 (4), 317–322.

27. Harden, R., Davis, M. and Crosby, J. (1997) The new Dundee Medical Curriculum: A Whole that is Greater than the Sum of the Parts. *Medical Teacher,* 31, 264–271.

28. Ket, F. (2001) Chapter 5: Integration. In J.A. Dent and R.M. Harden (Eds.), *A Practical Guide for Medical Teachers.* Edinburgh and London: Churchill Livingstone and Harcourt.

29. Ledingham, I.M. and Dent, J.A. (2001) Clinical Skill Centers. In J.A. Dent and R.M. Harden (Eds.), *A Practical Guide for Medical Teachers.* Edinburgh and London: Churchill Livingstone and Harcourt.

30. Lowry, S. (1993) *Medical Education.* London: BMJ Publishing Group.

31. Ludmerer, K.M. (1985) *Learning to Heal: The Development of American Medical Education.* New York: Basic Books.

32. Magzoub, M.E.M.A. and Schmidt, H.G. (1996) Community-Based Programs: What is their Impact? *Education for Health,* 9(2), 209–220.

33. Magzoub, M.E.M.A. and Schmidt, H.G. (2000) A Taxonomy of Community-based. *Medical Education,* 75 (7), 699–707.

34. Magzoub, M.E.M.A., Schmidt, H.G., Dolmans, D.H.J.M., & Abdel-Hameed, A.A. (1998) Assessing students in community settings: the role of peer evaluation. *Advances in Health Sciences Education,* 3, 3–13.

35. McGaghie, W., Miller, G., Sajid, A. and Telder, T. (1978) Competency-based Curriculum Development on Medical Education: An Introduction. *Public Health Paper,* 68, 11–91.

36. Newble, D., Stark, P., Bax, N. and Lawson, M. (2005) Developing an Outcome-focused Core Curriculum. *Medical Education,* 39, 680–687.

37. Norman, G.R. (1984) Standardized Patients. Paper presented at the Annual Meeting of the American Educational Research Association, New Orleans, LA.

38. Passi, V. Doug, M., Peile, E., Thistlethwaite, J. and Johnson, N. (2010) Developing Medical Professionalism in Future Doctors: a systematic review. *International Journal of Medical Education,* 1, 19–29.

39. Royal College of Physicians (2005) *Doctors in Society: Medical Professionalism in a Changing World.* London: Royal College of Physicians.

40. Royal College of Physicians and Surgeons in Canada (RCPSC) (2000) *Skills for the New Millennium CANMEDS 2000 Project.* Ottawa: Royal College of Physicians and Surgeons in Canada.

41. Schmidt, H.G., Neufeld, V.R., Noorman, M.Z. and Ogunbode, T. (1991) Network for Community-oriented Educational Institutions for the Health Sciences. *Academic Medicine,* 66, 259–263.

42. Simpson, J.G., Furnace, J., Crosby, J., Cumming, A.D., Evans, P.A., et al. (2002) The Scottish Doctor – Learning Outcomes for the Medical Undergraduate in Scotland: A Foundation for Competent and Reflective Practitioners. *Medical Teacher,* 24 (2), 136 –143.

43. Spady, W. (1994) *Outcomes-based Education: Critical Issues and Answers.* Arlington, VA: American Association of School Administrators.

44. Spencer, J.A. and Jordan, R.K. (1999) Learner Centered Approaches in Medical Education. *British Medical Journal,* 1280–1283.

45. Spencer, J., Blackmore, D., Heard, S., McCrorie, P., McHaffie, D., Scherpbier, A., Gupta, T.S., Singh, K. and Southgat, L. (2000) Patient-Oriented Learning: A Review of the Role of the Patient in the Education of Medical Students. *Medical Education,* 34 (10), 851–857.

46. Stacy, R. and Spencer, J. (1999) Patients as Teachers: A Qualitative Study of Patients' Views on their Role in a Community-based Undergraduate Project. *Medical Education,* 33 (9), 688–694.

47. Stark, P. (2006) Chapter I: Professionalism: In N. Cooper, K. Forrost and P. Cramp, *Essential Guides to Generic Skills. Massachusetts,* Wiley–Blackwell.

48. Stark, P., Hague, M. and Bax, N. (2009) Involving patients as educators: adding values to clinical experience. *International Journal of Clinical Skills,* 3 (2), 64–69.

49. Stern, D.T. and Papadakis, M. (2007) Medical Education – Professionalism. *New England Journal of Medicine,* 356 (6), 639–641.

50. Stern, D.T. and Papadakis, M. (2006) Medical Education: The Developing Physician; Becoming a Professional. *New England Journal of Medicine,* 355, 1794–1799.

51. Terry, P.M. (1996) Outcome-based Education: Is it Mastery Learning all over Again, or is it Revolution to the Reform Movement? 7th Annual Midwest Education Society (CIES) Conference, Indiana.

52. Van Dalen, J., Zuidweg, J. and Collet, J. (1989) The Curriculum of Communication Skills Teaching at Maastricht Medical School. *Medical Education,* 23(1), 55–61.

53. World Federation for Medical Education (WFME) (2003) WFME Global Standards in Medical Education; Status and Perspectives following the 2003 WFME World Conference. *Medical Education,* 37, 1050–1054.

54. World Federation for Medical Education (WFME) (1993) The Changing Medical Profession: Implications for Medical Education. *Medical Education,* 27, 1–2.

55. World Federation for Medical Education (WFME) (1998) International Standards in Medical Education: Assessment and Accreditation of Medical Schools' Educational Programs. A WFME Position. *Medical Education*, 32, 592–558.

56. Wykurz, G. (1999) Patients in Medical Education: from Passive Participants to Active Partners. *Medical Education*, 33 (9), 634–636.

57. Zaini, R.G., BinAbdulrahman, K.A., Al-Khotani, A.A. et al. (2010) Saudi Meds (unpublished work).

Chapter 4

Standards in Medical Education

John Hamilton

Objectives

By the end of this chapter, you will be able to:
- Understand what are the standards in medical education.
- Know what the "Curriculum" is.
- Be familiar with "Accreditation".
- Identify the process of accreditation between the Australian Medical Council (AMC) and the World Federation for Medical Education (WFME).

Introduction

The focus of this chapter is on how to evaluate the standards of medical education to ensure that graduates are safe and competent and have the capacity to remain so for the rest of their professional lives. We shall look at this issue through the principles and practice of medical school accreditation, which illustrates all the factors involved.

What do we mean by standards?

The International Federation of Medical Students' Associations (IFMSA) describes *Standards* in basic medical education as "Both a goal and a measure of progress towards that goal."[1]

- The *goal* (or outcome) is that graduates are fit to practice effectively, safely, and with relevance to the needs of patients, families, health services, and communities.
- The measure of progress relates to the curriculum, the program of activities (or process) which medical schools must arrange and with which students must comply to achieve the goal.

What do we mean by curriculum?

Nowadays when we speak of "the curriculum" we include not just the content, but the entire experience of the student. This includes:

- What the university or medical school prescribes to be learned and developed in knowledge skills and attitudes.
- The experience made available in the university, in the healthcare system, and in the community.
- The quality and number of teachers, mentors, and role models.
- The criteria and means for selection of students.
- The means of teaching and learning.
- The "hidden curriculum" of the real-world experience within the health system: "the set of influences that function at the level of organizational structure and culture including, for example, implicit rules to survive in the institution such as customs, rituals, and aspects that are taken for granted. They are not planned, are rarely annotated or assessed, but may have a profound effect on the values and attitude of graduates, for good and for bad."[2] We shall return to this later.

Other chapters in this handbook deal with how the several components of a curriculum should be developed and implemented, and will deal with standards specific to that component. In this chapter we shall adopt a perspective across the entire experience of medical education from the perspective of "accreditation."

What do we mean by accreditation?

Accreditation is the system of inspection and evaluation of medical schools that many countries use to assure government and the public that they are fulfilling their legal responsibility to produce safe and competent doctors. There are two aspects:

- The legal responsibility to inspect and evaluate standards of all individual schools and to rule on accreditation.
- A wider and longer-term role to improve the quality of medical education. This is done by consultations and workshops dealing with issues that arise during accreditations, and most of all by wide participation of teachers, medical educators, and other stakeholders at all levels of the process. Not all authorities undertake this second and longer-term role, but the two described below do:

2010 is the Centenary Year of Abraham Flexner's 1910 landmark report on the standards of medical education in the United States of America and Canada.[3] He created an early system for accreditation. He defined standards and titled them "The Proper Basis of Medical Education." They dealt with content, quality of staff, laboratories and hospitals and means of learning. He visited all 150 medical schools to assess whether the curriculum matched the standards. Large numbers did not, and were declared to be inadequate. Many soon shut down.

We shall look at two examples of the modern system of accreditation to illustrate how standards are set and described, how assessment of a medical school is conducted, and how recommendations for accreditation are updated and revised as a means of raising standards. These are the Australian Medical Council and the World Federation for Medical Education.

National Standards for Medical Education:
the Australian Medical Council

The author was founding chairman of the AMC Accreditation Committee, established in 1984.[4] The Committee's roles are:

- To develop guidelines, and policy and procedures, for the accreditation of medical schools and medical courses.
- To oversee the program of accreditation and make recommendations.
- To encourage improvements in medical education that respond to evolving health needs, practices, educational and scientific developments.
- The basis for the third role, to improve medical education, was established in early policy statements:

[Accreditation] *should strike a balance between its statutory supervisory role and its consultative and creative role in medical education.*

While it is the present standards of medical education that will be the immediate concern of the Accreditation Committee, it will also be mindful of the need to prepare successive generations of educators to sustain a high quality of medical education in the future. The Committee will also take into account the responsibility of medical schools to provide for their staff, the opportunity of coherent and rigorous academic and educational development.

The Accreditation Committee supports diversity in teaching approaches, provided schools evaluate their own approaches.

Clearly, even a detailed review of written curriculum and assessment would not be sufficient; a full range of support and enabling capacities of the school and its partner organizations would have to be reviewed. A wide range of stakeholders have a responsibility for standards and they must also be held to account. This was illustrated by the decision of the very first AMC accreditation in 1987. It awarded only a limited period of accreditation. The curriculum itself would benefit from stronger integration but was nevertheless producing competent graduates. It was the prospects for the future that caused the main concern. Key elements of that concern were:

- Difficulty in recruitment and retention of staff in the medical school – in part because of the following two problems.

- Failure to address longstanding difficulties in arrangements with teaching hospitals.
- Poor research cooperation between hospitals and universities.

It was not within the power of the faculty alone to solve these problems; the responsibility rested also with the universities, hospitals, clinicians, and the Department of Health. Prompt action was taken by all stakeholders, the issues were resolved, and the future welfare of the school assured.

The process of AMC accreditation

The current process is detailed in the AMC website:[5]

- Guidelines and standards are issued by AMC and are revised from time to time.
- Prior to accreditation, the school is required to provide a detailed description of the curriculum as support capacity.
- The school is also required to undertake an extensive internal review and to report on its strengths, weaknesses, opportunities and threats (a SWAT analysis). They relate this both to AMC guidelines and to the school's own aims and objectives. Plans must be prepared to address deficits and to respond to the evolving needs of patients, health systems, and students.
- An Assessment Team visits the school for five days; visits all sites and meets with staff and students and government officials. The team bases its inquiry on the report of the internal review. The inquiry is conducted in a collegiate manner that includes consultation and advice.
- From the very outset, the contribution of students gave some of the most perceptive insights about how the curriculum was working in reality. A confidential commentary by students is now sent directly to the AMC, unseen by the school.
- The essence of the evaluation is given verbally to the school to ensure immediacy, but the recommendation on accreditation is not provided, because it is the exclusive responsibility of the Council.
- The team prepares a report for the Accreditation Committee, which reviews it to ensure the grounds for the recommendations are sound. This is then referred on to the Council itself to approve the final recommendation and decision on accreditation. The decision and the full report are placed in the public record and are accessible to all.

The process is respected, strongly supported by Deans of Medicine who are all involved in the process, and the comments and recommendations are received as valid and constructive.

Guidelines appropriate to national needs

For the guidelines to respond to the needs of the nation, a review of those needs would be essential. In 1988, the AMC was given helpful direction by a national review of Australian workforce education and future needs, commissioned by the Ministry of Health and chaired by Professor Ralph Doherty.[6] This independent review consulted widely and AMC contributed to it. The review gave an ideal basis for a well-founded response through medical education to the health needs of Australia, and AMC revised its guidelines to match. Thereafter, as new priorities have emerged in healthcare or in education, these are reflected in regular revision of guidelines. Priorities have included:

- The need to reduce errors and to improve safety in healthcare in response to the national study of adverse outcomes in healthcare.
- The decision to widen the criteria for selection of students as a result of concerns of the public and the profession about personal qualities.
- To strengthen the curriculum in indigenous health and to recruit indigenous students to address the lamentable state of health of indigenous populations.
- The need for clinician practice to be based upon evidence.
- The opportunity to capitalize upon modern IT technology in healthcare and in education.
- The recognition of the importance of clinical and social experience in community and primary care.
- The need for better skills in readiness for internship.

Standards therefore are dynamic, evolving in scope and priority. The response to evolving priorities requires a contribution from stakeholders inside and outside the medical school. A curriculum with no attention to these new areas would be judged to be of insufficient standard.

The involvement of stakeholders and the collegial approach to accreditation enables the AMC to fulfill the mandate *"To encourage improvements in medical education that respond to evolving health needs and practices, and educational and scientific developments."* It has indeed made a strong contribution to the dynamic development of Australian medical education in the past two decades.

Global standards for medical education: the World Federation of Medical Education (WFME)

The AMC deals primarily with the needs of Australia and, more recently, New Zealand. The British General Medical Council and the United States Liaison Committee on Medical Education (LCME) and other national bodies have similar responsibilities.

Many countries do not have an equivalent system, relying only on university autonomy and internal quality control. This is less effective in supporting overall national standards and renewal.

Globalization of health and healthcare is growing. There is a high level of migration of medical graduates and movement of populations across cultural boundaries, changing health patterns. There is a rapid exchange and spread of knowledge, educational methods, pharmaceuticals, and equipment. It is recognized that there is a need for global standards in medical education.

In 1998, the World Federation of Medical Education launched an extensive international consultation among experts to produce the "WFME Global Standards for Quality Improvement."[7] The guidelines have been tested and found to be helpful and effective in a wide range of circumstances.

WFME guidelines, like those of the AMC, reflect the wide range of influences and stakeholders in medical education. They are grouped under nine headings:

1   Mission and Objectives
2   Educational Program
3   Assessment of Students
4   Students
5   Academic Staff/Faculty
6   Educational Resources
7   Program Evaluation
8   Continuous Renewal
9   Governance and Administration

To accommodate wide global differences in resources and systems of healthcare, each standard is written and defined at two levels: one obligatory, and one at a higher level:

- Basic Standards which must be fulfilled by all institutions to achieve a basic minimum standard of graduate outcome.
- Standards for Quality Development which ideally should demonstrate a capacity to improve and to respond to emerging needs.

These standards have been tested in schools in widely differing circumstance and found useable and constructive.

WFME does not claim a regulatory role but, within its overall mandate to improve medical education worldwide, offers the role of advisor and support to schools, countries and national accrediting agencies worldwide. In this, it has joined forces with the World Health Organization.

How can guidelines be used and by whom?

So far, we have considered the use of guidelines in establishing a national capacity in accreditation or at the invitation of individual schools. But they can also be used internally by staff or students to evaluate the standard of their own school. This can be done without the involvement of an external agency or with the assistance of one or more external advisors.

The full detail of the scope and standards for each guideline is found at the WFME website,[7] which should be consulted alongside this brief account. We shall look at three examples below:

Statement No. 1 – Mission and Objectives

This should state the overarching aims in educating and training doctors and should reflect the priorities of the medical school in the wider context of health services, community, and students.

It is easy to become cynical that such overarching statements have no bearing on reality either because there is no institutional commitment or no focus within the curriculum, or no assessment appropriate to the stated priorities; if that is so, then they are in effect ignored. Competent accreditation should identify that, as indeed should an internal review, and formulate plans to fulfill the priority. For instance:

– If the Mission is to prepare doctors who understand and can adapt their care to disadvantaged communities, then that must be demonstrably achievable through the curriculum, with opportunity to learn from the community and to gain experience within it.
– If it is these graduates who are to be educators of patients and their colleagues, then there should be a clear sequence of experiences and training and assessment to that end.

Statement No. 4 – Students

It is essential that the school have a clear policy on how it will assist students in their professional development and ensure that their skills match the needs of the community. This should cover:

• Student selection. The public sees personal qualities, motivation and commitment as important as pure academic achievement. Some schools ask students to be selectors. When we select students we create a community of scholars, hopefully diverse, with the capacity to learn together and to contribute to the continuing improvement of the school.
• The size of the class to match facilities and the number of patients they can access. There is a reciprocal need to explore alternative sources of clinical experience.
• The environment of learning, characterized by opportunity for discovery, accepting responsibility and opportunity to reflect and to grow.
• Student support and counseling. Medicine is a challenging field; support should not only be available in time of trouble but also as a positive facilitation of professional and personal growth. Many schools have a stream of curriculum committed to this, often linked to ethics and medical humanities,

and supported by mentors who themselves are role models of professional maturity.

- Student representation on committees and other bodies. Consultation and feedback must be a serious priority for the school and also for students. Students are adults and benefit from the challenge of responsibility.
- Staff must accept a responsibility in this, to be role models for good practice. It is here that the "hidden curriculum," mentioned above, is at work. Seeing how senior colleagues or the system of healthcare actually provide healthcare gives a strong message, for positive gain or for negative loss of motivation and commitment. So this requires the school, together with the health service and individual clinicians, to provide an experience that facilitates and reinforces positive professional development. A poor experience through the hidden curriculum causes students to lose their altruism and motivation.

Statement No. 8 – Continuous Renewal

A reliable system of course evaluation, involving student opinion and looking at outcomes through assessment and the advice of external examiners, is vital to maintenance of quality, provided the lessons learned are acted upon. This provides for continuous maintenance and improvement of quality. The following also have to be done to keep staff and students up to the mark:

- Ensure all staff and students are aware of educational principles and new trends through staff and student development.
- Use an understanding of learning to optimize students' opportunities and effectiveness as learners, and monitor the processes and outcomes of learning in all settings.
- Incorporate new technologies within the achievable scope of the institution.
- Refresh and adapt student assessment and course evaluation to the aims of the curriculum.
- Continue consulting with stakeholders.
- Support students and establish regular two-way communication.
- Share ideas and experience with other institutions, both nationally and internationally.

This is important, but it does not achieve the much larger aim of "renewal," which gives new profile and scope to what standards mean and takes into account the experience and expectations of all stakeholders.

A robust renewal requires the school to look again at the context of its community, or the experience of graduates, or the emerging requirements of the health service, or the experience of learning of its graduates, or the examples of other schools, to consider developing cooperation with other schools with similar challenges.

It is often in new schools with an open mandate that major innovation can emerge, providing new patterns of education for others to consider. Here are a few examples:

- *McMaster, Canada.* A new school, opened in 1969, developed problem-based learning (PBL).[8] In time this was implemented and adapted by others. PBL has solid foundations in principles of learning and requires careful planning and tutoring. It is not a format to be applied without understanding and preparation. A few schools have hastened into the format without attention to the principles, creating problems for students and staff. Innovation is not necessarily renewal.
- *Newcastle, Australia.* A school was set up with a specific mandate to explore and implement new approaches to medical education, student selection, an orientation to community care and social factors in health and healthcare.[9]
- *Ilorin, Nigeria.* A school was set up to fulfill a government policy that new schools should be community oriented through primary care.[10] The school's program of community-oriented education and service (COBES) gave direction to other schools. In relation to this, some of the best leads have been given by developing countries.

Schools already established can take equally bold steps in renewal. One example will suffice:

- *New Mexico, USA.* A school was established as the first medical school in the state and run on entirely conservative lines. After a few years the school realized, especially through its Department of General Practice, that neither the curriculum nor student experience was bearing any close relation to the real social and health needs of those living in the State of New Mexico. This was a community of cultural and historic diversity, poverty, migration, and disadvantage. The school also realized its curriculum was didactic and not centered on student learning needs. The result was a comprehensive renewal of learning, a focus on community, the use of remote communities for learning, and engagement with the community in joint action on health and welfare. What started in the undergraduate curriculum was soon taken up in postgraduate education, making the school a leader from which others could learn and from which government policy on medical education could take a lead.

All these examples are from members of the Network – Towards Unity for Health. The network's website[11] provides many examples of renewal from around the globe and the dynamic of students themselves in this endeavor.

References

1. International Federation of Medical Students' Associations (IFMSA): Policy on Implementing International Standards in Basic Medical Education. 2008.

http://www.ifmsa.org/index.php?option=com_content&view=article&id=68:policyposition-on-implementing-international-standards-in-basic-medical-education&catid=26:general&Itemid=41 Accessed 19.09.2009.

2. Lempp H, Searle C: *Brit Med J*, 2008, *336*, 718–721.

3. Flexner A: Medical Education in the United States and Canada. Carnegie Foundation. 1910.

4. Hamilton JD, Vandewerdt JM: The Accreditation of Undergraduate Medical Education in Australia. *Med J Aust*, 1990, *153*, 541–545.

5. Australian Medical Council. Assessing Basic Medical Education. http://www.amc.org.au/index.php/ar/bme. Accessed10.09.2009.

6. Doherty RL (Chairman): Australian Medical Education and Workforce into the 21st Century. Commonwealth of Australia,1988.

7. World Federation for Medical Education (WFME): Basic Medical Education. In *WFME Standards for Quality Improvement*. WFME Office, University of Copenhagen, Denmark. http://www.wfme.org. Accessed 19.09.2009.

8. Hamilton JD: The McMaster curriculum: a critique. *Brit Med J,* 1976, *1*, 1191–1196.

9. Hamilton JD: A Community and Population-Oriented Medical School: Newcastle, Australia. In KL White and JE Connelly (eds): *The Medical School's Mission and the Population's Health: Medical Education in Canada, The United Kingdom, The United States and Australia,* Chap 6., New York: Springer-Verlag, 1992.

10. Hamilton JD, Ogunbode O: Medical education in the community: a Nigerian experience. *The Lancet*, 1991, *338*, 99–102.

11. Network – Towards Unity for Health, <www.the-networktufh.org> Accessed 19.09.2009.

Chapter 5

Problem-based Learning

Henk G. Schmidt and Willem de Grave

Objectives

- To provide an overview of the problem-based approach to learning and instruction.
- To review some of the reasons that lead to this approach.
- To describe the mechanics of PBL as illustrated by an example of a tutorial group organizing its learning around a problem.

Introduction

Problem-based learning is a fairly new and, in some ways, revolutionary approach to learning and instruction. Although initially developed for medical education, it carries the promise of being able to solve some persistent problems that, for years, have plagued education in general. Before discussing some of these issues, we will briefly describe the approach.

What is problem-based learning and how does it work?

Problem-based learning can be described as a method of learning in which small groups of six to ten students work on "problems," guided by a tutor. The tutor is often a teacher, but in many cases senior students play that role. Problems are sometimes derived from professional practice (as is the case with problem-based medical curricula); often they are based on theoretical issues, important to the domain of study.

An example of such a problem, used in a problem-based curriculum, is the following:

Miraculous rescue

For more than 15 minutes an eight year old boy, Maurice, was lifelessly floating around in water colder than 60°F. Fortunately, a passerby succeeded in bringing him out of the water. Mouth-to-mouth resuscitation was applied immediately. Everyone was astonished to notice that the boy was still alive. Presently, Maurice is on the intensive care ward of the local hospital and is out of danger. According to his doctor he is expected to recover completely. Explain why this is possible.

Students initially discuss such a problem using prior knowledge, which, if the problem is carefully calibrated to the students' level of knowledge, will be insufficiently extended to help them comprehend it in full. Because their knowledge falls short, "learning issues" are raised in the course of discussion that act as guides for further individual self-directed learning activities.

After a period of self-study, the tutorial group meets again and reviews what has been learned in relation to the problem. Does one now have a better understanding of the problem and its causes? Is one better able to explain why some people display excessive fear responses to innocent stimuli? Are the physiological origins of fear clearly understood, etc.? Having completed the present problem in a satisfactory fashion, the tutorial group moves on to a subsequent, related, problem and the learning cycle starts all over again.

Reasons for developing problem-based learning as an approach to learning and instruction

Problem-based learning is an offshoot of approaches to instruction that emphasize active, self-directed and independent learning. It was developed initially in the context of medical education but is now applied in domains such as psychology, economics, law, physics, and secondary education. The introduction of problem-based learning in the late 1960s at McMaster University, Hamilton, Canada, was a comprehensive attempt to deal with a number of issues that bothered those involved in the attempt. We will briefly review these issues here. The concerns were formulated almost thirty years ago; all of them, however, seem as relevant today as they were thirty years ago.

- Students often perceive instruction as insufficiently relevant to their personal goals. For instance, a young woman who decides to study medicine is often primarily motivated by the idea that she will acquire knowledge and skills that will enable her to help other people by restoring and maintaining health. Such students are often disappointed by the emphasis on normal physiological and biochemical functioning of the human body in the first years of medical education. Although an understanding of these topics may be relevant to understanding malfunction, this relevance is not perceived as such. Hence, medical students often complain about the first part of their training.
- Acquisition of knowledge, gaining a deeper understanding of the world, is not seen as a possible end in itself, but simply as a means to pass examinations, or to acquire other goods such as a diploma or a well-paid job. Although these goals make perfectly good sense, they are hardly sufficient to maintain an acceptable level of intrinsic interest in subject matter to be studied on a

day-to-day basis. In fact, there are indications that external rewards impede intrinsic motivation.

- Failure to recognize learning as a partial social endeavor.
- Education seen as dull, not cool.
- Premature drop-out.
- Emphasis on abstract knowledge rather than emphasis on the contextuality of learning.
- Lack of emphasis on professional skills and attitudes.
- Lack of emphasis on the development of skills for lifelong, self-regulatory learning.
- Lectures as ineffective methods for transmitting information.
- Lack of integration among different knowledge domains.
- Discrepancy between existing educational practices and emerging beliefs that learning is the first requirement for all acquisition of knowledge.
- Massification of education; increased loneliness of students.
- Failure to develop authentic methods of assessment.
- Students often display minimalist, shallow, surface-level learning strategies, possibly as a consequence of the first and second points above. Educational researchers agree that good students are characterized by the use of deep-level strategies, suggesting that a comprehensive understanding of a domain can only be acquired through deep processing of topics studied.
- Students sometimes display an inability to use the knowledge they have acquired. They have the knowledge but are unable to use this knowledge when appropriate. The educational literature is replete with examples of this phenomenon. Studies in the social sciences, for instance, have demonstrated an alarming lack of theoretical concepts acquired during education in the master theses of graduates. Even in a very simple situation, students are often not able to apply their knowledge. In cognitive psychology, this is called the "competence–performance paradox." Human beings may possess the competencies, but are unable to demonstrate them while performing a competency-relevant task.

Let me give you an example: Imagine that I throw a coin into the air. The coin describes a certain trajectory, as indicated in Figure 5.1. Imagine the coin at position P. What forces exert their influence on the coin at position P?

Let me help you a little. Figure 5.2 offers four possibilities.

The first possibility is that two forces exert their influence on the movement of the coin at position P: the force of the hand (F_h) or the force of gravity (F_g). Both forces are equally large, as exemplified by the length of the line. The second possibility is that the force exerted by the hand is larger than gravity. The third possibility is just the other way around; the force of gravity is larger than the force of the hand; and the fourth possibility is that only the force of gravity exerts its influence on the coin at position P. What would be your answer? Possibility B? Wrong, but you are in good company. A group of students of an Ivy League college in the United States were required to solve this problem as part of an

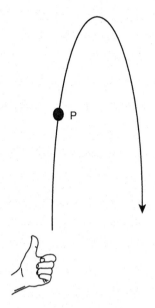

FIGURE 5.1   The author's hand throws a coin

introductory course in mechanics. These students, who were to major in Physics, had completed an introductory course in Newtonian mechanics and had a working knowledge of concepts such as force, velocity, acceleration and impulse. These were the concepts they used when required to justify their choice. Nevertheless, just like yourself, more than eighty percent of these students chose B, whereas the correct answer is the alternative D. According to Newton, the only force necessary to explain the behavior of the coin at position P is gravity.

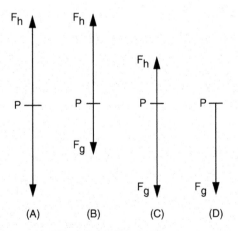

FIGURE 5.2   Which forces exert influence on the coin at point P?

Thus, although these students possessed the required knowledge, they were unable to use that knowledge to explain a seemingly simple situation.

A second and third example

Gonella et al.[3] monitored the care of a group of patients suspected of having a urinary tract infection. They noted in which of the cases the physicians (resident or fully trained) conducted critical evaluations with respect to the problems and what additional information was acquired, given the suspicion of pyelonephritis (an infection of the upper urinary tract). In only about 50% of the cases had the staff actually acquired information relevant to bacteriuria from the patients concerned. After completing this monitoring of care in an unobtrusive way, Gonella and colleagues asked the physicians involved to complete a multiple-choice examination dealing with diagnosis, treatment and follow-up of patients with urinary tract infection. The mean score of correct answers on the multiple-choice test pertaining to that same subject was 82%. These findings suggest that the physicians involved had knowledge they were unable to use when faced with a task relevant to that knowledge base.

Willems[5] established essentially the same phenomenon in investigations among students of law, social geography, planning science, and sociology. When writing a report on some topic or when solving problems, these students hardly ever used the concepts they must have had acquired previously; they simply seemed to be unable to use this knowledge.

Why is this so? Why does knowledge gained through books and lectures not translate itself into a useful instrument for practicing a profession or solving real-life problems? According to recent conceps of learning and instruction, of which we will come to speak in the next chapter, this is because students are not given sufficient opportunity to apply their knowledge in real-life situations. By institutionalizing learning in schools, we have stripped knowledge from its context, from its concrete here-and-now properties. The organization of learning in schools rather than through everyday practice has enabled us to give our students access to our culture's knowledge more than any other civilization has been able to accomplish, but possibly at the expense of the utility of this knowledge in daily life.

With the massification of higher education in the late 1960s, universities and other institutes for advanced learning have become hostile environments for many students. Since much of the training in these institutes is lecture-based, students are forced to spend much of their time in lecture theaters, sometimes together with hundreds of other students, the majority of whom they do not know and never will get to know personally. In this environment, they are, in some cases, confronted with teachers who are highly skilled and engaging, but they more often find teachers who are somewhat mediocre and generally uninteresting. In studies based on students' perception of lectures, it has been demonstrated again and again that students consider these lectures on average dull and uninspiring. Certainly, this is not the fault of the average teacher. Being able to attract the attention of a large audience and keep them interested in the subject of one's lecture requires the combined skills of the great comedians and story tellers of our time. Of course, we all remember the one exceptional teacher, the one who made you sit on the tip of your chair, the one who made you want to scream "More!" The fact that everyone remembers this teacher is a clear indication that the many forgotten teachers were less able to achieve this result. Again, this is not their fault. Listening to someone speak for more than twenty minutes is usually more than most human beings can bear. For that matter, lecturing is a somewhat old-fashioned and cumbersome way of transmitting information from one person to another. We have the book, remember? On average, people grasp ideas almost three times as quickly when they read about it rather than when they hear about it. This is simply because people can read faster than lecturers can speak. Books and other student-centered materials, in addition, have the advantage that one can easily review materials that were not understood the first time; a facility that a lecturer can only simulate by rehearsing the materials presented a number of times, an activity perhaps necessary for some students, but not for others.[1]

This problem becomes even more pertinent in situations where students view the acquisition of knowledge as a necessary but rather uninteresting means to a more interesting end, namely, having an interesting job, earning a good salary, and generally living a good life.

The process of problem-based learning: an example

There have been several attempts to deal with the problems as outlined above. One of these attempts is problem-based learning. The remainder of this chapter is intended to give you a "feel" of what problem-based learning is, how it works and what instructional measures are involved to make it work. We will endeavor to accomplish this by presenting a case history of problem-based learning. In doing so, we hope that you will arrive at a basic understanding of the approach so that you may appreciate the chapters that are to follow.

All learning in a problem-based curriculum starts with a problem such as this:

A stinging incident

Mr Laeven practices a hobby that most of us find rather scary to say the least. At the back of his yard, he has a number of beehives. He always visits his bees first thing in the morning. One morning, when he arrives at the back of the yard, he stumbles and hits a hive. No need of telling what happened. He hardly manages to reach the house and alarms his wife, who calls their family physician. Mr Laeven's sting wounds are seriously aching and after some five minutes he feels dizzy and almost fainting. He is in a cold sweat and is getting sick.

---

[1] Of course, this is a somewhat exaggerated, caricatural view of lectures as a method of teaching, to precede and enable the introduction of problem-based learning to shortly glow and shine.

The family physician arrives after 15 minutes. She sees a conscious looking man with a regular breath. The physician counts a pulse rate of 88 beats a minute and takes the blood pressure: 120/80 mmHg. After five minutes, she takes the pulse rate, 104 beats/minute, the blood pressure then being 115/80 mmHg. After another five minutes, Mr Laeven has a pulse rate of 120 beats per minute and a blood pressure of 85/55 mmHg. The acra are hot. The family physician injects adrenaline intravenously.

Explain what is happening to Mr Laeven.

A problem such as this has been written by a teacher, or team of teachers, with the aim of guiding students towards certain subject matter. The problem text usually describes some phenomena or events that can be observed in daily life, but can also consist of the description of an important theoretical or practical issue. The problem is presented to students for small group discussion. A group is generally made up of six to ten students, supported by a staff member known as a "tutor." Usually the students are to explain the phenomena or events described in terms of their underlying mechanisms, principles, or processes. The students do not prepare themselves for the initial discussion of the problem. They come into the situation equipped only with their prior knowledge. This knowledge may have been acquired through formal education, but also through the mass media, or derived from their own personal experiences of a similar situation. What is important is that the problem comes first.

The following is an excerpt of a discussion between first-year medical students of the University of Limburg, Maastricht, the Netherlands, dealing with the problem as presented above. The excerpts are slightly edited for readability.

Students start by reading the text silently and finding out whether there are words used in the problem that they do not know. One of the students, Sabine, acts as the chairperson.

Sabine (chair):	Have you all read the text? (short silence) Did you come across difficult words?
Erica:	Yes, what are acra?
Chairperson:	Nobody knows what acra are?
Janneke:	I think acra are the sites where stings are located, but I am not sure.
Bas:	I do not know.
Chairperson:	Well, that means we have to look up this concept, or ask the tutor.
Tutor:	Acra are...
Chairperson:	Are there any other difficult concepts?
Astrid:	No.

After this check on understanding of the text, the students proceed in trying to figure out what exactly needs to be explained by them. They call this part of the discussion the problem formulation phase.

Chairperson:	Then we can now start with the formulation of a problem definition. Does anybody have a suggestion for a problem definition?
Astrid:	What happens after a bee sting?
Janneke:	We should specifically elaborate on the effects of the venom injected into the body during a bee sting.
Erik:	Is venom actually being released during a bee sting?
Monica:	Yes, I think so.
Chairperson:	So, what happens, i.e., how does the body respond to a bee sting?
Erik:	I do not understand why Mr Laeven's pulse rate increases so late.
Erica:	Yes, it happens on the family doctor's arrival; only after some 25 minutes does the body show a dramatic response.
Chairperson:	So, our first question is: What happens after a multitude of bee stings? And why does the blood pressure change only after 25 minutes? And what are you supposed to do then?
Janneke:	You mean both blood pressure and pulse rate?
Erica:	Yes, I assume they are interrelated.
Chairperson:	Why do blood pressure and pulse rate change only after 25 minutes?
Erik:	Why are the acra hot? And what is the use of injecting adrenaline here?
Monica:	What other symptoms do we need to explain?
Astrid:	That man feeling fainted and getting dizzy and being in a cold sweat. He seems to be conscious all right.
Chairperson:	Is that all there is?
Monica:	Perhaps it is important that the adrenaline is injected intravenously.
Erica:	That is to allow a quick absorption.
Monica:	All right, I do not suppose the bee's venom enters the veins directly.
Chairperson:	You may add this one to the problem definition concerning the adrenaline: why is it injected intravenously?

Here the chairperson speaks to the secretary, a student who keeps track of the discussion on the blackboard. Students often consult his or her writings to check to what extent they have accomplished the task set and as a memory aid for things still to do. At this point in the discussion, the following can be read on the blackboard:

1. Difficult words: acra (limbs?)
2. Problem definitions
   • What reaction takes place in the body after a bee sting?
   • What happens after a multitude of stings?

- What causes the first symptoms: faint, dizziness, and sweat?
- Why do blood pressure and pulse rate change only after 25 minutes?
- How do blood pressure and pulse rate interrelate?
- Why are acra hot?
- What is the effect of adrenaline (why intravenously?)?

The students now have agreed on what is to be explained. They are ready to construct a theory of what has been going on in the body of Mr Laeven, based on whatever prior knowledge they have or on further ideas that may be produced. They call this phase "brainstorming."

Chairperson:	Let us continue with the brainstorming. The first question was: which physical reaction is caused by a bee sting?
Janneke:	I am not sure, but we also discussed bee stings in the first or second block. I believed it had something to do with histamine.
Erik:	Does a bee's venom contain histamine?
Janneke:	No, I thought it is produced by the body as an immune response.
Erik:	Yes, and the release of histamine causes an inflammatory lesion or something like that.
Erik:	That means the blood vessels dilate somewhat, leaking tissue fluid.
Tutor:	Please try to keep to the chain of causal relations for a while.
Chairperson:	So it starts with a sting, venom being injected into the body. The body contains mast cells that release histamine as an immune response. This causes an inflammatory lesion meaning dilation of the blood vessel wall. The vessels then release tissue fluid, which results in distension. This distension....
Bas:	(interrupts) what causes this distension?
Monica:	Well, vasodilatation causes fluid to leak into the tissue.
Erica:	It occurs to me that vasodilatation has nothing to do with distension.
Janneke:	Histamine makes the blood vessel wall more permeable, is it not?
Monica:	I think histamine is only a messenger that tells something has entered the body. It dilates the blood vessel wall, yet histamine and venom do not react.
Erik:	No, histamine evokes inflammatory lesion. This reaction brings white blood cells in the tissues to break down the venom.
	(...)

Chairperson:	That will do for the first problem definition. What reaction takes place in the body after a bee sting? Can we now continue with the question of what happens if you get a lot of bee stings?
Erica:	Let us just say suppose it happens that your body contains much histamine, enough to call for a doctor. What is the effect of this histamine, apart from vasodilatation?
Erik:	Does histamine affect the same receptors as adrenaline?
Janneke:	Yes, it has something to do with neurotransmitters and the like.
Bas:	An antagonist of adrenaline, histamine causes sympathetic activity.
Bas:	Could histamine be a competitive agonist of adrenaline?
Janneke:	If it is an agonist, why does the physician inject adrenaline? I suppose histamine is an antagonist after all.
Erik:	But you do not know. An adrenaline injection provides an excess of adrenaline, making the histamine ineffective.
	(...)
Chairperson:	We already suggested that histamine dilates the blood vessels, thus allowing fluid to leak. I believe it affects the blood pressure and pulse rate. Yes, for if fluid leaks from the vessels into the tissue, the blood pressure will diminish.

At this stage, the following text has appeared on the blackboard (the numbers refer to the original problem formulations; the arrows indicate a causal influence or temporal order of events):

---

1) histamine → defence of body

sting → poison → activation of mast cells →

histamine → vasodilatation

inflammatory lesion: vasodilatation → release of tissue fluid →
   swelling and redness → blood vessels more permeable.
   white blood cells remove venom
   Is histamine adrenaline's agonist or antagonist?

2) many stings → more histamine → blood pressure/
   pulse rate?

The group proceeds with a discussion of the causes of the pain, the dizziness and the sweating. We skip this part of the discussion here. It results in the following text on the blackboard:

> 3) pain from inflammatory lesion, sting
> faint, much pain, substance to brain,
> energy, insufficient in brain
> > protection against pain, feeling
> > weak; poison: paralyzing
> > substance
> > certain substances??
> sweat: fear, inflammatory lesion, energy
> sickness: pain

Tutor: Considering the available time, it seems wise to concentrate on the changes in blood pressure and pulse rate.

Chairperson: Yes, these changes taking place after 25 minutes. I believe we already have some idea.

A brief discussion follows in which one of the students argues that histamine activates the sympathetic nervous system by activating the adrenaline receptors in the heart.

Chairperson: Anyway, histamine dilates the blood vessels. If large arteries are equally affected, the blood pressure will of course change.

Janneke: I thought an increased pulse rate is a reaction of the body to maintain a steady blood pressure.

Tutor: Do you mean that explains why in the beginning blood pressure and pulse rate are normal, changes occurring only under the influence of histamine?

Janneke: Yes, fluid leaks from the blood vessels into the tissue, which diminishes the blood volume in the arteries. Subsequently, the heartbeat increases so as to maintain a steady pressure in the arteries. At some point, however, the pulse rate is not able to maintain a steady blood pressure because the blood vessels have grown too wide. No matter how hard the heart pumps, the blood pressure will drop. Let me show you, first the heartbeat rises at a constant blood pressure. Only after 25 minutes the blood pressure drops. I think that is how it works, yet I do not know if it explains the delayed drop in blood pressure.

Bas: I do not get it at all.

Erica:	Well, we first assumed that histamine dilates the vessels.
Erica:	And this vasodilatation makes the blood pressure drop.
Erik:	Why?
Monica:	Because the blood volume in the blood vessels has diminished; first, a higher pulse rate will ensure a steady blood pressure.
Erik:	I thought the blood pressure will drop first.
Monica:	Yes, but here it almost happens at the same time.
Bas:	You do not know that for sure. It takes 15 minutes before the physician arrives.
Bas:	You do not know what happened to the blood pressure in the meantime.
Chairperson:	That is true, but we assume it takes a while before histamine gets into the blood vessels. It first enters the skin; only after a while does it dilate the wall of the blood vessels, making fluid leak and the blood pressure drop.
Erica:	In my opinion, the pulse rate first rises so as to avoid the blood pressure from falling.
Janneke:	All right, but only if the blood pressure has slightly dropped. What about these baro-receptors that measure the pressure in the vessels? If the pressure drops, they will probably increase the heart rate. But, it may of course also happen that this histamine activates the adrenaline receptors. The heart also has adrenaline receptors. They increase the heart rate if activated by adrenaline. If histamine is an agonist to adrenaline, it may also be responsible for the higher pulse rate.
Astrid:	But of course the pulse rate does not only depend on the blood pressure. It involves more. I believe an inflammatory lesion always results in an increased heartbeat. Consequently, the body will have to work harder to accomplish the extrusion of waste matter.
Chairperson:	What will be the fourth problem definition? The blood pressure drops because of vasodilatation or sympathetic stimulation. We have not solved sympathetic stimulation by means of histamine yet. And we still have these baro-receptors, which measure the pressure. They can send impulses which may lead to changes as well. Adrenaline receptors alter the heart rate and might be sensitive to histamine as well. And an inflammatory lesion alters the pulse rate anyhow. Is that about it?

This is what can be read on the blackboard after completing this part of the discussion:

> 4) and 5 explanations for changes in blood
>   pressure/pulse rate
> histamine activates adrenaline receptors → impede/
>   activate?
>
> blood pressure follows pulse rate
> histamine → vasodilatation → baroreceptors measure
>   pressure → adrenaline → increased heartbeat.
>   Histamine probably has the same effect.
>
> blood pressure drops because of vasodilatation or
> parasympathetic stimulation

Chairperson:	All right, let us discuss the sixth problem definition: why do the acra feel so hot?
Janneke:	Because of the inflammatory lesions.
Chairperson:	Yes, that seems logical to me too. I suppose most of these stings are located on the limbs.
Bas:	But why do they get hot?
Chairperson:	I would say because more blood is circulating and because these inflammations take energy.
Erica:	An inflammatory lesion usually increases the temperature.
Erik:	What is the purpose of it?
Monica + Erik:	It improves recovery.
Chairperson:	Does this clarify these hot spots?
	(..........)
Chairperson:	The last question: What is the function of adrenaline here? We already discussed the fact that histamine may be an agonist or antagonist to adrenaline.
Erica:	What is the effect of adrenaline on the blood vessels? I thought it constricts them.
Janneke:	Yes, as far as skin vessels are concerned. But the effect of adrenaline on coronary vessels is dilation rather than constriction.
Tutor:	It seems to me that, in general, vasoconstriction leads to high blood pressure.
Astrid:	Yes, but if vasoconstriction does not take place, adrenaline has no effect at all.
Erica:	No, I mean the vessels in general, if all vessels are constricted.
Astrid:	Well, I think that is exactly what adrenaline does not do.
Janneke:	What is the effect of adrenaline on the heart?
Erica:	I thought that it affects the B-receptors, resulting in high blood pressure and pulse rate.

Erica:	And expansion of the heart-minute volume.
Janneke:	Yes, but expansion of the heart-minute volume means much more blood is pumped, which leads to high blood pressure.
Astrid:	But if you develop a serious vasoconstriction, the blood pressure should easily rise again.
Tutor:	So in your opinion, the blood pressure is a vital threat in Mr Laeven's case?
All:	I guess so.
Janneke:	When my grandfather died he suffered from dramatic changes in blood pressure at a diastolic pressure of 50 and a systolic pressure of 250. He received adrenaline to maintain a steady blood pressure. I do not know why it worked, but I do know that this was the reason for injecting adrenaline.
Erik:	Perhaps adrenaline has another effect as well.
Astrid:	Adrenaline regulates the blood pressure somehow.
Chairperson:	And why does adrenaline have to be injected intravenously?
Erik:	In this way it will have a greater effect on the heart than the blood vessels in the skin.
Erik:	All right, but what about this histamine, is it an agonist or antagonist?
Chairperson:	I guess we will have to look this one up.
Erik:	We cannot argue just like that.
Janneke:	As far as I am concerned, and I thought we all agreed, histamine dilates the blood vessels, as does adrenaline, at least some of them.
Erica:	Is it possible that histamine is a typical antagonist to adrenaline, yet only locally?
Bas:	You mean in relation to the distinction between A and B receptors?
Janneke:	Yes, for example, perhaps histamine only activates A receptors.
Chairperson:	Yes, we will have to consult the literature.

In the words of the secretary:

---

7) Adrenaline constricts skin vessels and dilates larger vessels. It also increases the heart rate

> → Heart-minute volume blood pressure

up   → maintaining steady blood pressure. How?

Intravenous injection: to reach the heart faster?

Subsequently, the students try to integrate what they have produced so far in terms of tentative explanations for the phenomena described in the problem. This phase can be considered the "model construction phase." It results in a diagram that summarizes the main conclusions reached. It looks like this:

> Histamine → inflammatory lesion → pulse
> activated? (same effect
> ↓   as adrenaline at
>   increased pulse rate?
>   vasodilatation
>
> ↓
>
> drop in blood pressure
> ↓
>
> activation of baroreceptors
> ↓
>
> higher pulse rate
> ↓
>
> expansion heart-minute → however, after
>   volume   some time cannot
>   keep up with falling
>   blood pressure
>
> adrenaline injection
> ↓
>
> vasodilatation: constriction only in skin
> ↓
>
> Increased blood pressure, expansion heart-minute
> volume and quicker breakdown of venom

The discussion is completed with the formulation of goals for self-study.

Chairperson: Shall we now formulate learning objectives?
Erik: Let us have a look at the results of the brainstorm.
Janneke: I want to know what actually happens when someone gets a
                 bee sting.
Chairperson: What physical reactions take place anyway?
Janneke: What happens in your body?
Erica: Where do we start?
Chairperson: Physical reactions.

Erica:	Particularly when someone gets a lot of bee stings at the same time.
Monica:	Yes, but we also have to verify that story of those mast cells and histamine.
Tutor:	So also the inflammatory lesion?
Tutor:	And particularly those points mentioned, let us see if they are true.
Chairperson:	Do we also need to formulate a learning objective about the venom? All I think it is part of the first learning objective.
Erik:	What is the effect of adrenaline and histamine?
Astrid:	Shall we investigate whether histamine influences blood pressure or heart rate?
Erik:	And what is the effect of adrenaline on blood pressure and pulse rate?
Chairperson + Erik:	Yes, and how does it affect sympathetic and parasym-pathetic processes?
Astrid:	Perhaps we should first have a look at the normal blood regulation and the regulation of the heartbeat.
Chairperson:	There may be other factors involved.
Tutor:	Do you mean that we have to look more generally; not only this specific case?
Chairperson:	Yes, the regulation of both blood pressure and pulse rate.
Monica:	And also whether histamine is an agonist or antagonist to adrenaline.
Chairperson:	Yes, what is the relation between adrenaline and histamine?
Monica:	And then we should just relate our findings to the problem.
Chairperson:	Shall we discuss the regulation of blood pressure as the first and most important issue?
Tutor:	Let us not spend too much time on the bee sting itself.
Tutor + all:	Well, all right, that is about it.

Again, in the words of the secretary:

Learning issues:

1. What physical reactions took place after a bee sting? (many stings?)

2. What is the effect of histamine? (pulse rate, blood pressure, (para)sympathetic)

3. What is the effect of adrenaline?

4. Blood pressure regulation

5. Pulse rate regulation

6. What is the relation between adrenaline and histamine?

Some explanatory elaborations

Once you have studied the student interchanges carefully, you may have noticed a number of things. First, the students work on the problem in a systematic fashion. There is a chairperson whose task is to ensure that the meeting proceeds in an orderly manner by introducing new topics for discussion, summarizing the students' contributions and making certain that the group achieves its goal. There is also a secretary who is responsible for recording the discussions. He notes on a blackboard issues that arise during the exchange of ideas and that he considers important. If the ideas are disproved, he would then erase them and replace them with new ones. In addition, he keeps a record of questions that arise and issues that still need to be solved or understood. While discussing a problem, the group employs a specific procedure which they have been taught. This procedure is called "the seven jump" and guides them from the initial clarification of terms through a phase of brainstorming, through a phase where ideas are critically evaluated, and finally to the formulation of learning issues for self-directed study. Thus, small group discussion of a problem is not a spontaneous ad hoc process, but proceeds along prescribed lines.

The second observation you may have made is that what the students are really engaged in is the construction of a theory explaining the phenomena described in a problem, in much the same way as a scientist tries to make sense out of reality. They produce tentative explanations that may or may not satisfactorily clarify the situation as described in the problem. For instance, they formulate the hypothesis that histamine dilates the blood vessels and then spend considerable time interpreting the empirical evidence supporting or refuting this hypothesis. Thus, while discussing the problem, the students build a "shared mental model" of the situation. This model is first tested against the problem at hand and, subsequently, elaborated upon through problem-oriented learning activities, of which we will come to speak further down the line. What may at first appear to be a disorganized way of playing with ideas is, in fact, a concerted attempt at understanding. While doing so, students mobilize and apply whatever knowledge they have available in order to make sense out of what initially appears them to be a chaotic situation.

Third, if you have background knowledge of the bee sting problem, you may have noticed that students are often incorrect and, if their ideas are not completely wrong, they tend to be fairly global. In the first encounter with the problem, there is no detailed and comprehensive understanding of the physiological processes that influence the phenomena described in the problem. This is the way it should be. If students were able to provide a comprehensive account of these processes, there would be no need for further learning, would there? The loose ends of the discussion, the question marks and the uncertainties displayed, form the fertile soil for self-directed learning. In fact, it is assumed that an awareness of one's own lack of knowledge is a strong stimulator for activities aimed at closing the gap between what one knows and what one still needs to know. This process is called intrinsic motivation.[1, 4]

Fourth, you may have noticed that students do not assign different tasks to individual members. Contrary to popular belief, there is no division of labor among the participants of a tutorial group. There is a simple explanation for this: Imagine that you, as a member of a tutorial group, have undertaken the assignment to study topic A, and let us assume that it took you about half a day to fully understand that topic. Let us further assume that your peers each have studied one different topic, B, C, D, E, or F. However, to acquire a fair, in-depth understanding of the problem, every student needs to understand topics A to F. The next session dedicated to the problem would then, theoretically, consist of the exchange of information gathered, in order to acquaint each of the students with all of the topics. Given six students and one hour of time for discussion, you would have, on average, exactly ten minutes in which to acquaint your peers with what you, and you alone, have understood from topic A. So, while you had four hours of self-directed learning in which to master the topic, your peers would have no more than ten minutes to comprehend the same. This example clearly shows why everyone cannot do much else than to study the same topics.

An early study[2] investigated the effect of division of labor in tutorial groups on achievement and satisfaction. The study required half of the participating tutorial groups to divide the work, whereas the other half of the groups were required to study all of the learning issues produced. Although they failed to find differences in achievement (which they attributed to the lack of sensitivity of the measuring instrument), they found large differences in satisfaction, the division-of-labor groups being far more dissatisfied with the whole exercise than the groups that did not divide tasks. In addition, they observed that students from the division of labor groups would deal individually with the remainder of the learning issues once the exercise had been completed.

This does not exclude the possibility that a student might also follow his/her individual interests to pursue a particular goal and share his/her findings with fellow students. In fact, this is often the case in tutorial groups. The students design a core curriculum together, as exemplified by the learning goals produced through the small group analysis of the problem, but, in addition, some students may have developed an individual agenda of issues that bother them without being of general interest to the group as a whole.

The tutor's role in the discussion is that of facilitator and, if necessary, devil's advocate. His contributions are geared towards challenging the students to clarify their own ideas, to look for inconsistencies and consider alternatives. By doing so, he helps the students to resolve their miscomprehensions.

How does the learning proceed?

When everything has been said and the issues requiring further study have been defined, it is time to break up. A period of self-directed learning activity has now begun. In most cases, the unit guide that contains the problem(s) also includes a number of relevant references to textbooks or other sources such as articles in scientific journals, videotapes, computer programs or slide shows. For the problem discussed, the references were:

1. Bernards en Bouman: *Fysiologie van de mens* (Human Physiology). Bohn, Scheltema en Holkema, Utrecht, the Netherlands, 5th print, 1988.
2. Sodeman and Sodeman: *Pathologic Physiology*. Saunders, Philadelphia, 7th print, 1985.
3. Guyton: *Textbook of Medical Physiology*. Saunders, Philadelphia, 8th print, 1991.
4. Schmidt and Thews: *Human Physiology*. Springer Verlag, New York, 1989.
5. Ganong: *Review of Medical Physiology*. Appleton and Lange, 13th print, 1987.
6. Roitt, Brostoff, Male: *Immunology*, Chapter 1, Churchill Livingstone, London, 3rd print, 1993.
7. Van der Linden: Anafylaxie, een overmatige reactie op insectesteken (Anaphylaxis, an overreaction to insect bites). *Modern Medicine*, 4, 265–273, 1994.
8. Videotape: The pathogenesis of shock (The tape shows the three forms of shock: cardiogenic, hypobolemic and anaphylactic.)

These references are only suggestions. Students are encouraged to search for additional sources by taking advantage of the facilities offered by a modern library. Students are also encouraged to read material from at least two separate sources concerned with the topic at hand. This deepens the students' comprehension and makes one sensitive to potential differences of opinion in the literature. It teaches students that scientific knowledge is not God-given and absolute, but rather human-made and tentative. One student has put it this way:

Gabriel (a second-year health sciences student): *One of the largest differences between problem-based learning and high school education is that one discovers that science is not just a bunch of facts. Science is about theories and these theories may fall short in explaining some phenomena or simply may be wrong. Problem-based learning enables one to confront different points of view with regard to the topic at hand and to find out which point of view seems most reasonable given the evidence. In one group, we even developed some experiments to test the differences between two theories!*

After about two days of self-directed learning, students return to their tutorial group. At the beginning of the session, students compare notes on the nature of the sources used. Disclosing the names of the books and chapters from which he or she has gathered information; which articles had been read and which audiovisual aids had been used; was an invention of the students themselves in the early years. The purpose is twofold: First, it provides advance clarification of the different perspectives from which each of the students has tackled the learning issues.

Second, it informs fellow students about the availability of interesting resources not previously found. An implicit, non-stated objective of this kind of exchange is, however, to monitor whether everybody has completed what was agreed upon. It is one of the mechanisms of social influence exerted by peers to help individuals keep up with their fellow students. Subsequently, students begin to discuss their findings in relation to the original problem. The goal here is to make sure that they now have gained a better, deeper and more detailed understanding of the causal mechanisms or processes underlying the problem. There is no need to discuss the students' findings related to the bee-sting problem here in detail.

The follow-up discussion of the bee-sting problem fulfills several objectives. It enables students to check whether their understanding of the subject matter studied is accurate. It provides opportunities for clarification by peers or by the tutor, and it provides opportunities to discuss the implications of the subject matter studied for similar problems or for future professional practice. Shared theory construction here finds its natural end. It is time to move to the next problem. We will, however, not follow this group any further on its road to understanding but, rather, concentrate on the broader educational context within which problem-based learning takes place.

Figure 5.3 shows the problem-based learning "cycle."[5] Arrows indicate the direction of the process; the dashed arrow signifies the possible cyclical nature of the ongoing learning.

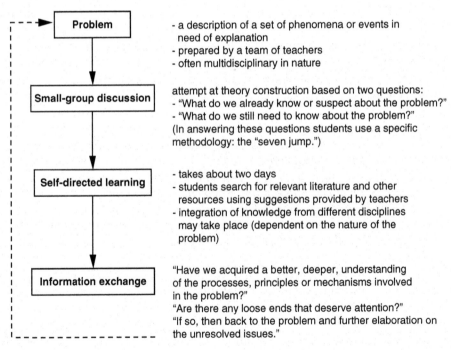

FIGURE 5.3 The problem-based learning cycle

---

[2] Since students may go back to the original problem for further analysis and – possibly – additional learning issues for self-directed learning, problem-based learning is sometimes described as a learning cycle.

Summary

1. This chapter has presented you with an overview of the process of problem-based learning and how this process is embedded in a curriculum.

2. We have attempted to demonstrate that students, in problem-based learning, work in a rational way towards the understanding of relevant problems, using their prior knowledge and whatever other information or ideas they can come up with.

3. We have also provided you with a glimpse of what a problem-based curriculum could look like. By doing so, we have briefly introduced you to some of the topics that will be the focus of this book.

References

1. Berlyne, D.E. (1978). Curiosity and learning. *Motivation and Emotion*, 2, 97–175.
2. Bouhuijs, P.A.J. and Schmidt, H.G. (1977). *Effecten van taakverdeling binnen onderwijs-groepen op leerresultaat en satisfactie bij studenten* (Effects of division of labor in educational groups on achievement and satisfaction of students). Maastricht, the Netherlands: University of Limburg.
3. Gonella, J.S., Goran, M.J., Williamson, J.S. and Cotsonas, N.J. (1970). Evaulation of patient care, an approach. *Journal of the American Medical Association*, 214(11), 2040–2043.
4. Hunt, J. McV. (1971). Intrinsic motivation: information and circumstances. In H.M. Schroder and P. Suefeld (Eds). *Personality Theory and Information Processing*. New York, NY: Ronald.
5. Willems, J. (1981). Problem-based (group) teaching: a cognitive science approach to using available knowledge. *Instructional Science*, 10, 5–21.

Chapter 6

The Student as a Valuable Source in Medical Education

Fadi Munshi and Peter H. Harasym

Objectives

- To understand the significance of students as stakeholders in medical education.
- To identify the roles medical students can perform during their educational experiences within the medical school.

Discussion 1

A discussion between Dr Wright, Dean of the Faculty of Medicine, and Dr Brain, a faculty member, was taking place at the corridor at Comeck University:

Dr Wright: Good morning, Dr Brain. How is the progress with the accreditation?

Dr Brain: Good morning, sir, we are at the initial stage of identifying and involving various stakeholders in the accreditation process.

Dr Wright: May I ask, whom did you identify as stakeholders?

Dr Brain: The higher administrators at the ministry and at the university, staff, and members of the community.

Dr Wright: Did you forget any important stakeholders?

Dr Brain: I am sure we have all the important stakeholders involved.

Dr Wright: Dr Brain, the forgotten stakeholders are the students!

Dr Brain: STUDENTS?? What value can students add to an accreditation process? They barely pass their courses. Over that they are always complaining about the curriculum, the teaching, and the exams. They are too young to be involved in such a major project.

Dr Wright: Oh Dr Brain. If you only heard, responded, and acted upon what you deem as student complaints, you would recognize the value of students' opinions and feedback. Students are a valuable source in medical education. I am sorry but I will have to ask you to step down from your current position in the evaluation and accreditation committee.

Why are students important stakeholders in medical education?

A stakeholder is an individual or group interested in the success of an organization. Medical students are usually the brightest individuals selected from a group of intelligent applicants. A medical student is usually eager to improve the quality of medical education. A famous quote states "Quality is in the eye of the beholder." As students are beholders of their education, they are a rich source in educational development, assessment, and improvement.

Discussion 2

Dr Wright: I am glad that you accepted the offer to lead the evaluation and accreditation committee, Dr Heart.

Dr Heart: It's a privilege to lead this committee.

Dr Wright: From your extended experience in education and accreditation, what roles can students take within an educational organization?

Dr Heart: As you know, I have been teaching for 25 years and I have been the pacemaker for many accreditation processes within medical schools. Students are valuable resources in medical education. A student is a teacher, learner, assessor, leader, and quality controller (Figure 6.1).

Dr Wright: Could you elaborate more on each role.

Dr Heart: Sure. I will discuss each role in detail.

The student as a learner

Learning is a life-long, voluntary, and self-motivated process. Starting from the early developmental stages of a human, learning is not a passive knowledge acquisition course. Babies and children actively process information received by senses and integrate them with previous knowledge.[1] Past experiences are a rich resource for learning. A child that experiences touching a hot teapot will link the pot with the hot burning sensation.

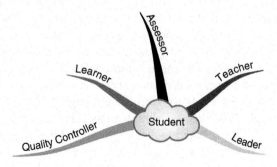

FIGURE 6.1   The roles of a medical student

As part of maturing, the need and capacity to be a self-directed learner grows. The driving force is an internal motivation which can be in the form of a desire, urge, need, curiosity, or satisfaction. With the daily advancement of research and knowledge, no curricular content can keep a professional up to date. Specifically, health professionals require continuous professional education. Students should be encouraged and prepared to be life-long learners.

Self-directed learning has been defined as "a process in which individuals take the initiative, with or without the help of others," to diagnose their learning needs, formulate learning goals, identify resources for learning, select and implement learning strategies, and evaluate learning outcomes.[2] From the definition, self-directedness is the active role the learner exerts to define what should be learned, what resources are used, and how the outcomes will be measured. Total self-directedness is not possible within educational institutes. A degree of guidance for learning is needed more during the initial years of a program. With progress, the increase and compilation of prior knowledge becomes the source of "internal" guidance.[3]

The student as a teacher

Many faculties worldwide assign medical students to roles as facilitators, tutors in basic sciences classes, or as clinical skills teachers. Student teachers in general are evaluated highly with regard to participants' satisfaction with the teaching.[4] Student teachers are good at understanding the learning difficulties of peers, and provide informative feedback. Student teachers can be as good as associate professors in teaching clinical skills. Teaching should be introduced and practiced in medical school as it is an important skill for future residency training and practice.[5] An integral part of being a physician is teaching.

The student as an assessor

A student is a valuable source of self- and peer assessments. Student assessments are viewed from two different perspectives. The first is viewing students' self-assessment as a reliable tool for gaining insight into their level of understanding. In this perspective students are considered to know what they need to know. In contrast, a different perspective is that students do not know that they do not know.[6] They are not familiar with the broad and big picture within a discipline; therefore they are unable to recognize their knowledge gaps and the sufficient quality of skills needed. Students' tendency to over- or underestimate gradually evolves with experience, maturity, and practice. The more common direction of change with experience is towards increased under-estimation and decreased over-estimation.[7]

Peer assessment helps students gain insight into their own level of understanding within a topic. It is considered both an assessment process and a learning experience. Peers judge structured tasks or provide global ratings of colleagues. The quality of peer assessments is influenced by reliability, relationships, and stakes. Factors affecting reliability are the number of performances observed, number of peers involved, and number of aspects of competence that have been evaluated.[8] Relationships between students can influence peer ratings. Competing students may tend to underrate each other, while overrating can occur with personal friends. Also, in high stakes assessments, peers are likely to inflate estimates of performance. A useful method to overcome this overestimating is to ensure the anonymity of the assessors.

The student as a leader

The roles and responsibilities of a physician are many within a healthcare system. High-quality clinical practice requires a physician to be a member, and often a leader, of a team. In medical schools, little importance is given to developing leadership skills in students. Common leadership skills need to be identified first, and then integrated within the curriculum. Physician leadership qualities that are deemed important are vision, ability to sacrifice, and courage.[9] Medical schools must target these qualities in admission procedures, incorporate their practice within the curriculum, and train medical students to be future leaders.[10]

A form of leadership development and practice currently followed in many medical schools is student body representation in various committees. These committees include, but are not limited to, curriculum, assessment, evaluation, and accreditation committees. Involving students in these committees benefits both the students and the committees. The students benefit in maturing their leadership skills, while the committees benefit from gaining insight into students' perspectives.

The student as a quality controller

Healthcare systems are characterized by a multidisciplinary team approach. It is essential that these clinical settings monitor and maintain standards of patient care. When students are taught in these clinical settings, they can effectively contribute to the quality assurance program.[11]

As Zusman suggests, "all should be involved in continuous quality improvement teams, seeking and maintaining improved performance, everyone from the Chief Executive Officer to the cleaner," let alone the students.[12] Within healthcare settings, medical students can contribute to the quality assurance processes during their educational experiences. For example, in a surgical operating ward, students can identify quality assurance issues and suggest solutions. Quality assurance problems with pre-operative, intra-operative, and recovery room care can be identified by students. Experience and knowledge are two main factors that contribute to students being a good quality controller.

Conclusion

Students can provide invaluable feedback in the following general areas:[13]

- Accessibility of dean(s) and faculty members.
- Participation of students in medical school committees.

- Curriculum, including workload, quality of required courses and clerkships, instructional formats, balance between scheduled class time and time for independent learning.
- Student assessment, including the grading system, and amounts and timeliness of feedback.
- System for the evaluation of courses or clerkships and teachers, and whether identified problems are corrected.
- Student support services and counseling systems (personal, academic, career, financial aid), including their accessibility and adequacy.
- Student health services, including adequacy, availability, cost, and confidentiality, and availability and cost of health and disability insurance.
- The learning environment, including policies and procedures to prevent or respond to harassment or abuse.
- Facilities, including quality of educational space, availability of study and relaxation space, security on campus and at affiliated clinical sites.
- Library facilities and IT resources, including access and quality of holdings, and information technology resources.
- All recipients are an invaluable resource of the quality of the delivery system. For example, patients are an invaluable resource of the quality of the health-care system. Likewise, students are an invaluable resource of the quality of the medical educational system. To improve on quality within a system, it is essential that the recipients be used as a valuable source of information. They will provide insights for improvement that are unavailable by any other means.

Discussion 3

Dr Wright: Well, Dr Heart, it is obvious that you clearly have your heart and mind in this accreditation process.

Dr Heart: Students can provide useful feedback, not just during the accreditation process but all year long. For example, end-of-course evaluations, if structured and analyzed properly, can improve the quality of teaching.

Dr Wright: Students are filling questionnaires at the end of each course but we never take their feedback seriously.

Dr Heart: Not appreciating or acting upon students' feedback is not just a waste of a valuable resource but it also de-motivates students to further provide constructive feedback.

Dr Wright: Thank you, Dr Heart, its very clear that students are a valuable source.

References

1. Sylva K. Critical periods in childhood learning. *British Medical Bulletin* 1997 Jan 1;53(1):185–197.
2. Knowles M. *Self-Directed Learning: A Guide for Learners and Teachers*. New York: Association Press, 1975.
3. Kirschner PA, Sweller J, Clark RE. Why Minimal Guidance during Instruction does not Work: An analysis of the failure of constructivist, discovery, problem-based, experiential, and inquiry-based teaching. *Educational Psychologist* 2006 Jun 1;41(2):75–86.
4. Tolsgaard MG, Gustafsson A, Rasmussen MB, Hooiby P, Muuller CG, Ringsted C. Student teachers can be as good as associate professors in teaching clinical skills. *Med Teach* 2007 Jan 1;29(6):553–557
5. Amorosa JMH, Mellman LA, Graham MJ. Medical students as teachers: How preclinical teaching opportunities can create an early awareness of the role of physician as teacher. *MedicalTeacher* 2011 Jan 28;33(2):137–144.
6. Langendyk V. Not knowing that they do not know: self-assessment accuracy of third-year medical students. *Medical Education* 2006;40(2):173–179.
7. Frye AW, Richards BF, Bradley EW, Philp JR. The consistency of students' self-assessments in short-essay subject matter examinations. *Medical Education* 1992;26(4):310–316.
8. Norcini JJ. Peer assessment of competence. *Medical Education* 2003;37(6):539–543.
9. Kt W. Physician leadership. *Singapore Medical Journal* 2007;48(12).
10. Chadi N. Medical leadership: doctors at the helm of change. *McGill Journal of Medicine (MJM)* 2009 Jan;12(1):52–57.
11. Rudkin GE, O`Driscoll MCE, Limb R. Can medical students contribute to quality assurance programmes in day surgery? *Medical Education* 1999;33(7):509–514.
12. Zusman J. Moving from quality assurance to continuous quality improvement. *Physician executive* 1992;18(4):3–8.
13. The Role of Students in the Accreditation of Medical Education Programs in the U.S. and Canada. *LCME Publications* 2010 Jul.

II

STUDY SKILLS

Chapter 7

Reading Skills

Rana Faisal Kattan and Hanan Balkhy

Objectives

- To know the importance of reading.
- To be able to read efficiently and effectively.
- To learn reading strategies and skills.

Introduction

Victor Hugo once said "To learn to read, is to light a fire; every syllable that is spelled out is a spark."[1] Reading is the mind's exercise. It opens the door to many areas of knowledge. In Islam, the first revelation fortified and illustrated the importance of reading.

Definition of reading

In English literature, reading has many meanings:

- To look at and understand the meaning of written or printed matter by interpreting characters or symbols.
- To speak written or printed words from a passage, text or sign.
- To understand or interpret the nature or significance of the reading material.

Importance of reading

Reading expands one's knowledge by facilitating the understanding of science and medicine. It also promotes critical thinking and clinical reasoning. Furthermore, it enriches the individual's experience and ability to critically appraise and analyze literature.[2] Reading also enhances the ability to process information, which is essential for medical and science students.[2] Later in this chapter we will discuss active learning in detail.

Reading English as a foreign language

English is a second language for many students around the world. Consequently, students may face difficulty in their first year of college, because most of the scientific materials are in English. One of the main obstacles that students face is that of reading scientific material in the same way they read fiction, i.e. by trying to comprehend each word, thereby missing the exact meaning of the text. This is referred to as the decoding–comprehension relationship.[3–4]

Colleges report that Arabic students face several obstacles in their understanding of written English. One such example is the failure to understand hidden meanings, treating words separately, not understanding the correct meaning of words and failure to integrate words into the whole context. They also reported failure to connect paragraphs together to understand the larger idea.

Solutions

Students try several methods in an effort to overcome these setbacks. These methods may include translating into Arabic, using an English dictionary, or utilizing text features such as tables and figures to help comprehend the material at hand. In addition, intensive English courses are of great help.[3, 5–6] Web-based courses are excellent teaching methods to help strengthen students' language skills.

Skilled reader

Who is a skilled reader?

A skilled reader is one "who, relative to a given age group, shows comprehension and reading rates that is at least average."[4] A different definition of skilled reading is "the ability to read all or most of the words on a page, read words quickly and use context cues only minimally for word recognition, which is primarily driven by using letters to access sounds."[4]

The two main characteristics of a skilled reader are: (1) speed in reading; (2) ability to comprehend text by planning, self-monitoring and self-evaluation.

- *Planning* – deciding on the purpose of reading.
- *Self-monitoring* – deciding on the appropriate reading strategies.
- *Self-evaluating* – deciding if your reading strategies are appropriate or need to be changed.

Reading strategies

Nowadays, science is expanding rapidly and information is expanding and being updated frequently. This makes it challenging to keep track of all the information. Students are forced to increase their effort throughout their college years, in order to catch up with the enormous amount of daily reading required of them.

To do this, they are encouraged to adopt certain methods. The following are some strategies that have proven useful.

1. Decide the purpose of your reading. You need to establish what you need to know. What information is required to finish your project? In what areas are you deficient? Asking these questions will keep you more focused and efficient and will save your time.
   Solution – Read the abstract of an article, introduction of a book chapter, and the headings. This should provide a summary of the material.
2. Decide what information you need. Your next step is to decide how deeply and thoroughly you need to read to understand the topic.
   Solution – If you want basic information, quickly scanning the introduction and conclusion is the best method. If you need more details, include the paragraph headings; if you still need more details, then you need to read the entire material.[7]
3. *Active reading.* This is an important concept that students need to embrace. To read actively is to activate prior knowledge using cognition awareness.[8] The first step in active reading is to have post-it notes and a pen nearby. Throughout your reading, jot down your questions and comments. You can highlight or underline the important parts of the material, as demonstrated in Table 7.1. You can refer to your comments later if you need more information or explanation, or you can read and memorize the highlighted parts when studying for an exam.[7]
4. *Critical reading.* When reading an article, it is of critical importance to judge its strength and value by careful reading. Keep a worksheet nearby for critical appraisal to decide whether the article is useful or not. There are several websites for critical appraisal of scientific articles, such as www.CASAP.org.

Speed reading. Several factors may affect reading speed. For example, it will depend on whether the text is in the native language of the student.[4] Furthermore,

TABLE 7.1 Cornell note format.[7]

Subject:	Date :
Main ideas	Details
Summary:	

the reader's level of experience greatly influences the speed of reading. For example, senior students who are more expert tend to read faster and more efficiently than junior students.[3]

Solution – Try to read in blocks, increasing the number of words you read in each block. Also, try to decrease the amount of time you need to read each block. Lastly, decrease the number of times you revisit a paragraph.[7] *Another technique to increase reading speed is RSOSR:*

- **R**emember previous knowledge, to activate it and compare it to new information.
- **S**can reading material to decide whether it will answer your question and serve your objectives.
- **O**rganize your knowledge and categorize it to be aware of areas of deficiency, and structure a plan for reading.
- **S**kim the material to get the information you need.
- **R**epeat the process (if needed) to answer all your questions.

These are some websites on reading skills:
http://www.mindtools.com/speedrd.html
http://www.spreeder.com/
http://www.readingsoft.com/

Reading skills

Active reading – we return to active reading, as it is a cornerstone of reading skills and is essential for every student to master. When you start, you need to read with a purpose and specific aim in mind and be aware of what you wish to achieve. A good way of doing this is by looking through headings and sub-headings to see whether this material best serves your purpose.[7]

Intensive thinking – when you go through the text, relate the material to your main goal and purpose or to previous readings that might be useful. You can accomplish this by examining the structure of the material and selecting relevant information.[7]

SQ3R strategy – a strategy to ensure that all students read in a critical manner. It is not the amount of reading that is important. Instead, it is the way of doing it that truly matters. One of the techniques used to facilitate active reading is the SQ3R technique:

- Survey: set a timeline to read a selected part of the materials.[7]
- Question: build and construct a set of questions. The easiest way to do this is by altering the meaning of the headlines to convert the headings into questions. There are several types of questions:
  1) Fundamental questions related to definitions.
  2) Part-whole-connection questions. These connected questions relate steps, reasons and analysis of the overall concept of the material.

3) Hypothesis questions. Using knowledge to understand how to deal with a situation.
4) Critical questions. These questions judge the material (York University, 2010).

- *3Rs:*
  1) Reading.
  2) Reciting. After reading, try to recall (either verbally or in writing) what was read. This will show how much you were concentrating.[7]
  3) Reviewing. This serves two purposes: (a) it will keep the material fresh in your mind, and (b) it will allow you to connect it with other reading materials. Schedule a regular time for reviewing.[7]

How should you start reading?

A key factor that allows these strategies to work is to apply them early, i.e. at the beginning of each subject or module. Know the main objectives and the primary references that you should read to meet the objectives. In order to benefit from the experience of previous students, it may be helpful to ask them what sources they found helpful and how they navigated this module. Start reading from day one; it is never too early to start. The sooner you begin, the less reading will accumulate. You should arrange a fixed time to read, with a scheduled break (keeping in mind that the adult concentration span is 25 minutes). You should study in a well-lit, quiet room with a comfortable chair and desk. Do not worry if you feel that you cannot concentrate. Stop and take a break, and then come back when you are fresh. It is not useful to read passively when you are unable to concentrate; you will spend more time on the subject and, more than likely, not remember most of it. Finally, many students forget the importance of a healthy lifestyle. The importance of healthy food, regular exercise and avoidance of smoking cannot be over-emphasized.

Conclusion

Reading is important for your education and later your career. One must be motivated and master the skills needed to read in order to succeed in life.

Summary

- Reading in English literature means understanding the meaning of the written words.
- Reading enhances critical thinking and clinical reasoning.
- Reading and studying in a second language requires hard work.
- The skilled reader has two main features: (1) he/she reads fast; (2) has the ability to comprehend text by planning, self-monitoring and self-evaluation.
- Use the Cornell note format as a reading strategy.

- Use mnemonic RSOSR for speed-reading: remember, scan, organize, skim, and repeat.
- Active reading: use the SQ3R strategy.

References

1. Hugo *V. Think, exist* [cited 24 April 2011]; available from: http://en.thinkexist.com/search/searchquotation.asp?search=reading&q=author%3A%22Victor+Hugo%22.
2. Chen F-C, Lin M-C. Effects of nursing literature reading course on promoting critical thinking in two-years nursing program students. *Journal of Nursing Research* 2003;11(2):137–147.
3. Malcolm D. Reading strategy awareness of Arabic-speaking medical students studying in English. *System* 2009;37:640–651.
4. Jackson NE. Are university students' component reading skills related to their text comprehension and academic achievement, learning and individual differences? 2005;15:113–139.
5. Bitchener J, Basturkmen H. Perceptions of the difficulties of postgraduate L2 thesis students writing the discussion section. *Journal of English for Academic Purposes* 2006;5:4–18.
6. Tanyeli N. The efficiency of online English language instruction on students' reading skills. *Procedia Social and Behavioral Sciences* 2009:564–567.
7. Centre CAD. *Reading Skills for Universities*. Toronto, Ontario: York University, 2008; available from: http://www.yorku.ca/cdc/lsp/skillbuilding/reading.html.
8. *Tool m*. Reading strategies 2011; available from: http://www.mindtools.com/rdstratq.html.

Chapter 8

Writing Skills

Rana Faisal Kattan and Hanan Balkhy

Objectives

- To know the definition of professional writing.
- To understand the importance of professional writing.
- To know the basic rules of professional writing.
- To identify the most common problems in writing.

Introduction

Skillful writing is probably one of the most important tools for the healthcare professional. Through writing we document patients' condition, management, and hospital course. The importance of writing cannot be overemphasized, and mastering it is challenging. In this chapter, we will elaborate on different styles of writing, their relevance to clinical practice, and on ways we can improve our writing skills.

Professional writing

Professional writing in the medical field consists mainly of writing patients' case presentations, follow-up notes and case summaries, in addition to concise medical reports and discharge summaries. It also includes more formal written work, such as research proposals and grants, publishable case reports, and highly technical research publications.

Why is writing important?

Writing is an ancient art that developed in the earliest civilizations, and through it extinct empires and cultures are documented. In the past, clinicians practiced medicine and documented their achievements through writings. This can be seen in the books of Ibn Siena, Jabber Ibn Hayan, and other Muslim scientists.

Learning and mastering the art of writing is critical for one's career and future. For example, when applying to college, seeking a job, or requesting promotion, a well-crafted written work is essential. Students in the medical field are taught various types of writing. This mainly takes place at the beginning of clinical rotations in medical school, where one of the first skills taught is how to conduct patient histories and physical examinations. This is the core of medicine, without which accurate diagnoses cannot be made. It is here that the importance of writing becomes clear. In the healthcare profession, writing is like a master key that can open a number of doors behind which opportunities lie. It will distinguish you from your colleagues and improve your chances of earning rewards. It will also allow you to track newly published articles and apply such developments to your career.

At this point, we may ask why some medical professionals do not write. Reasons are abundant: some claim that there are not enough hours in the day to finish their duties and still have time to write; or they have no supporting staff to aid them in data collection when starting a new research project; some simply hate writing. Others do not know how to start and lack confidence in their abilities; or they think that most topics have already been published and discussed. I agree that writing can be overwhelming, and to some it poses seemingly insurmountable barriers. To address these issues we need to know the rules for proper writing.[1]

Basic rules for writing

What do we need to know when starting to write? There are general guidelines that one needs to master before beginning to write: these include grammar, proper spelling, and ability to construct a well-formed sentence. For example, when writing case presentations, one must narrate, as if telling a story, not merely list factual information, so as to grab the reader's attention and to ensure that all aspects of the case history are covered.

1. *Decide on your topic*
   Your first step in writing is to decide on a topic that interests you. Keep a small journal in your pocket when you are doing your daily rounds, and you may encounter a question that interests you enough to merit further research. You will be surprised at the number of questions that you will write down. Another way to choose a topic is by picking an issue in which you might want to specialize and are interested in investigating. You also need to keep in mind the goal of your work: why should people read it, and what new information will you add to existing knowledge? It is important not to do research that has been already replicated repeatedly by others, and should be kept in mind when choosing case presentations.[2]
2. *Goals and objectives*
   After deciding on your topic, you need to have a clear vision: why did you choose this topic? Why should others read your writing, and what is your objective? What are the take-home messages and new information to be taken from this article? When you have a clear goal and objective, you will

become more focused and be able to perform better and with fewer distractions. Writing without a clear vision is like driving a car without a clear
destination – one might end up in an unwanted place.

3. *Literature review*

After deciding on your topic, you need to search the medical literature for
previous work on your topic. Has it been extensively reviewed, or is there
something new on the horizon? This will help you in refining your research
and directing it appropriately.

4. *Resources*

To make your writing smooth, you will need to have on-hand English and
medical dictionaries to help you with your writing. Using the internet and
electronic databases makes searches much easier and more effective.

5. *Grammar and spelling*

This is a critical step, as it can ruin your work if you neglect it. Before
you start, you need to know how to write proper English. Nowadays, this is
made easier by the automatic spell- and grammar-checkers in Microsoft
Word. In order to write fluent and interesting sentences, some researchers
say that reading poetry and literature will help to enrich your self-expression
in English.

6. *Rules and regulations*

Once you reach this step, you need to follow specific guidelines for the type
of writing in which you are engaging. For example, for a review article you
need to know the general layout of the target journal in which you wish
to publish your work. This will increase the chances of your work being
published and will help avert unwanted criticism.

7. *Protected time*

Once you are ready to start writing, you need to choose a suitable time in
which to write. This time should be protected and free of interruption; it can
be in the morning or at night, according to your schedule. Most researchers
agree that at least twenty minutes per day is the minimal time needed for
writing. This is an individual matter, though, and varies from one person to
another.

8. *Working space*

You need to clear a space in which to work, with a desk, a comfortable
chair and good illumination. It is suggested that you write directly on your
computer in order to save your work and to be able to perform spell and
grammar checks. Various software programs have been developed to facilitate your writing, including Software Engineer, Bookends Software and
Professional Communication[3] (see Figure 8.1).

After carrying out the above steps, you are now ready to start writing. In the
next paragraph we will discuss some of the most common types of professional
writing that you are likely to encounter during your career.

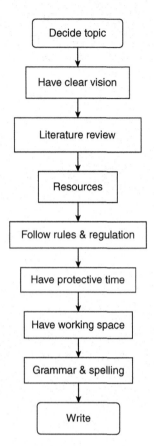

FIGURE 8.1   Flowchart to start writing

Types of professional writing

There are several types of professional writing. Some of the main ones that you may wish to produce are review articles and case presentations.

Personal statement

A personal statement is an essay designed to persuade the other party that you are worthy of a promotion, job, or research grant. A personal statement is attached to the curriculum vitae (CV); this can be tricky as one tends to make it an addendum to the CV. A personal statement is your opportunity to pull the information in the CV together into a theme, to provide information that does not easily fit into a CV, or to explain things that you think might seem worrisome to a reviewer. One pitfall is the tendency to make the statement overly long; this may cause the reviewer to overlook some of your important academic achievements or projects. Furthermore, you should avoid embellishment, as it will look unprofessional.[4]

Review article

A review article is like a book chapter that includes the most up-to-date information on a topic. In addition, the author may or may not include personal data and opinions in the review. This format has several subtypes, such as literature review, meta-analysis, and evidence-based clinical review. A literature review or state-of-the-art survey serves several purposes and mainly summarizes the searches done on a topic for knowledge and future research. A meta-analysis is a "method of several results of several studies into a summary conclusion, using quantitative strategies that will allow consideration of data in diverse research reports."[5] An evidence-based clinical review is a "special type of meta-analysis that focuses on clinically relevant questions with emphasis on evidence-based medicine."[5]

Case presentation

You will first encounter case presentations during your clinical rotations; the key to success is first to be familiar with all the elements that should be included in your history and physical examination. Then, when you write all the information taken from the patient himself and/or the patient's caregiver, you need to narrate the history as if you were telling a story rather than stringing together a list of facts. By doing so you will not miss any details in your history and your audience will be more engaged. When you reach the assessment part of your presentation, which is the part that shows your intellect and your critical thinking and reasoning, you should list the three most likely diagnoses, along with supporting information that led you to those conclusions. When another colleague reads your chart later, he will have a clear impression of the patient's condition and the initial assessment of the medical team; this helps in maintaining continuity of patient care. Finally, you should clearly document your plan of care for the patient.

Problems in writing

There are several pitfalls that you may face when starting to write; knowing about them will help you to avoid them. The following are some common problems that you may face.

- Plagiarism
  Plagiarism is using other people's work without proper reference to them; it includes words, figures or tables and can happen either intentionally or unintentionally. To avoid plagiarizing, you need to cite your references properly, and, when using an author's exact words, they must be put within quotation marks. It may also be helpful to ask a colleague to review your text. This also applies if you need to use your own words that have been previously published, as you must secure copyright permission from the publisher.[6]
- Abbreviations
  Abbreviations should be avoided as much as possible. If necessary, it is best to use an internationally accepted abbreviation, and you should include the full word along with the abbreviation the first time it is used in your text.

Conclusion

Writing is a joyful act that one should enjoy doing. It requires a lot of hard work and dedication, but the rewards are worth it. In this chapter, we talked about the basic principles of writing and the main rules and guidelines to be followed. We also talked about the main types of professional writing that you may face during your career, especially during the college years. Hopefully, when you reach the end of this chapter, you will be encouraged to write and eager to publish an article.

- Professional writing is an important skill that the medical professional should master.
- The basic rules for writing are: decide the topic, formulate goals and objectives, review the literature, utilize your resources, check grammar and spelling, obey rules and regulations, protect your time, and create a working space.
- Types of professional writing include personal statements, review articles and case presentations.

References

1. Pololi L, Knight S, Dunn K. Facilitating scholarly writing in academic medicine. *J Gen Intern Med*. 2004 Jan;19(1):64–68.
2. Price A. Professional writing: collective purpose. *Nurse Stand*. 2001 Apr 4–10;15(29):42–44.
3. Stepanski LM. Becoming a nurse-writer: advice on writing for professional publication. *J Infus Nurs*. 2002 Mar–Apr;25(2):134–140.
4. Wenger D. The Five Minutes Mentor: What shall I put in a personal statement? *Academic Physician & Scientists* 2007:8–9.
5. Taylor RB. *The Clinician's Guide to Medical Writing*. USA: Springer 2005.
6. Cronin SN. The problem of plagiarism. *Dimens Crit Care Nurs*. 2007 Nov–Dec;26(6): 244–245.
7. Campanelli PC, Feferman R, Keane C, Lieberman HJ, Roberson D. An advanced practice psychiatric nurse's guide to professional writing. *Perspective Psychiatry Care*. 2007 Oct;43(4):163–173.
8. Goodman N, Edwards M. *Getting Started in Medical Writing*. Third edition. New York: Cambridge 2006.
9. Katz JK, Morahan PS. The cover letter road map to a successful reading of your CV and executive summary. *Academic Physician & Scientists*. 2005:2–3.
10. Liller KD, Liller DA. Practicing public health: the important role of professional writing. *J Public Health Manag Pract*. 2007 Jan–Feb;13(1):1–2.
11. Morgan PR. 10 steps toward professional writing. *J School Health* 1996;66(10):353–354.
12. Smyth J, Nazarian D, Aigo D. Expressive writing in clinical practice. In: Vingerhoets Aea, editor.: Springer, 2008. pp. 215–233.

Chapter 9

Managing Time

Mohammed Zamakshary, Tariq Al Tokhais,
Mohi Eldin Magzoub, and Margaret Elzubeir

Objectives

By the end of this chapter students will be able to:
- Describe the importance of effective time management in medical education.
- Describe helpful tips on how best to manage your time, balance multiple priorities, and manage your life effectively.
- Review and describe common obstacles to effective time management.

Introduction

Anything becomes urgent if you wait long enough. – Danny Cox, *Leadership When the Heat is on.*[1]

It is universally agreed that time management for students is important generally, and due to the nature and volume of workload typically encountered, even more important for medical students. Studying for exams, preparing assignments, attending seminars, participating in various college activities, patient contact activities, etc. are among some of the many tasks expected of you. Furthermore, you may be a mature student with a family, have interests outside of medicine which you need to maintain and therefore have to also manage the social aspects of your life to maintain a healthy academic and social life balance. The benefits to practicing good time management are therefore significant, not least of which is a reduction in your stress and anxiety levels[2].

Managing time entails identifying your responsibilities, carefully prioritizing their importance, making choices about how to use your time most effectively and monitoring your performance. It is a combination of skills that will be useful throughout your lifelong learning careers and can be developed by thinking and acting strategically. In this chapter, we will discuss problems arising from ineffective time management, and principals that might contribute to your ability to function at a higher level and achieve more.

The problem

> The more important an item, the less likely it is urgent, and the more urgent an item, the less likely it is important. – Dwight Eisenhower (1890–1969) 34th President of the United States.

Common mistakes in time management

> Don't say you don't have enough time. You have exactly the same number of hours per day that were given to Helen Keller, Pasteur, Michelangelo, Mother Teresa, Leonardo da Vinci, Thomas Jefferson, and Albert Einstein. – H. Jackson Brown[4], author of "Life's Little Instruction Book"

Undoubtedly, some people are capable of getting so much more done not necessarily because they have more time but because of their superior ability to manage their time effectively. In order to manage your time more effectively, you should avoid some common mistakes:

- Not having a plan. Starting the your day without a specific plan is likely lead to compromising your productivity for the whole day.
- Not choosing an appropriate place to carry out/address each task. For example, not choosing an appropriate place for study is likely to impede effective study because there may be multiple distractions leading to lack of concentration and compromising your productivity.
- Not getting enough sleep. Students have a tendency to compromise sleeping time, especially, for example, as you approach deadlines or examinations. However, sleeping well is an important pre-requisite for effectively enhancing your productivity.
- Not accounting for peripheral activities that are essentially "time stealers" These include Emails, phone calls, chatting, and visitors. These "time stealers," if not taken into consideration, will significantly cut into your productivity, as they tend to have a cumulative effect on efficient utilization of time.
- Procrastination. We all tend to put off important tasks over and over again, for various reasons. Key to controlling this damaging habit is to have some emotional intelligence[3] (i.e. having self awareness and understanding); recognize when you start procrastinating, and take positive action to overcome it.
- Trying to be a perfectionist. Nobody is perfect and we have to face this fact. Although there is nothing wrong with aiming to be the best you can be in all aspects of your personal and professional life, we strongly believe that you are much better off aiming to effectively perform all tasks that are required of you, as opposed to perfecting just one task.
- Wasting time worrying about what you have to do. Some people use multiple "To-Do" lists and hardly ever address any of the items. However, remember that approaching what you have to do systematically, and getting busy working on it is extremely important.

- Over scheduling. We all aspire to be multi-taskers. However, we sometimes take on more than we can handle; whether its extra courses, extracurricular activities, job responsibilities, etc. Make sure you do not create conflicts by scheduling activities at the same time. Learning to say "NO" if it affects your schedule is a skill you will need to develop. Indeed, according to Helene Lerner[4] *"Saying 'No' to someone else, is like saying 'Yes' to yourself"*.

The above are just some common barriers to enhancing your productivity. Reflect and examine them closely; you may be able to come up with other mistakes or poor practices that you have found compromise *your personal productivity.*

Guidelines for effective time management time management

> Time is the most, scarce resource of the manager; if it is not managed, nothing else can be managed. – Peter Drucker, Management Guru and Author (1909–2005)

These tips, although discussed separately, are interconnected and are recommended practice:

Determine your goals

If you don't know where to go, definitely you will reach somewhere else and even you may not know it. A goal is a purpose or an end towards which you direct your intentions and efforts to achieve it. The important criteria for good goals are being specific, feasible, measurable, and should be motivating and linked to a time frame. Without setting goals, we would just drift along.

Know what you want to achieve in a day, a week, a semester or a year. Make it your concern and priority. You can start with listing down all the things you are supposed to do. Then you can categorize in groups familiar to you, for instance, academic, professional, social etc. You may also want to classify them further into short term intermediate and long term goals. Then you can break down your goals into specific objectives that can be achieved within a certain time frame. Completing objectives on time increases your motivation and satisfaction and keep goal achievement on schedule. Furthermore goal setting will put you in a position to be proactive rather than just being reactive.

Prioritize your goals

Remember the fact that all goals are not of equal importance. Once your goals have been determined, the next step is to prioritize them according to certain criteria. These criteria may include importance to your overall goal, relevance and urgency. Once you finish this step, you need to identify the tasks that you should perform in achieving each goal. At this stage you will always know exactly what needs to be done next.

Plan before you implement

Each day you will discover that you have plenty of activities that you need to perform. Invest at least twenty minutes daily to plan and organize what you are going to do. Based on your overall goals and objectives A "To-Do" list is an effective method of planning your daily activities, tasks and priorities[6]. Always remember that bad ink is better than good memory therefore, putting goals, strategies to achieve them in writing is very important to achieve organization and productivity.

Schedule your activities

At this stage it is important to schedule your activities. Scheduling is of utmost importance and considered as an effective skill you can utilize. Appropriate scheduling reduces stress, avoid crisis management and maximize your effectiveness. A good schedule should be flexible enough to accommodate unforeseen events and other surprises that cannot be anticipated. These events should never affect your plans; make you lose control; and push your agenda off-track. A good schedule may include an alternative or plan B. Creating a schedule that caters for different possible scenarios is crucial. To make an effective schedule, you need an effective scheduling system. Different forms of arranging a schedule include a diary, calendar or paper-based organizer. You can make use of the recent advances in technology such as smart phones, IPADs personal computers etc. Scheduling is best done on a regular basis, for example at the start of every week. To avoid time pressure and unnecessary stress, always allow enough or more time for each task to be completed[7-8].

Write down your tasks

Experts in time management consider writing down a list of tasks is the key to effectiveness. Written lists help you organize your goals, strategies, responsibilities, objectives and tasks. An old Arabic saying is that time is like gold when efficiently utilized and like a sword when it is wasted. Effective time management is less about saving time at any cost, than using the time you have efficiently.

Lists have various advantages. First, they are great motivators. Time management experts agree that nothing brings motivation and satisfaction to most people more than deleting things off a "To-Do" list[6]. Second, lists are expected to improve your outcomes. Writing down your goals, priorities, plans, and schedule on a List, helps you remember even the smallest details of your activities to be accomplished towards reaching an objective. Last, making lists also is expected to help you organize your thinking, which is of utmost importance for effective time management. Scattered thinking wastes time to a great extent. It is strongly recommended to write down important dates for exams, events, and other deadlines. You need to review your "To-Do" list on a regular basis. If you really want to manage your time in an effective way, recognize that it will take a major effort to overcome inefficient habits that may have become ingrained. But it is also true that the first step toward change may be as easy as getting out a piece of paper and starting your "To-Do" list right now.

Time selection

Timing and proper selection of time is an important requirement for achievement. The most productive time of the day varies from one individual to another. Choose the time of the day that you believe your energy levels are highest. Every moment is important, so make use of extra time appropriately. When you waste a minute it will not come actually, it is gone forever.

A recommended strategy is to combine related activities together to utilize time properly. Socialize with peers and friends whenever you get the chance. Sound ideas would not necessarily come to mind every time. Keep listening to others and try to male role models for you from their good habits or practices they follow. You will face a time when you develop the feeling that 24 hours is not enough to finish your work in a day, Do not panic or get frustrated simply, apply and practice your time management skills. In this case you will survive the time rush and pressure. Sound time management practices are intended to make you capable of controlling both your life and your work. By proper planning in protecting your work time and scheduling your activities, you will be in better position to make equilibrium in your work and personal life.

The take home message out of this chapter is to enjoy your student life to the maximum extent through managing your time effectively. Learning this skill during your study time is expected to successfully accomplish the tasks and duties set out for you as a future professional!

Good and poor time management practice

Good time management practice	Poor time management practice
• Write things down.	• Relying on memory alone to remember important notes.
• Adjust priorities as necessary.	
• Allow yourself more time than you think you need to perform necessary tasks.	• Letting distractions sabotage your list of tasks.
• Designate a specific time of the day to handle emails.	• Letting emails accumulate in and clutter your inbox. Delete or file them after you have dealt with them.
• Take important calls and schedule time for the rest.	
• Let others know that you are busy, but do not forget that others are busy, too.	• Falling into time traps, like private net surfing or excessive chatting with friends.
• Be prepared for crises and catastrophes. Schedule time for them.	• Procrastinating.
	• Neglecting to have a Plan B in case of unforeseen emergencies.

References

1. Cox D, Hoover J. *Leadership When the Heat's On*. Second edition. McGraw-Hill 2007.
2. Macan TH, Shahani C, Dipboye RL, Phillips AP. College students' time management: Correlations with academic performance and stress. *Journal of Educational Psychology*. 1990: 760–768.
3. Covey SR, Merrill RA, Merrill RR. *First Things First*. Simon & Schuster 1994.
4. Brown HJ, Spizman RB. *Life's Little Instruction*. Rutledge Hill Press 2000.
5. Lerner H, *Time for Me*. Sourcebooks Inc 2005.
6. Drucker P. *The Practice of Management*. New York: Harper 1954.
7. Misra R, McKean M. College students' academic stress and its relation to their anxiety, time management and leisure satisfaction. *American Journal of Health Studies*. 2000: 16(1).
8. D'Zurilla TJ, Sheedy CF. Relation between social problem-solving ability and subsequent level of psychological stress in college students. *Journal of Personality and Social Psychology*. 1991: 61(5), 841–846.

Chapter 10

Guide to Literature Search for Medical Students

Hana M. A. Fakhoury and Ali H. Hajeer

Objectives

Reading this chapter will give you tips on how to:
- Select the best source for your literature search
- Specify search terms and form a search statement
- Filter your search
- Find your article of interest
- Keep up to date with My NCBI from PubMed
- Search EBM Resources such as PubMed Clinical Queries, UpToDate, and DynaMed

Section 1: The Six Steps to a Successful Literature Search

No matter what literature you are searching for, it is essential to learn the basics of effective searching. Listed below are six steps to help you find the correct literature for your search terms.

Step One: Select the Best Sources for your Search

- Depending on your search, you might need to access a range of relevant databases and sources of information.
- PubMed is a suitable source to start with (http://www.pubmed.com); it is free and can be accessed from anywhere.
- If you decide to search other databases, your own institution might have a digital library with access to a number of databases. For example, at King Saud bin Abdulaziz University for Health Sciences digital library, (http://www.ac-knowledge.net/ngha/), there are several databases to choose from such as: OVID, McGraw Hill collection, EBM databases, e-Journals, and e-Books.
- If you are looking for a quick updated review of the literature, UpToDate database is your best resource (http://www.uptodate.com/). It must be said however, that this database is only available for subscribers.

Step Two: Specify your Search Terms

List the terms you need to search for, keeping in mind the following points:

- A broader term or terms might be more useful (e.g. using viral hepatitis instead of HCV). Always ask yourself if there are any related words which might be more interesting.
- To build a detailed search, we advise you to use MeSH term (Medical Subject Headings) database in PubMed. MeSH terms are arranged in a hierarchical manner. Using this database will help you build a very precise search with your subheadings of interest.
- Remember to start broadly, then focus your search by using filters or search history (see Step four).

Step Three: Form a Search Statement

Use the Boolean operators (OR, AND, NOT); they are very useful in combining terms to retrieve the results from a database. Use of phrase searching can be useful sometimes. Although databases vary slightly in how they apply these operators, they can be used in most literature databases. Phrase searching allows you to search for a group of words exactly as you type them.

"Truncation"replaces the end of a word with a symbol such as * to pick up variant endings.

"OR" allow you to include synonyms or related ideas in a search.

"AND" allows you to combine two ideas in a search, narrowing it down.

"NOT" allows you to search for one term but not the other.

Details option in PubMed allows you to check exactly what PubMed engine searched for when it ran your query. Review the details of the search in order to revise, modify or keep your terms.

For example: searching for pulmon* (truncation) will result in searching for more than 600 versions of the word. You can use the "Details" option to see for yourself what PubMed looked for.

pulmon[All Fields] OR pulmon'alis[All Fields] OR pulmon'e[All Fields] OR pulmon'es[All Fields] OR pulmona[All Fields] OR pulmonaal[All Fields] OR pulmonaalihypertensio[All Fields] OR pulmonaalihypertension[All Fields] OR pulmonaalihypertensiosta[All Fields] OR pulmonaalstenose[All Fields] OR pulmonaalvenen[All Fields] OR pulmonaary[All Fields] OR pulmonabiol[All Fields] OR pulmonable[All Fields] OR pulmonados[All Fields] OR pulmonae [All Fields] OR pulmonaery[All Fields] OR pulmonai[All Fields] OR pulmonaie [All Fields] OR pulmonaiere[All Fields] OR

Step Four: Filter your search

The result of your search will probably contain too many hits, so you will need to refine or filter the search. In PubMed, you can use "Limits" to filter your search and apply certain criteria to reduce the number of results to a manageable list (Figures 10.1 and 10.2). You can limit by:

- Type of Article
- Languages

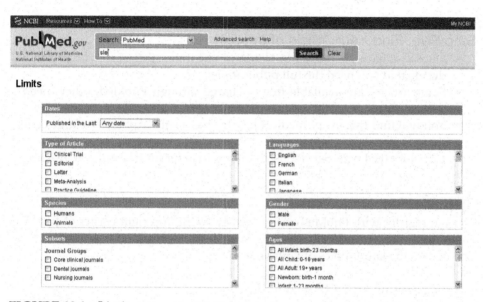

FIGURE 10.1 Limits page

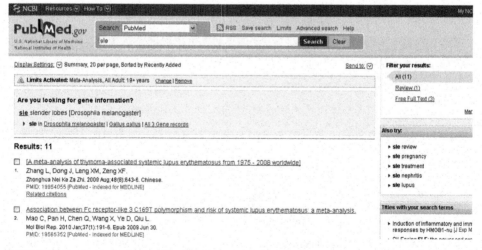

FIGURE 10.2 Search was limited by age and meta-analysis

- Gender
- Ages
- Journal Groups

Several search engines have facilities to help you revise your search. In PubMed for instance, History can be very helpful. Search history is usually kept on the used computer for up to eight hours. This is a very useful facility in PubMed, as it allows you to combine searches with the Boolean operators (OR, AND, NOT) by clicking the left hand button of the mouse on the search number.

Step Five: Find Your Article of Interest
- Once you have succeeded in obtaining the interesting abstracts, you might decide that you need the full publications.
- Some articles are available free of charge through PubMed; others need a subscription.
- You will find that every medical Library has a subscription to a large collection of journals.
- Inter-Library Loans Service, is another source for finding full text articles.

Step Six: Keep up to Date
You can register with PubMed, using the My NCBI (top right corner of PubMed page) (http://www.ncbi.nlm.nih.gov/sites/myncbi/register/) in order to be updated on the latest topics of your choice.

- Log in using My NCBI (Figure 10.3)
- Do any search using simple or complex terms
- Click on save search (Figure 10.4)

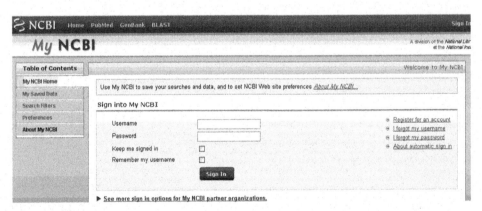

FIGURE 10.3   Sign in for saving any search term you want PubMed to update you with

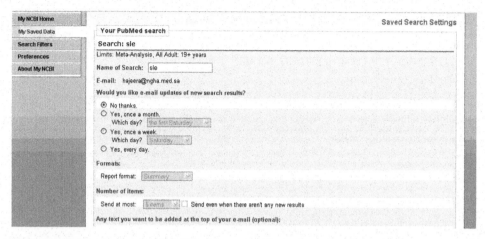

FIGURE 10.4 Save search and select your terms for receiving updates

- Select the terms of the update that you want PubMed to email you the results of
- You can perform and save as many searches as you want

The basics of effective searching:

- There are specialist databases for particular types of literature. "PubMed" is a suitable source to start with. If you are looking for a quick updated review of the literature, "UpToDate" database is your best resource.
- You can use MeSH database in PubMed to build a very precise search.
- Use the Boolean operators (OR, AND, NOT); they are useful in combining terms to retrieve the results from a database.
- Remember to start broadly, then focus your search by using filters or search history.
- In PubMed you can use "Limits" to refine your search.
- Some articles are available free of charge through PubMed. Others might be available through your own medical library or through Inter Library Loans Service.
- You can register with PubMed to be updated on the latest topics of your choice. This service is called My NCBI.

Section 2: Searching EBM Resources

PubMed

You can search PubMed for EBM resources. This is done through the PubMed Clinical Queries (Figure 10.5). You can search citations that correspond to a specific

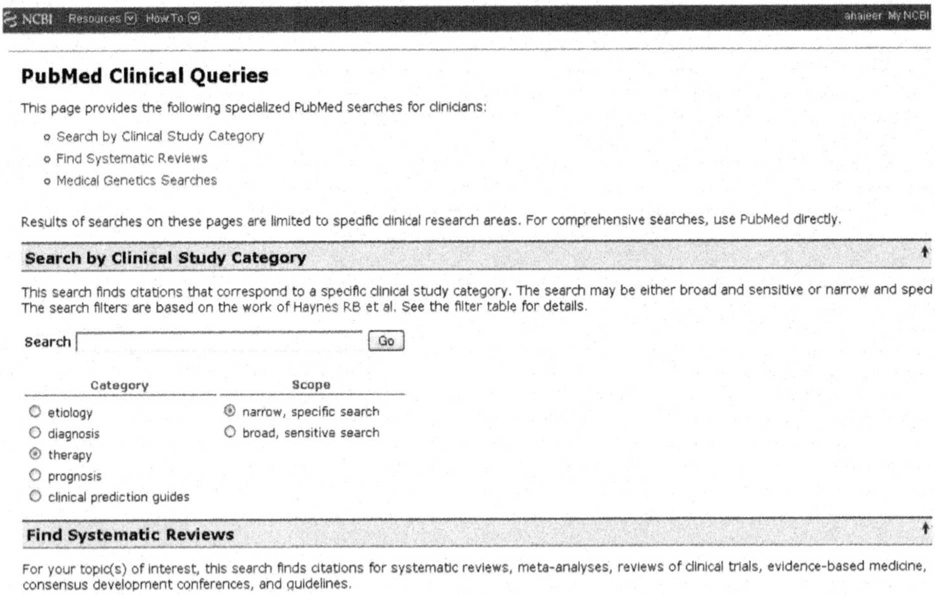

NCBI   Resources ⊡ How To ⊡   ahajeer My NCBI

PubMed Clinical Queries

This page provides the following specialized PubMed searches for clinicians:

- o Search by Clinical Study Category
- o Find Systematic Reviews
- o Medical Genetics Searches

Results of searches on these pages are limited to specific clinical research areas. For comprehensive searches, use PubMed directly.

Search by Clinical Study Category   ↑

This search finds citations that correspond to a specific clinical study category. The search may be either broad and sensitive or narrow and speci
The search filters are based on the work of Haynes RB et al. See the filter table for details.

Search [   ] [Go]

Category	Scope
○ etiology	◉ narrow, specific search
○ diagnosis	○ broad, sensitive search
◉ therapy	
○ prognosis	
○ clinical prediction guides	

Find Systematic Reviews   ↑

For your topic(s) of interest, this search finds citations for systematic reviews, meta-analyses, reviews of clinical trials, evidence-based medicine,
consensus development conferences, and guidelines.

FIGURE 10.5   PubMed Clinical Queries

clinical study category such as therapy, diagnosis, prognosis, etiology and clinical prediction guides. You can also search from this page for systematic reviews, meta-analyses, reviews of clinical trials, evidence-based medicine, consensus development conferences, and guidelines (Figure 10.6).

UpToDate

UpToDate is an evidence-based, peer-reviewed database of disease and drug interactions. It can be searched through the search box, which will result in a list of topics that can be prioritized by "adult, pediatric and patient topics".

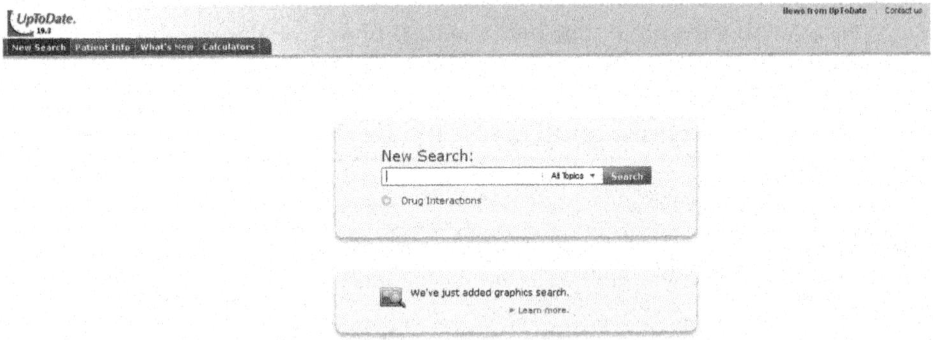

UpToDate.   News from UpToDate   Contact us
  19.3
New Search Patient Info What's New Calculators

New Search:
[   ] All Topics ▾ [Search]
○ Drug Interactions

We've just added graphics search.
► Learn more.

FIGURE 10.6   UpToDate search page

UpToDate can answer questions quickly so as to increase your clinical knowledge and improve your patient care. Topics are reviewed by analyzing the latest evidence and producing specific recommendations.

One or more terms can be searched in the search box. Just after writing the first three letters, UpToDate, automatically displays a list of possible matches.

UpToDate also includes a comprehensive drug database that includes information on drug dosing, interactions and adverse effects. Drug names can be searched in a similar way to searching for any medical term in UpToDate. Searching will return information from both the drug information database and any other topic in UpToDate. You can search the drug interaction database for a single drug name of two or more, and link them together by clicking "analyze button" to get the specific information on their interactions (Figure 10.7).

DynaMed

DynaMed is a reference tool for clinicians at the bedside, or at 'point-of-care'. It includes clinically-organized summaries of more than 3,000 topics. DynaMed is designed to answer with evidence, most clinical questions during practice. It is updated daily, with reviews from more than 500 medical journals.

DynaMed's menu summarizes diseases or conditions, with overall conclusions, representing a synthesis of the best available evidence (Figures 10.8 and 10.9).

Results on diseases are categorized under the following headings:

- ICD-9 and 10 Codes
- Causes and risk factors
- History
- Physical
- Diagnosis
- Prognosis
- Treatment
- Prevention and screening
- Quality improvement
- References

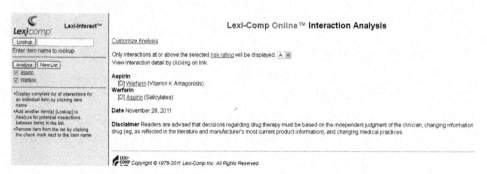

FIGURE 10.7   Drug interactions database in UpToDate

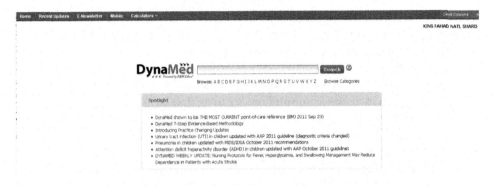

FIGURE 10.8 DynaMed homepage

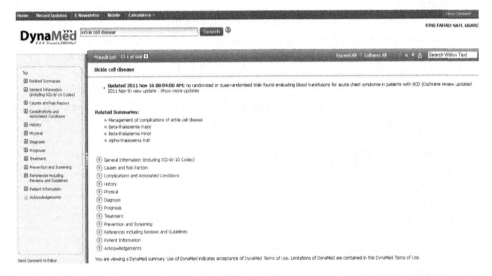

FIGURE 10.9 Topics reviewed in DynaMed

It describes in detail the following valuable tools for medical students and practicing doctors:

- How to take a history;
- How to perform a physical examination;
- How to diagnose a disease.

In addition, DynaMed can be searched for more than 800 topic summaries on Drug Information. It is a very comprehensive database that gives summaries on:

- Dosage and administration
- Cautions and adverse effects

- Interactions
- Warnings
- Stability and compatibility
- References

DynaMed is available in a PDA version for Palm OS and Microsoft Mobile devices. Information on technical requirements and installation instructions for using DynaMed on a PDA device can be found on this site: http://www.epnet.com/dynamed/technical.php

- Other EBM resources
  - PICO Linguist http://babelmesh.nlm.nih.gov/pico.php
  - Turning Research Into Practice (Tripdatabase) http://www.tripdatabase.com/index.html
  - SUMSearch http://sumsearch.uthscsa.edu/
  - The Cochrane library http://www3.interscience.wiley.com/cgi-bin/mrwhome/106568753/HOME?CRETRY=1&S
  - Curbside.MD. http://www.curbside.md/

Basics of EBM search

- You can search "PubMed" for EBM resources. This is done through the "PubMed Clinical Queries"
- "UpToDate" is an evidence-based, peer-reviewed database of disease and drug interactions.
- "DynaMed" is a reference tool for clinicians at the bedside or at the point-of-care. "DynaMed" is designed to answer with evidence, most clinical questions during practice.

Bibliography

1. Tuttle BD, Von Isenburg M, Schardt C, Powers A. PubMed instruction for medical students: searching for a better way. *Med Ref Serv Q*. 2009:199–210.
2. Hoogendam A, Stalenhoef AF, Robbé PF, Overbeke AJ. Answers to questions posed during daily patient care are more likely to be answered by UpToDate than PubMed. *J Med Internet Res*. 2008: 10(4):e29.
3. Goodyear-Smith F, Kerse N, Warren J, Arroll B. Evaluation of e-textbooks. DynaMed, MD Consult and UpToDate. *Aust Fam Physician*. 2008: 37(10):878–82.
4. Alper BS. DynaMed is evidence based. *Fam Med*. 2003: 35(8):540–1.
5. Hajeer AH, AlKnawy BA. *Doctor's Guide to Evidence-Based Medicine*. Riyadh: Alasr Printing Company 2006:160.

Chapter 11

Research Skills

Hani Tamim

Objectives

After reading this chapter, you will be able to:
- Learn important research skills required by medical students.
- Learn how to carry out a literature review.
- Learn how to write a proposal.
- Gain knowledge on collecting and analyzing data.

Introduction

One of the aims of medical curricula is to graduate medical practitioners who are able to utilize their research skills in selecting best evidence-based practices, and more importantly are capable of being actively involved in producing scholarly medical research. Thus, future medical practitioners should be capable of communicating advances in biomedical research that in turn will translate into major advances on the health of the society. Direct participation in research by medical students is widely regarded as a valuable component of medical education and as a stimulus to a career in scientific research.[1] Within the medical field, and particularly in light of the escalating importance of Evidence Based Medicine (EBM) practice, a strong understanding of research methodologies and processes through practice is essential for the success of medical doctors and their ability to become researchers or to critically judge the relevance of publications.[2]

The aim of this chapter is to highlight the important research skills required by medical students. This is done in a simplified manner, following the sequence usually adopted by medical researchers. The different sections involved in this chapter are:

- identifying a research question;
- carrying out a literature review;
- writing a proposal;
- collecting data;
- entering, cleaning, and managing data;
- analyzing data; and
- publishing results.

In the following subsections, details of each of the above steps will be provided.

Identifying a research question

A research question is the question the student wishes to study or the hypothesis he/she wishes to test. The selection of the research question needs to be given special attention, as it will drive the whole research project. The student has to identify the areas that needs further study, and this could be identified through observations, reading, etc. The research question should attempt to fill a gap in knowledge. Moreover, it would be the basis for developing and conducting the research project. It should also be specific enough to be answerable and researchable.

A good research question should be relevant and should avoid duplication of previous work. Moreover, it should be feasible and cost-effective and, more importantly, it should be doable within a specified time frame allocated for the student's research program. Finally, any research project that needs to be studied needs to meet the minimum ethical standards.

Carrying out a literature review

A literature review consists of different tasks that the student has to go through. Such tasks include:

- reading;
- analyzing; and
- summarizing what scholars and other researchers have done and reported on the specific topic the student is interested in.

The need for a literature review is highlighted for different reasons. One reason for doing a thorough literature review is to reveal existing knowledge about a certain topic. Through this process, the student will be able to identify areas of consensus and debate among different researchers on the topic. More importantly, the student will be able to identify the gaps in knowledge that exist in the literature, which in turn justifies carrying out the research project. Through carrying out a thorough literature review, the student will be able to identify approaches to research design and methodology. Finally, the student will be able to identify other researchers who share the same research interests, who might act as support for future queries.

The characteristics of a good literature search are:

- searching;
- assessing; and
- integrating.

The student has to develop good searching expertise, which will allow him/her to efficiently search the available resources through the different electronic search engines. Once the student identifies the relevant articles, he/she has to have enough expertise to assess the content of the article in terms of relevance, validity, etc.

Finally, the student has to be able to integrate the important and relevant work into his/her own research project, specifically from the methodology and results point of view. This is usually a tough task, as most of the available research usually exhibits apparent contradictions.

Writing a proposal

A proposal is a very important step in the process of research, as it is a summary of the suggested process to be used to answer the research question. A research proposal is a time-consuming process, and enough time should be devoted for it. It should be done through gathering information, reading, integrating, organizing ideas, and planning. The proposal should include all key elements involved in the proposed research process and enough information for readers to evaluate the process. Moreover, it is intended to convince the reader that the investigator has an important research question to be answered, as well as that he/she has the competence to carry out the project.

The main reason why a research proposal is essential is that it draws the road map for the research project. Moreover, Institutional Review Board (IRB) approval is essential for conducting research and it requires submission of a detailed research proposal. Finally, in some cases, research needs financial support to be carried out, and thus a research proposal will be the application based on which the funding agency will grant a fund to the researcher to carry out the study.

Briefly, the research proposal should answer the following questions:

- What do you want to do?
- Why do you want to do it?
- How are you going to do it?
- And when are you going to do it?

More specifically, any research proposal should include specific sections, such as background information, literature review, purpose, methods, references, time-line, and ethical considerations. The format is dependent on the institution at which the study will be carried out, but the key point is to adhere to the specific format required.

Under the background information, the student has to provide information about the name of the principal investigator, as well as the co-investigators, their affiliations, and contact information. Moreover, the principal investigator and the department head at which the study will be carried out should sign the form indicating knowledge and approval for the conduct of the study.

For the literature review, the student has to provide the reader with background information for the research, which acts as a framework for the proposed research, as well as establishing the link with other reported studies. More specifically, the literature review section should be written in such a way as to create interest about the topic, and lay the broad foundation for the problem that leads to the proposed study. Moreover, it should clearly identify the gap in knowledge that needs to be filled through the proposed study. This should in fact answer the question: why is this study needed? Finally, it highlights the student's expertise and knowledge about the area in which the study will be carried out.

The purpose of the study should be very clearly specified in a sentence or two that summarizes the research question to be answered by the proposed research. The purpose of the study should be clear to the student before an attempt is made to put it in words.

The methods section of the proposal is the heart of the proposal. It should be as detailed as possible, as it will be the main section that will be assessed by the reviewers. The methods section is expected to provide logical continuity. Following are some important subsections that a reviewer expects to find in the methods section, keeping in mind that all the subsections should be directly related to the objectives of the study:

- The setting of the study, in terms of Person (the population to be studied), Time (the time frame of the study), and Place (the location where the study will be carried out).
- The design of the study, which should identify the study design to be used to answer the research question.
- Inclusion and exclusion criteria should be specifically identified and justified.
- The sampling procedure through which the subjects to be included in the study will be selected.
- Detailed information about the data to be collected, which should include any questionnaire to be included in the study.
- Sample size calculation, which should be carried out appropriately and justified by proper statistical calculation.

The proposal should include a separate section about the proposed statistical analyses to be carried out, which should address univariate, bivariate, and multivariate analyses (if applicable). This should also include information about the program to be used for data entry and analyses.

A specific subsection should be included about ethical considerations. More specifically, the investigator has to provide information on how confidentiality and anonymity of the subjects would be maintained.

Finally the references used in the write-up of the proposal should be included as well. More specifically, only references that are cited in the text should be included. Moreover, the references used should be relevant to the topic, and should be updated.

A general tip for writing up the research proposal is to give the whole process enough time and not to do it in a rush and under pressure. Moreover, the student has to keep an open eye on the deadlines for submission of his/her proposal. The student has to know what he/she is trying to do before starting to put it into words. A good proposal would go through few rounds of writing and modification.

Collecting data

Data collection is a process through which information is collected about subjects included into the study. Data could be collected through many different methods depending on the study design, availability or electronic data in the institution where the study is to be carried out, available resources, etc. It could be carried out through data abstraction (chart review), interviews, or self-administered question-naires. The most important aspect in the data collection process is to select the relevant information needed to answer the research question, and discarding those that are not relevant. The development of the data collection form is a time-consuming process, and it should be given enough attention to make sure it is clear, valid, and reliable. It is advisable to use already existing tools that have been used and validated in different populations. Moreover, the data collection form has to be tested on a small sample of subjects to guarantee applicability, as well as to identify any potential problems in the tool.

Once the data collection form has been developed, the duration through which the actual data collection is carried out varies depending on the study design (whether prospective or retrospective), the sample size calculated, and the avail-able manpower doing the job.

The key point in the success of any research project is the validity of the data collected, since it is these data that will be used to answer the research question.

Entering, cleaning, and managing data

Once the data has been collected, it has to be entered into a spreadsheet which will allow further analysis. There is a variety of possible programs that could be used for this purpose, such as Microsoft Excel, Microsoft Access, Statistical Package for Social Sciences (SPSS), etc. Before the student can start to enter the data into the preferred program, he/she has to structure the program in a way that it will be compatible with the data collection form, a step that will facilitate the data collection process.

Special attention should be given to the process of entering the information from the paper format to the electronic format. This is a tiresome process but it should be done properly, as it is the data that is entered that will be used for the statistical analyses.

Once the data is entered into the program, another step of data cleaning should be carried out to make sure there are no mistakes in the dataset created. In other words, human error is highly probable when data is being entered into the com-puter, which makes it crucial to spend considerable time cleaning the dataset created. There are two types of data entry mistakes that could have taken place during the process.

The first type is those mistakes that fall outside the logical range of possible answers. For example, assume that one of the inclusion criteria for a certain study was that the subject should be below 80 years of age, and thus any age which is above 80 should be checked. These types of mistakes are easily identified by looking at the frequency distribution of that variable.

The second type of mistakes would be those that are within the expected range, for instance, if a subject's age is 76 and the entry was 16. Unlike the previous type of mistake, such errors are hard to identify, and more sophisticated data analyses are needed to identify them.

Once a mistake has been identified, efforts have to be employed to identify the source of the mistake and make sure the value is corrected.

Once the data is cleaned, another stage is crucial to prepare the final dataset that is ready for the data analyses. Data management is a step where manipulation of the information collected is done. For instance, the student might have collected information regarding the weight and height, but what would be really needed for the statistical analyses would be the body mass index (BMI), which needs to be calculated from the weight and height information.

Analyzing data

Statistics is the systematic collection, organization, analysis, and interpretation of numerical data, which is divided into two main types: **descriptive and inferential statistics**. Before addressing these two types of statistics, it is important to identify the different types of variables. A variable is an attribute that is characteristic of a subject included in a research project, which includes any piece of information collected on this subject. There are two types of variables: *categorical* and *continuous*.

A *categorical variable* is composed of categories into which a subject would fall, for example gender, marital status, disease status, etc. On the other hand, a *continuous variable* can take on any of a range of values. It is important to differentiate between these types, as different statistical analyses are carried out for different types of variables.

Descriptive statistics are the techniques used to describe the main features of a sample. A categorical variable is described by calculating the number and percentage for each of the different levels of the categorical variable. Moreover, a categorical variable is graphically summarized by constructing either a bar chart or a pie chart. On the other hand, a continuous variable is described by providing a measure of central tendency and a measure of dispersion. A measure of central tendency could be one of three measures: *mean, median,* or *mode*. Measures of dispersion could be the range, variance, or standard deviation. Similarly, a continuous variable could be graphically presented as a histogram or a line chart.

On the other hand, *inferential statistics* are the techniques used to draw conclusions on certain questions about the population from information collected from a sample. There are two types of inferential statistics: a *confidence interval* and a *hypothesis testing*.

A *confidence interval* is an interval consisting of two numerical values which define a range of values that includes the parameter being estimated, with a specified degree of confidence. Most confidence intervals calculated are 95%.

A *hypothesis test* is another method to carry out inferential statistics. There are two types of hypotheses, a *null hypothesis* which is a statement consistent with "no difference," and an *alternative hypothesis* which is a statement consistent with "a difference." Based on the data collected from the sample, either one of those two hypotheses will be accepted. A p-value, which is a probability of obtaining the observed difference due to chance, will be calculated. If the p-value ≤ 0.05, then reject the null hypothesis and accept the alternative (thus there is a statistically significant difference), whereas if the p-value > 0.05 then do not reject the null hypothesis (thus there is no statistically significant difference). Different statistical tests are available to calculate p-value, which depends on the types of the variables tested. Such tests include the Chi-square test, the Student's t-test, etc.

Publishing results

After finalizing the data analyses for the research project, it is crucial to publish the results so that other healthcare workers and researchers can have access to the work the student has done. Publishing the results of the research project could take different forms, such as an abstract in a conference, a report, etc., the most important of which is a manuscript to be published in a medical journal.

Preparing a manuscript might not be an easy task the first time it is done. Thus, following is a suggestion of a sequence of items to be prepared which might facilitate preparation of the manuscript:

- Prepare the tables and figures. This organizes the findings, as well as highlighting any missing analyses that have to be carried out.
- Go back to the literature review carried out at the proposal stage and update it, since there might be new studies published in the same area. You will have to critically evaluate the literature in light of the results you found in the study.
- On the basis of the literature review, you may have to go back to the analyses stage and further analyze the data according to the findings reported by the literature.
- Once the final tables and results have been prepared, you will need to write the manuscript. One important advice is to get the work organized within a detailed, structured outline. Preparing and presenting the findings of the research project might be of great help to you in organizing your thoughts.
- You will have to identify the journal to which you are planning to submit the manuscript. Almost all medical journals have "instructions to authors" documents on their websites, covering details such as the length, format, style, etc., that will help you prepare the manuscript in its proper form.,

Most medical journals require the manuscript to be structured according to the following sections: *abstract, introduction, methods, results, discussion,* and *conclusion.* Both the *introduction* and the *methods* section have been prepared earlier for the proposal; nevertheless, the student has to update the literature review, as well as to modify the methods section according to what methods actually were used for carrying out the study.

On the other hand, the *results* section is a summary of results found which should be presented in tables and graphs. The *discussion* section is the overall evaluation of the study from the student's point of view, and should include comparison between similar studies and the present one, strengths and limitations of the present study, etc. Finally, the *conclusion* section is where the student summarizes the main message drawn from the research project, as well as any recommendations and proposals for future research.

References

1. Kemph JP, Claybrook JR, Sodeman WA, Sr.: Summer research program for medical students. *J Med Educ* 1984, 59(9):708–713.
2. Windish D, Huot S, Green M: Medicine residents' understanding of the biostatistics and results in the medical literature. *JAMA* 2007, 298:1010–1022.

Chapter 12

Presentation Skills

Ibrahim Al Alwan

Objectives

- Define elements involved in a successful presentation.
- Describe, in detail, the elements involved in a presentation.
- List of general rules for a high quality presentation.

Introduction

A "presentation" can be defined as *a speech delivered in front of an audience*. The presentation's central purpose, whether it is written, oral or visual, is to communicate a topic effectively. A good presentation should be simple, concise, and delivered in an interesting manner.

There are four elements that influence a presentation, each of which affects its quality and success:

- **The presenter**
  The first element of a high-quality presentation is the presenter. The best presenter is one who has an engaging personality, as well as the following characteristics:
  - Knows when to talk and when to stop.
  - Talks about the important issues that the audience came to hear.
  - Uses simple language.
  - Uses normal body gestures.
  - Engages the audience emotionally and visually.

  These characteristics can be achieved by both verbal and visual methods:
  - *Verbal methods:* This involves the ability to verbally deliver the presentation in such a manner that it is clear and understandable to the whole audience. The language should be clear, with a smooth flow. Speech is dynamic with variable tones and several pauses. These are needed to stress a point, start a new or important point, and to retain the attention of the audience. The presenter should stress the presentation's important points, repeat them and then provide a summary of these points. The basic law of delivering a presentation is to: "Tell them what you are going to tell them, tell them, and then tell them what you told them."

○ *Visual methods:* The visual part of the presentation includes the presenter's body language and dress, as well as the visual aids used. The presenter should be animated and dynamic but not overly so. Appropriate attire for the occasion should be worn. The presenter should be energetic, enthusiastic and excited about the topic being delivered to the target audience.

• **The presentation**

The second element of a good presentation is the presentation itself, which has two content issues:

○ quality of the presentation, and

○ quantity of the presentation.

The quality and quantity should be based on the length of the presentation and the make-up of the audience, with the expectation that most are knowledgeable in the field and the remainder comprises either experts or novices on the topic. The introduction and summary of the presentation should target the entire audience, with the body of the presentation focused for the majority, who are field knowledgeable. The quantity of the presentation should be based on the time allocated for the presentation.

The audience, as a rule, will only remember three things from the presentation, so you should plan what these three points will be in advance. Decide the key message at the start of the planning process and build the presentation around these key points. Lists should be used wherever possible in the presentation – and remember, "Less is more." Keep the points limited to three, and keep the content varied to include the entire audience.

The quality of the visual aids used, whether as part of a slide or a video presentation, should include basic colors and simple backgrounds, with clear and simple text, clear illustrations and focused points. If the presentation is video based, the video should have clear sound.

The following guidelines should be followed for PowerPoint slide preparation:

○ *Background color:* Should be dark; commonly used colors are dark blue, black or dark green.

○ *Text color:* Should be light; usually white or yellow work well. Red and pink should be avoided as these colors are usually not visible.

○ *Content:* Each slide should have no more than seven words per line and no more than seven lines per page.

○ *Font:* Font size used should be 30–45 for the title and 18–24 for the text. Most commonly used font types are Ariel or Times New Roman. Intricate or ultra-contemporary font types should be avoided as the audience may find them difficult to read.

○ *Illustrations:* should be used liberally, but should be simple, uncluttered, and cropped.

Examples of good and bad slide presentations are shown in Figures 12.1, 12.2 and 12.3.

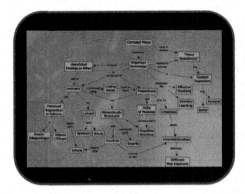 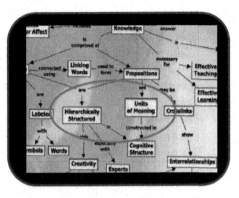

Bad Scanned Document   Well-Cropped Scanned Document

FIGURE 12.1   Example of a (left) badly scanned and (right) well scanned, well cropped document

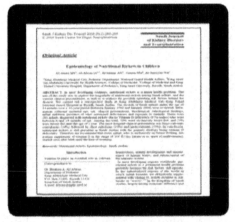 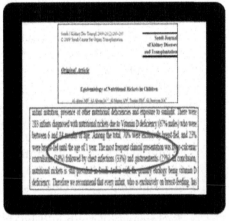

Full Page Manuscript - Illegible   Pertinent Extract e.g. Title, Name of Author,
Publication Date & highlighted Points only

FIGURE 12.2   Extract from manuscript: (left) illegible; (right) legible and pertinent, showing title, author, publication date, and just one highlighted point

- **The audience**
  - *Type:* The audience will vary by age and comprise people from different backgrounds, i.e. nurses, medical students, physicians, sub-specialized physicians, and administrative staff. It is important to know the audience, their background and their level of awareness of the topic and the message to be delivered.

Good presenters may complete questionnaires prior to their presentation in order to understand audience deficiencies and identify the questions the audience needs to have answered.

○ *Number:* The number of attendees is important since this can range from a small group of less than 25 people to a larger group of more than 25.

Small groups have their own special presentation needs compared to audiences of more than 25. Small groups need eye-to-eye contact during most of the presentation. It is advisable for the speaker to stop periodically and ask questions directly to the audience, or to answer their questions.

Large groups of more than 25 people have two important elements that presenters must maintain. First, the presenter needs to be seen by the entire audience; second, the presenter needs to be heard by the entire audience, especially by those sitting in the back row.

- **The time and place of the presentation**

  Presenters must be aware of the time of the presentation. A morning presentation where everyone is rested and awake, with more energy and alertness, is different from an evening or afternoon presentation, or after a large meal.

  A good presenter visits the presentation venue (if possible), knows the seating plan, the type of seating available, the podium location and what visual aids will be used. The presenter may be able to make a test run of the presentation in the actual room where it will be given. However, if the presenter is not physically able to visit the venue, then a full description of the room – chairs, laptop, screen, and audio system available in the room – should be requested.

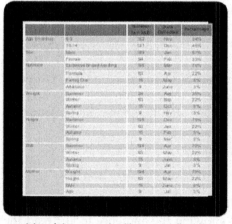

A lot of data squashed into a small table   Well presented table with clear legible data

FIGURE 12.3   (left) A lot of data squashed into a small table; (right) well presented table with clear, legible data

General rules

General rules for good presenters may be summarized as three Ps:

- **Prepare**
  The presentation should be prepared keeping in mind the four elements (Presenter, Presentation, Audience, and the Time and Place). You should be well prepared and have suitable content ready. Take time to perform a good search, plan the presentation based on the content, review the time allocated for the presentation, and identify the number of the audience, the variety of the audience and the venue of the presentation. Prepare to answer appropriate questions for your presentation, and allow time for this.
- **Practice**
  After preparing well, practice the delivery of the presentation, either in front of a mirror or in front of colleagues or family. A good presenter may rehearse the presentation more than five times for one presentation. Presentation skills must be practiced to obtain the desired result, but these skills will be clearly evident in future presentations as they improve.
- **Present**
  Finally, make your presentation. It should follow the following format:
  ○ Title
  ○ Objectives for the presentation
  ○ Core subject
  ○ Summary, with home messages.

Each section of the presentation needs to be linked to each other by using transitions. It is always advisable to summarize while you are presenting and repeat points so that the audience will understand. A good presentation needs to be in context, with the presentation including either a story for each section or the use of examples or proverbs that link the ideas that are being delivered.

Start by planning what you will do in each section. The beginning is ideal for an attention grabber or an ice breaker. The end is the right place to wrap things up or to end with a grand finale.

It may be a repeat presentation, but it will not be identical to previous presentations. By varying the content to be current and relevant for each audience, the presentation will be different for each audience and, therefore, the presentation quality will be different.

- Mistakes to avoid during your presentation:
  ○ Rushing slides
  ○ Skipping slides
  ○ Errors in spelling, grammar, and legibility
  ○ Giving incomplete sentences and allowing the audience to just read the slides
  ○ Misalignment between what you verbally present and what is written on the slide
  ○ Reading constantly from the computer or projection screen

- Playing with the laser pointer
- Apologizing for any shortcomings during your presentation, e.g.:
  - Sorry, I did not prepare
  - Sorry, I forgot
  - Sorry . . .

In some references, you may find these points listed as *5 Ps:*

1. Planning
2. Preparation
3. Pattern
4. Presentation
5. Performance evaluation

Performance evaluation

The quality of your presentations will improve over time through feedback and evaluations by peers or other presenters. Be enthusiastic to hear and receive audience feedback, and use their critiques to overcome any deficiencies identified and enhance the quality of the presentation.

References

1. Hill MD. *Oral Presentation Advice.* University of Wisconsin–Madison; April 1992 [updated January 1997; cited 2011, 15 March]. Available from: http://pages.cs.wisc.edu/~markhill/conference-talk.html.
2. Patterson DA. *How to Give a Bad Talk.* University of California–Berkeley; 1983 [cited 2011, 15 March]. Available from: http://pages.cs.wisc.edu/~markhill/conference-talk.html.
3. Wertheim EG. *Making Effective Oral Presentations.* Northeastern University, College of Business Administration [cited 2011, 15 March]. Available from: http://www.honors.vcu.edu/pdfs/MakingEffectiveOralPresentations.doc.

Further reading: Books

1. How to Run Seminars & Workshops: Presentation Skills for Consultants, Trainers & Teachers by Robert L. Jolles: John Wiley & Sons Inc. 02 September 2005.
2. Maximize Your Presentation Skills: How to speak, Look and Act on Your Way to the Top by Ellen Kaye: Random House USA Inc. 19 December 2002.
3. Effective Presentation Skills: A Practical Guide for Better Speaking by Steve Mandel: Crisp Learning, January 2000.
4. Powerful Presentation Skills: How to get a Group's Attention, Hold People's Interest and Persuade Them to Act by Debra Smith (Audio Book) – HYPERLINK "http://www.amazon.com/" www.amazon.com

III

LEARNING IN THE CLASSROOM

Chapter 13

Learning in Small Groups in PBL

Diana H.J.M. Dolmans, Floris van Blankenstein, and Rachelle Kamp

Objectives

- To outline some characteristics of small group learning in PBL.
- To explain the three phases involved in PBL group learning.
- To outline different roles in PBL group learning.
- To provide tips for students about effective PBL.

Characteristics of small group learning in PBL

Student learning in higher education has been dominated many years by lecturing. Lectures can have their function, but small group learning also has many advantages for students and is nowadays successfully implemented in many curricula in higher education. One of the successful implementations of small group learning is problem-based learning (PBL). PBL is very popular in medical education. In this chapter it will be explained what the advantages are of small group learning, which problems students may experience with PBL and tips for effective group functioning will be given.

Description of small group learning in PBL

One of the main characteristics of problem-based learning (PBL) is that students work together in small groups while discussing problems. During the discussion students activate their prior knowledge about the subject under discussion and detect which issues need further study. These issues, so called student-generated learning issues, are subsequently studied by students during individual study. In the next small group meeting, students meet again to further discuss what they have learnt about the problem during self-study.

The small group usually consists of about 6 to 10 students who meet twice a week during a two hour session. A teacher, a so-called tutor, participates in the tutorial group meeting. One of the students is discussion leader and another student is the scribe. During the first part of the tutorial group meeting students usually discuss the subject that they studied, during the second part of the tutorial group meeting, students discuss about a new problem. In most medical PBL schools student groups stay together for six or ten weeks and thereafter the groups are rearranged.

A problem to be discussed in the tutorial group could be as follows:

> The past few years, Ellen has grown much taller very fast. She has always been a tall girl, but at the age of 11 years and a height of five feet, four inches, she is head and shoulders above her age group. People always take her to be older, which can be quite wearisome.

When students discuss this problem in the small tutorial group they may discuss about hormones and genetics and how they influence growth. But during the discussion issues will also be raised that cannot be answered yet, such as what are normal and abnormal growth rates, which factors influence growth and how do they influence growth or what are the possible psychological effects of being too tall? These issues are formulated as student-generated learning issues that need further study.

Why small group learning in PBL?

Learning in small groups fits with current insights about effective learning. These insights emphasize that group learning or collaborative learning has several advantages from a cognitive and motivational perspective.[2]

From a cognitive perspective, a group provides opportunities to the group members to ask questions, to answer questions, to reason with each other, to discuss contradictions, to explain in own words, to correct misconceptions and to give feedback to each other which leads to better learning.[3-5] Especially active engagement, such as reasoning aloud during the discussion, leads to better knowledge retention on the long term.[6] Group learning is considered superior to individual learning when the learning task is complex.[7, 8]

From a motivational perspective, a group is assumed to motivate the individual within the group because of two reasons. First, because a group develops team spirit due to which the group members want the group to succeed. Second, because an individual within the group can only succeed if the group succeeds. Students in a group also learn to work together which may help them become better collaborators.[9]

Effective cognitive behaviours in the tutorial group

- Ask questions to other group members
- Answer questions of other group members
- Reason with each other
- Discuss contradictions with each other
- Explain in own words
- Give feedback to each other
- Correct misconceptions

Three phases in group learning in PBL

Group learning in PBL is organized around three phases: the brainstorming phase, the self-study phase and the reporting phase.

During the first phase, the brainstorming phase, students discuss about a problem, e.g. about a tall girl, as given in the example above. During this phase students activate or mobilize their prior knowledge on a particular subject. E.g. students discuss about what they know about factors influencing growth, such as hormones and genetics. The brainstorming phase is a very important phase, because students use the knowledge that they have already acquired to interpret and understand new information. By stimulating students to make connections between their previously acquired knowledge and the new knowledge, they will better understand and comprehend the new information.[10] During this phase it will also become clear which issues need further self-study. These are the student-generated learning issues that were mentioned before. A student-generated learning issue could be "What are normal patterns of growth and which factors influence growth?

In the second phase, the self-study phase, students spend time on self-study in order to better understand the subject discussed during the brainstorming phase. During this phase students work individually and study materials related to the subject under discussion. It is important that each student spends a considerable amount of time on studying since time spent on studying and even time available for self-study is a positive predictor for student performance.[11] It is important that the student does not only study those topics that were discussed during the brainstorm or only those topics that were formulated as student-generated learning issues. A broadening approach should be encouraged. This means that the student should also study issues that are related to the subject under discussion, in other words related to one's own interest or knowledge gaps. It has been shown that students who studied beyond the self-generated learning issues and spend more time on self-study, performed better on tests.[12] Finally, although the self-study phase is often done individually, working together during parts of this phase may also have a positive effect on learning, because students can help each other to clarify issues that are unclear and can support and motivate each other.[13, 14]

In the third phase, the reporting phase, students discuss the subject studied in the group. During this phase students synthesize their acquired knowledge by verbalizing in their own words what they have learnt, by asking questions about issues that are unclear or by discussing contradictions. During this phase it is important that students clearly link the new information acquired. Furthermore it is important that the acquired knowledge is applied to the problem under discussion. During the reporting phase the student can compare his own acquired knowledge with the knowledge that other students report during the discussion and will discover what he or she did not yet understand well or certain knowledge gaps. If it is difficult for a student to follow the discussion during the reporting phase, the student should spend some extra self-study time on the subject discussed.

Three phases	Main activities
Brainstorming	Activate prior knowledge
	Make connections between prior knowledge
Self-study	Study in-depth and broadly
Reporting	Verbalize in own words
	Make connections between prior and new knowledge
	Make connections between new knowledge
	Apply knowledge to the problem under discussion

Different roles in tutorial groups in PBL

In PBL different roles are fulfilled by students in the group, such as group member, discussion leader and scribe.[15, 16] Furthermore a teacher or so-called tutor is available for the students in each group.

Group member

All members that participate in a group are of course group members. Each group member is expected to join all group meetings, to adequately prepare all the group meetings, to arrive on time, to participate actively in the group and to share information. It is important to make clear appointments about these issues at the start of the group meeting. Preferably between 6 and 8 group members participate, otherwise it will be difficult to ensure active engagement of all students in the group. In order to make a group successful it is important that the group members encourage each other to exchange information and to challenge each other's reasoning. Group members should hold each other responsible for their contribution to the group and promote each others' efforts in the group.[7]

Discussion leader

One of the students is the discussion leader for the group meeting. For each group meeting another student can be assigned as the discussion leader. The discussion leader plays an important role in the group. The discussion leader leads the discussion, ensures that all students can and do participate in the discussion and ensures that the most relevant topics are discussed within the available time. The discussion leader also ensures that clear learning issues are generated, that group members clearly explain the subject and that they relate the information to each other. In addition, the discussion leader summarizes the main issues discussed by the group. Leading the discussion is not an easy role. Students should receive training in how to lead a group discussion. Leading a group discussion in PBL is a skill that is also of importance during professional practice later on. Studies have demonstrated that collaborating in small groups in PBL facilitates the acquisition of interpersonal skills, such as discussion leading skills.[17]

Scribe

During the discussions in the group notes should be made on a blackboard or flip-over. The scribe can help the group members and the discussion leader because he or she summarizes the main issues to be discussed. The scribe should also clearly write down the student-generated learning issues that are formulated by the group. In some occasions it is helpful if the scribe makes a scheme on the blackboard or flip-over to structure the discussion. An effective scribe listens well to the group members and checks whether the information that is written down is a correct summary of the discussion.

Tutor

The tutor, or teacher within the group, should facilitate the discussion at the content and process level. The tutor should encourage the students to interact deeply with each other.[18] The tutor should stimulate student learning by asking questions and encouraging deep discussions. There has been a debate in the literature, whether a tutor should be a content-expert or not. Research has however demonstrated that a tutor needs some content expertise, but also needs to know how to use this expertise during the group work; i.e. the tutor should not transmit the knowledge but should ask thought-provoking questions to be answered by the students.[19] Furthermore it is important that a tutor facilitates the group process, e.g. (s)he evaluates group functioning on a regular basis, intervenes when the discussion leader might not adequately lead the discussion and makes agreements to improve the group process if needed. For instance, the tutor could ask the students to evaluate the strengths and the weaknesses of the group and the tutor so far. Students could for example mention that the tutor should leave more room for the discussion leader to lead the discussion. From this feedback the tutor could learn that (s)he might perhaps wait a little bit longer before intervening, so that the discussion leader can better fulfil his role.

Role	Activity
Group member	Be actively engaged
Discussion leader	Lead discussion, ensure equal participation, monitor time, summarize, ensure the generation of clear learning issues, stimulate deep discussion
Scribe	Summarize discussion on blackboard
Tutor	Facilitate group discussion at the content and process level

Problems with small group work

Although group work can be very effective when discussing complex materials, in practice several problems are encountered by students. Main problems that are often experienced by students with group work are: uncertainty about the depth and breadth of studying the materials, unequal participation of students, and superficial discussions. The three problems are of course also related to each other.

Uncertainty about depth and breadth of studying the materials

One of the problems often reported by students when being confronted with their first PBL tutorials is that students do not know how deep or broad they need to understand the materials to be discussed in the tutorial group. One of the causes is that it is not exactly prescribed which chapters should be studied for each tutorial group meeting. However, as described before, during the reporting phase students will discover what their personal depth and breadth of understanding of the materials is in comparison with the other students within the group. If it is difficult for students to follow the discussion during the reporting phase they will discover that they need to study the materials more in-depth or more broadly.

Unequal participation

Another problem that is sometimes reported is that some students do not participate in the discussion; i.e. are very quiet or that some students dominate the discussion. These behaviors of unequal participation of students can lead to conflicts within the group. However, Hendry, Ryan and Harris (2003)[20] reported that a quiet student is perceived as being less hindering the group work than a dominant student, probably because students just ignore the quiet student. However, if too many students do not participate in the discussion actively, the group will not be effective. If a student dominates the discussion, this can lead to mini-lecturing and can also have a negative effect on the motivation of other students in the group to contribute actively to the group discussion.

A superficial discussion

One of the problems that are sometimes reported is that the group discussion just scratches the surface and is not really in-depth. This takes place when students for example do not, or only briefly, brainstorm, when students just read aloud their notes and do not summarize in their own words, when students skip issues to be discussed, when students studied the materials superficially or when some students are not well prepared.[20, 21] A superficial discussion can also take place when students divide the learning issues between the students and do not all study all learning issues that were generated. If not all students studied the materials in-depth it will be difficult to have a deep discussion. The behaviors described here that lead towards a superficial discussion are often caused by lack of motivation. A lack of depth in the discussion is perceived by students as having a strong negative impact on learning.[22]

Tips for students about effective group functioning in PBL

Acquire skills as a student about how to work in a group

Working as a student in a group is not easy and therefore requires student training. During these training sessions students should be provided with information about how to work in a group. They should also experience how to fulfill the role of discussion leader or scribe. Furthermore it is important that students learn how to receive and give feedback to each other in the group and how to deal with difficult situations, such as a dominant student in the group.

Make clear agreements at the start about how to work

At the first meeting of each group clear agreements should be made about how to work together.[23] What are the different roles in the group, who fulfills which role and when? But, appointments should also be made about what to do when being absent. Group members should explain to each other what they expect from each other. Furthermore, the students and the tutor should evaluate at a regular basis whether the group sticks to the agreements that have been made.

Be well prepared as a student for each group meeting

Each group member should prepare for the group meetings well. This means that a student should study all the learning issues in-depth and also from a broad perspective. Preferably the student makes use of different resources to study the materials and not only one resource, because this might enrich the discussion and depth of understanding. It is also important that the student after having studied the materials for the next group meeting checks whether all learning issues are covered and can be answered previous to the discussion in the group.

Summarize in own words

When students report in the tutorial group about what they have learnt during self-study they should be stimulated to summarize their knowledge in own words. It should be avoided that students read aloud their notes or parts of the literature. Furthermore, in order to ensure a well structured discussion and to avoid a haphazard discussion, at regular intervals the discussion should be summarized. These summaries can be given by the discussion leader, but also by another group member or the tutor. A summary makes clear what has been learnt so far, how different issues are related to each other and provides opportunities to check whether the subject is well understood. Furthermore, summaries make it easier for students to listen actively to the contributions of other group members.

Evaluate at a regular basis

At a regular basis the group work should be evaluated. The evaluation can focus both on the contents of the discussion (whether they have sufficient depth) and on the process of the group work (active participation of all members, preparedness). It is important that the group members give each other constructive and supportive feedback and focus on both strong and weak issues. But, it is also highly important to suggest alternatives or improvements. It is the responsibility of the discussion leader and the tutor to evaluate the group work at a regular basis, but each group member can initiate the evaluation when deemed necessary. The Maastricht Peer Activity Rating Scale is a valid and reliable instrument that can be used by students to evaluate each peer on the contributions made to the tutorial group discussion.[24] This instrument is aimed at measuring the students' constructive, collaborative and motivational contributions to the group. Peer evaluations of behaviours in group work are perceived as helpful by students.[25]

Take home message: Tips for effective group functioning in PBL

- Acquire skills as a student about how to work in a group
- Make clear agreements at the start about how to work in the group
- Be well prepared as a student for each group meeting
- Summarize in own words
- Evaluate on a regular basis

References

1. Slavin, R.E. (1996). Research on cooperative learning and achievement: What we know, what we need to know. *Contemporary Educational Psychology, 21,* 43–69.
2. Slavin, R. E., Hurley, E. A., & Chamberlain, A. (2003). Cooperative learning and achievement: Theory and research. In: G. E. Miller & W. M. Reynolds (Eds.), *Handbook of Psychology: Educational psychology* (Vol. 7, pp. 177–198). Hoboken, NJ, US: John Wiley & Sons Inc.
3. Van der Linden, J., Erkens, G., Schmidt, H. & Renshaw, P. (2000). Collaborative learning. In: R.J. Simons, J. van der Linden & T. Duffy. *New learning.* pp 37-54 Kluwer: Dordrecht.
4. Visschers-Pleijers, A.J.S.F., Dolmans, D.H.J.M., Wolfhagen, H.A.P., &Vleuten van der, C.P.M. (2005). Development and validation of a questionnaire to identify learning-oriented group interactions in PBL. *Medical Teacher, 27, 4,* 375–381.
5. Dolmans, D.H.J.M. & Schmidt, H.G. (2006). What do we know about cognitive and motivational effects of small group tutorials in problem-based Learning? *Advances in health Sciences Education, 11,* 321–336.
6. Van Blankenstein, F.M., Dolmans, D.H.J.M., Vleuten, van der, C.P.M. & Schmidt, H.G. (2011). Which cognitive processes support learning during small-group discussion? The role of providing explanations and listening to others. *Instructional Science, 39,* 189–204.
7. Johnson, D.W., Johnson, R.T. & Smith, K. (2007). The state of cooperative learning in Postsecondary and Professional settings. *Educational Psychology Review, 19,* 15–29.
8. Kirschner, F. Paas, F. & Kirschner, P.A. (2009). A cognitive load approach to collaborative learning: United brains for complex tasks. *Educational Psychology Review, 21,* 31–42.
9. Hmelo-Silver, C.E. (2004). Problem-based learning: What and how students learn. *Educational Psychology Review, 16, 3,* 235–66.
10. Schmidt, H. G. (1993). Foundations of problem-based learning: Some explanatory notes. *Medical Education, 27,* 422–432.
11. Schmidt, H.G., Cohen-Schotanus, J., Van der Molen, H.T., Splinter, T.A.W., Bulte, J., Holdrinet, R. & Van Rossum, H.J.M. (2009). Learning more by being taught less: a "time-for-self-study" theory explaining curricular effects on graduation rate and study duration. *Higher Education, 60, 3,* 287–300.
12. Van den Hurk, M.M., Wolfhagen, I.H.A.P., Dolmans, D.H.J.M. & Vleuten, van der, C.P.M. (1999). The Impact of student-generated learning issues on individual study time and academic achievement. *Medical Education, 33, 11,* 808–14.
13. Hendry, G.D., Hyde, S.J. & Davy, P. (2005). Independent study groups. *Medical Education, 39,* 672–679.
14. Moust, J., Roebertsen, H., Savelberg, H. & De Rijk, A. (2005). Revitalising PBL groups: Evaluating PBL with study teams. *Education for Health, 18, 1,* 62–73.
15. Van Til, C. & Van der Heijden, F. (1998). *PBL Study Skills on overview.* Maastricht: University of Maastricht.
16. Moust, J.H.C., Bouhuijs, P., A. & Schmidt, H. G. (2007). *Introduction to Problem-based learning. A guide for students.* The Netherlands: Noordhoff.
17. Schmidt, H.G., Van der Molen, H.T., Te Winkel, R. & Wijnen, W.H.F. (2009). Constructivist, problem-based learning does work: A meta-analysis of curricular comparisons involving a single medical school. *Educational Psychologist, 44, 4,* 227–249.
18. De Grave, W.S., Dolmans, D.H.J.M. & Vleuten, C.P.M. van der (1999). Profiles of effective tutors in problem-based learning: scaffolding student learning. *Medical Education, 33, 12,* 901–906.

19. Dolmans, D.H.J.M., Gijselaers, W.H., Moust, J., Grave, de, W., Wolfhagen, H.A.P. & Vleuten, van der, C.P.M. (2002). Trends in research on the tutor in problem-based learning: conclusions and implications for educational practice and research. *Medical Teacher, 24, 2, 173–180.*

20. Hendry, G.D., Ryan, G. & Harris, J. (2003). Group problems in problem-based learning. *Medical Teacher, 25, 6,* 609–616.

21. Houlden, R.L., Collier, C.P. & Frid, P.J. (2001). Problems identified by tutors in a hybrid problem-based learning curriculum. *Academic Medicine, 76, 1,* 81.

22. De Grave, W., Dolmans, D.H.J.M. & van der Vleuten, C.P.M. (2001). Student perceptions about the occurence of critical incidents in tutorial groups. *Medical Teacher, 23, 1, 49–54.*

23. Azer, S.A. (2004). Becoming a student in a PBL course: Twelve tips for succesful group discussion. *Medical Teacher, 26, 1,* 12–15.

24. Kamp, R.J.A., Dolmans, D.H.J.M., Van Berkel, H. & Schmidt, H.G. (2010). Can students adequately evaluate the activities of their peers in PBL? *Medical Teacher, 33, 2,* 145–150

25. Wigen, K., Holen, A. & Ellingsen, O. (2003). "Predicting academic success by group behaviour in PBL." *Medical Teacher, 25, 1,* 32–37.

Chapter 14

Interactive Lectures

Julie Browne and John Bligh

Objectives

After reading this chapter, you will be able to:
- Learn: what is a traditional lecture? Its advantages and disadvantages.
- Understand the place of lectures in medical schools, and whether these are effective.
- Know: what is active learning? And whether lecturing is compatible with active learning.
- Know what a lecturer could do to make lectures more interactive.
- Learn how a student can get the most out of a lecture.

Introduction

London: 1816. *The clinical lecturer stands behind a desk. Facing the lecturer, in rows of tiered seats, sits a group of over a hundred medical students. The lecturer is speaking, occasionally reading from notes to help structure his talk. Most of the students are quietly taking notes, although some are staring into space or doodling on their notebooks. One of those daydreaming medical students is the 20-year-old aspiring poet, John Keats. The flowery doodles in his notebook show that even one of the greatest minds of the 19th century struggled to maintain concentration during lectures.*

Your medical school: 2012. *The lecturer may be using an electronic slide presentation instead of notes. But the students are still quietly taking notes, daydreaming or doodling. There have been no fundamental changes for nearly 200 years.*

What is the place of lectures in medical schools?

All medical schools need on occasion to gather a large group of students together as a community and address them on matters concerning the knowledge they need to acquire as entrants to the profession. The most straightforward way of doing this is by staging a lecture.

The formal lecture is such a traditional feature of medical education that it is impossible to imagine a medical school anywhere that does not have at least one large auditorium where students congregate in a large group. Lectures are so fundamental a part of the medical curriculum that medical educators continue to be known as lecturers. All medical students expect to be taught in formal lectures for at least some of their course[1] and, as they continue into practice, they will encounter plenary sessions, keynote addresses and large-group presentations whenever they attend continuing professional development events and conferences.

Even in those medical schools where most teaching is delivered through practical sessions and small group discussions, lectures are still frequently used to introduce a new subject, to give overviews of a topic and to give advice on learning and the institutional processes that support it. Because lectures are so commonplace as a teaching method, however, it is easy to forget that getting the very best out of them takes skill, experience and concentration on the part of both lecturers and students.

Are lectures effective?

A great advantage of formal lectures is their economy of scale. They are easy to timetable and accommodate within the medical school's working day. A single lecturer can address large numbers of students, and since a lecturer's time is relatively expensive and in short supply and student numbers are increasing, it is unsurprising that medical schools see lectures as a cost-effective way of delivering teaching compared with small groups and seminars.[2]

But the cost effectiveness of any teaching format is entirely dependent on how successful it is at achieving its key goal, which is to stimulate students to acquire and retain new knowledge and to recall it later when needed.[3] This is a serious issue for medical schools, because although lectures are probably no worse than other methods for conveying information, they are relatively ineffective when it comes to promoting thought, inspiring and motivating interest in a subject, teaching professional values or changing students' attitudes.[4] Furthermore, they are known to be particularly poor at holding students' attention, and concentration starts to decline within about 20 minutes after the start of a formal lecture.[5]

Research done in the West has shown that medical students do not like formal lectures and consider them ineffective, boring and less relevant to clinical practice compared with more interactive teaching formats.[1, 6] Indeed, lecturers themselves believe that formal lecture formats are ineffective.[7, 8] The more tedious and irrelevant the lectures, the more likely students are to find excuses not to go at all unless compelled to do so, which further decreases their effectiveness.[9]

What is active learning?

The most serious problem with traditional lectures is that they are particularly ineffective in developing desirable attitudes to learning.[10] Lectures in which the students sit passively, receiving whatever information the lecturer thinks appropriate, encourage a *surface* approach to learning. Surface approaches lead students to learn facts by rote simply to pass exams, without much interest in or retention of content. But medical schools want students to develop *deep* approaches to learning, whereby learning is seen as an "active search for understanding."[11] Deep approaches to learning are associated with success in final examinations at medical school and are essential to effective clinical practice.[12,13]

Small group sessions and discussions involve the students in active learning, and are therefore specifically designed to develop deep learning approaches.[11] According to Michael Prince,[14] *"Active learning is generally defined as any instructional method that engages students in the learning process. In short, active learning requires students to do meaningful learning activities and think about what they are doing. ... The core elements of active learning are student activity and engagement in the learning process."* Active learning requires both teacher and student to work cooperatively to enhance the learning experience. Interactive formats, in which students are encouraged to 'own' their learning, are usually popular with students and, importantly, are also more effective at improving knowledge gain and recall. [15,16] Today's students expect and respond best to a more active, individualistic approach,[17] and they have a particular struggle with traditional lecture formats.

Is lecturing compatible with active learning?

Teaching and lecturing are an inevitable part of a professional's life. As a medical student, you will certainly be on the receiving end of many lectures over the course of your career, and you may well be asked to deliver them, too. Even while at medical school you may be expected to give lectures and make presentations to groups of your peers. This is becoming increasingly likely as medical school curricula recognize the need to offer students opportunities to develop teaching skills.[18]

Having accepted and understood the need to develop deeper learning approaches in students, many teachers are already responding in remarkably creative ways to the challenge of making their large group teaching sessions more interactive. They use every possible opportunity to ensure that students stay awake, pay attention, get involved and think for themselves, carefully tailoring the information in the lecture so that students can assimilate it into their existing knowledge frameworks, understand it properly and recall it later when they need to.

There are many good books advising lecturers on ways to make formal lectures more interesting and stimulating for the students (see *'Further reading'* for some examples, and your institution's library will also be able to help). But making lectures more interactive involves going a step further than just improving your style of delivery. It requires lecturers to offer activities that will actively engage the students, not just in listening and writing notes but also in other ways such as talking, questioning and thinking. Here are some ideas to get you started. You will develop more techniques of your own as you progress, since good teaching is all about developing scholarship, using literature, research and feedback to improve and adapt your teaching methods constantly.

What can a lecturer do to make lectures more interactive?

1. **The lecturer: it does not have to be just you!**

   1.1 Try delivering the lecture as part of a pair or team,[19] or invite guest lecturers.

   1.2 Invite patients, experts, senior students and others to join you. They can:
   - Deliver or contribute to parts of the lecture.
   - Form part of a 'round table' to answer questions from students.
   - Comment and feedback on what you have said.
   - Sit with students to share ideas during discussions.

2. **Introducing activity**

   2.1 Try asking the students beforehand to think about what they need to know, and ask for feedback.

   2.2 Introduce quizzes, tests and games. It can be particularly helpful to give a quiz early in the lecture so that students become aware of what they do not know and need to learn; and it can also help to reinforce what students have learned during the lecture.

   2.3 Invite comments and questions at regular intervals and, if possible, make yourself available after the session.

   2.4 Sub-divide the group and get them to work in pairs or teams on activities such as:
   - 'Brainstorming', where the students are set a problem or question and have a few minutes in which to come up with as many ideas as they can.
   - Buzz groups and small discussions where each group concentrates on a task and reports back to the whole group.
   - Snowball consultations where groups come up with ideas and then share them with other groups, which then share with another group and so on.
   - Nominal group technique where group members work together to reach a consensus on a set of ideas and to rank them on their perceived importance.
     (For more information on these and other techniques, see 'Further reading.')

   2.5 If the size of the group and difficulties with the venue make it impossible to introduce much activity or variety into your lecture, then simply getting your audience to stand up and stretch for two minutes every 20 minutes or so can improve learning.[14,20]

3. **Visual aids**

   3.1 Can you do practical demonstrations, experiments and role plays? Can you involve students in these? If the group is large, could you use technology to enable live demonstrations to be projected on screen?

   3.2 Slide shows, interactive white boards and electronic presentations are now ubiquitous: but make sure you know how to use them well, since a boring and confusing presentation is worse than useless. Why not try teaching your large group without an electronic slide presentation – just for fun? Or get them to design and present slides and materials?

3.3 One way of introducing interactivity in large groups is to use electronic polling systems, where the audience have small keypads that can be used to register votes. These are fun for multiple-choice quizzes or simply for polling audience opinions.

3.4 Videos, films and DVDs are fun, but should be used with caution as they can encourage passivity if overdone. Besides, if a film clip can nowadays be made available to the audience online before (or after) a session, why waste lecture time showing it?

3.5 Some lecturers reinforce learning by sending emails and texts to students after the event to remind them of key points and tips or to give them access to readings and texts. Today's students are comfortable with new technologies such as mobile phones and PDAs, and therefore it is worth exploring whether you can make use of the opportunities these offer to help them learn.

4. Notes and handouts

4.1 Handouts do not have to be a dull reiteration of the lecture. Try including activities such as diagrams, quizzes and sections for the students to complete. Try including sections for students to review what they have learned after the lecture.

4.2 Record the lecture and make it available afterwards. And if possible, make available other audio-visual material that supports your lecture.

4.3 Consider advising students on note taking during the lecture. For example, why not tell the students when you want them to make a particular note of something important? Or ask them to stop writing to ensure that they are paying full attention to an important explanation, then, having checked that they have understood it, give them time to write it up afterwards in their own words?

4.4 Seek student feedback so you can monitor and improve your own performance next time.

So how can a student get the most out of a lecture?

As we hope we have shown, it is much easier to learn in a lecture where the lecturer has tried to engage the audience's attention by providing a variety of activities, experience and teaching methods to encourage students to get actively involved in their own learning. But even in the most passive and dry environments, students can improve what they learn and retain by careful planning.

Here are some tips on how to make the most of a lecture:

1. *Prepare in advance.* If you know where the lecture fits into the course structure, you will find it easier to see why it is relevant to the overall course. Try to plan your reading so that you are not coming to a lecture completely cold.

If you have read the course guide and know something about the subject in advance, it will be easier to spot when the lecturer is saying something that isn't covered elsewhere. If the lecture is part of a series, review your notes from previous lectures to refresh your memory.

2. *Organize yourself.* It may sound obvious, but it is important to turn up on time – especially to large lectures – so that you have a comfortable seat where you can see and hear what is going on, and where potential distractions (e.g. late arrivals who disturb the class) are kept to a minimum. Come equipped with the things you may need during the lecture – especially paper, pens and notebooks. Develop a system for filing and storing notes, and if you can make backups of your notes in case you lose them, do so. Record the date of the lecture, the name of the lecturer, and number each page.

3. *Making notes: listen more, write less.* Some students try frantically to write down everything they hear. This is not only hard work, but it is ineffective if, at the end, all you have achieved is a great mass of scribbled longhand without shape or structure. Try using key words, lists and bullet points as much as possible so that the emphasis is on listening and understanding. There are several techniques that will help you make your notes clear and concise:

   - *Pay attention to the structure of the lecture.* Some lecturers provide you with a summary of the lecture before they start. But even where they do not do this, lecturers will almost certainly give you information about where the key points are. Listen out for phrases such as: "There are three main things I want to discuss . . .", "My next point concerns . . .", "On the other hand, it has been argued . . .", "Finally, . . .", "So, to sum up what has been said so far . . .". These structural pointers will help you maintain a sense of where you are going as the lecture progresses and find your bearings again if you lose the thread.

   - *Make note taking an active process.* To repeat, do not try to write a transcript of what the lecturer has said: your goal is to try to understand what the lecturer is saying, not to record every word. Summarize the lecture in your own words where possible. Use abbreviations – but be careful not to overdo this in case you have trouble reading them later. Have fun with space, color, symbols and images. You might like to try using mind maps rather than linear notes.[21] Consider technology such as using a digital note pad. You could also try recording the lecture. If you want to do this, ask the lecturer beforehand.

   - *Leave gaps.* If you miss a point or lose the thread, do not panic about it in case you get further behind. Just leave a gap and ask another student later.

   - *Pay particular attention to references.* If the lecturer refers to a book or paper, make careful note of the title. You may want to check it out, especially where you subsequently find you need more detail than the lecture was able to provide.

After the lecture

- *The question and answer session is important.* If other people ask questions, be polite and listen carefully. There may be vital information provided within the answers. If you need to ask a question yourself, keep it short, simple and clear, and pay attention to the response. The question and answer session is not the place for you to demand a private tutorial. If you need more than a short answer to your question, then speak to the lecturer separately.
- *Do not be too quick to leave.* Lecturers often leave important information and announcements to the very end of the class. If you are busy picking up your belongings and standing up, you may miss something important such as a date or an assignment, or the reply to another student's question.
- *Actively review your notes after the lecture.* Make additions and corrections as you read. It is most effective if you do this within 24 hours of the lecture, while it is fresh in your memory. Some people retype or rewrite their notes, which helps with review and also with organization, storage and recall.
- *Follow up.* If any questions arise during the review process, follow them up and look for the answers. Go and get that recommended text from the library. If directed to a website, go and look at it. Discuss issues – especially those on which you were unclear – with fellow students. Check whether you will be able to revisit the material in a seminar or tutorial.

In summary, lectures are a traditional feature of the medical school, and all medical students will attend, and possibly deliver, large group teaching sessions during their medical training and later career as a doctor. Lectures are not the most effective way of developing deep learning approaches in medical students and are frequently disliked. Nowadays, in response to the changing needs of modern students and the opportunities offered by modern technology, many lecturers are adopting more interactive approaches to lectures, and there are a variety of techniques that can be used to enliven and stimulate a large audience. Whatever the level of interactivity, however, students can enhance their learning experience and make the most of the available learning opportunities by adopting a more active and strategic approach before, during and after the lecture.

References

1. Sander P, Stevenson K, King M, Coates D. University students' expectations of teaching. *Studies in Higher Education* 2000; 25(3): 309–323.
2. Finucane P, Johnson SM, Prideaux DJ. Problem based learning: its rationale and efficiency. *Med J Aust* 1998; 168: 550–563.
3. Belfield C, Thomas H, Bullock A, Eynon R, Wall D. Measuring effectiveness for best evidence medical education: a discussion. *Medical Teacher* 2001; 23(2): 164–170.
4. Bligh DA. *What's the Use of Lectures?* 2000. New York: Jossey Bass.
5. Stuart J, Rutherford RJD. Medical student concentration during lectures. *The Lancet* 1978; 312: 514–516.
6. Bligh J. Problem based, small group learning. *BMJ* 1995; 311: 342–343.

7. Willcoxson L. The impact of academics' learning and teaching preferences on their teaching practices: a pilot study. *Studies in Higher Education* 23; 1: 59–70.
8. Burkill S, Dyer SR, Stone M. Lecturing in higher education in further education settings. *Journal of Further and Higher Education* 2008; 32: 321–331.
9. Mattick K, Crocker G, Bligh J. Medical Student Attendance at Non-compulsory Lectures. *Advances in Health Sciences Education.* 2007;12(2):201–210.
10. Morrision J. Where now for problem based learning? *The Lancet* 2004; 363: 174.
11. Spencer J, Jordan R. Learner centred approaches in medical education. *BMJ* 1999; 318: 1280–1283.
12. Dacre J, Fox RA. How should we be teaching our undergraduates? *Ann Rheum Dis* 2000; 59: 662–667.
13. McManus IC, Richards P, Winder BC, Sproston KA. Clinical experience, performance in final examinations and learning style in medical students: prospective study. *BMJ* 1998; 316: 345–349.
14. Prince M. Does active learning work? A review of the research. *J Eng Ed* 2004; 93(3): 223–231.
15. Norman G, Schmidt H. Effectiveness of problem-based learning curricula: theory, practice and paper darts. *Medical Education* 2000; 34: 721–728.
16. Vernon D, Blake R. Does problem-based learning work? A meta-analysis of evaluative research. *Academic Medicine* l993; 68(7).
17. Twenge JM. Generational changes and their impact in the classroom: teaching Generation Me. *Medical Education* 2009; 43(5): 398–405.
18. GMC. *Tomorrow's Doctors.* 2009. London: General Medical Council.
19. Hudson JN. A further example of paired-teacher lecturing to link theory to practice. *Medical Education* 2005; 39: 1254.
20. Ruhl KL, Hughes CA, Schloss PJ. Using the pause procedure to enhance lecture recall. *Teacher Education and Special Education* 1987; 10: 14–18.
21. Buzan T. *The Buzan Study Skills Handbook.*2006. London: BBC Active.

Further reading

1. Brown G, Edmunds S. Chapter 10: Lectures. In: Dent J, Harden R. *A Practical Guide for Medical Teachers.* 2009. London: Churchill Livingstone.
2. Gibbs G, Habeshaw S, Habeshaw T. *Fifty-three Interesting Things to Do in Your Lectures.* 1988. Trowbridge: The Cromwell Press.
3. Long A, Lock B. *Understanding Medical Education: Lectures and Large Groups.* 2008. Edinburgh: Association for the Study of Medical Education.
4. Newble D, Cannon R. *A Handbook for Teachers in Universities and Colleges: A guide to improving teaching methods* (3rd edn). 1995. London: Kogan Page.

Chapter 15

Learning in Teams;
Working in Teams

Emily Hall, Melinda Perlo, and Boyd Richards

Objectives

After reading this chapter, you will be able to:
- Understand why team training is important in medical education and clinical practice.
- Know why team-based learning is an effective method of learning.
- Learn what is the team-based learning method and its difference from problem-based learning.
- Know the educational theory behind the team-based learning method and identify potential challenges in the use of the technique.
- Learn how to make team-based learning an effective learning experience.

Introduction: Why do teams matter?

As a medical student new to the hospital wards, Jamal was still unsure of his clinical skills. But when his resident demanded that Jamal take a blood pressure on their patient – a middle-aged man complaining of severe chest pain – he jumped to the task. The blood pressure in the left arm was normal: 123/85, which Jamal reported to his resident. The resident nodded. Then the nurse in the room spoke up: "When I took his blood pressure five minutes ago, it was 170 over 100."

The resident asked Jamal to take the blood pressure again. After a few moments, Jamal nervously reported that the pressures were the same as before: 125/85. But the nurse firmly and politely voiced her concern and requested that she take the blood pressure again. She reached across the bed and took the sphigmanometer from Jamal and took the patient's blood pressure in his other arm. "It is still very high," she stated firmly as she released the cuff, "170/105."

The resident realized that both Jamal and the nurse were right – the patient had different blood pressures in different arms for a reason – and their willingness to speak up in turn helped save the patient's life. After an emergency CT scan demonstrated an aortic dissection, the patient was rushed to surgery.

The hospital ward is an intense and often hierarchical environment where people with diverse levels of skill and knowledge are asked to work together. The above clinical scenario demonstrates how a clinical group can work well together for the benefit of the patient. Learning to work in teams is a critical skill in the education of healthcare professionals. Therefore, many medical educators are recognizing that "the required educational programs for all physicians, including medical students as future physicians, will need to incorporate the theory and practice of teams and teamwork."[1]

But what is a team and how is it different from other groups? Fundamentally, a group retains individual accountability for each member and evaluates work completed by individuals – work that is delegated to members. But a team works together to produce a collective product – an outcome that holds both individual and mutual accountability. This effort to transform groups of students into functioning teams is the bedrock of the team-based learning technique, which we introduce in this chapter.

Team-based learning is a teaching technique developed in the 1980s and 1990s by Larry Michaelsen, PhD, while teaching large classes of business students. Since the late 1990s it has been adapted and applied in health sciences education, and has gained popularity with faculties that want to use active teaching methods in large classes.

This chapter will describe the basic elements of team-based learning, explain the theoretical rationale for its use, highlight potential challenges you may experience, and provide tips to facilitate your learning using the method. Finally, there will be a brief examination of ways you can benefit from team-based learning strategies and principles outside of a team-based learning course.

Just what is team-based learning?

By the time you finished your post-secondary education, you had probably experienced some form of group learning. But you, like many students, may have found this experience lacking, since "group work" can often devolve into individuals dividing up tasks and then working alone. Or, even worse, "team assignments" can sometimes result in one or two people shouldering the burden for the whole group. Neither of these experiences does much (if anything) to foster team skills, and both can leave students with a deeply negative impression about group work.

Team-based learning, by contrast, is designed to take student groups and transform them into "high-performance teams."[2] The technique helps students actively learn and apply material and, in the process, teaches them that they can accomplish more as a team than as individuals.

Team-based learning may seem complex at first but becomes increasingly understandable once you become comfortable with the strategy. It involves a series of three repeating steps.

Before beginning the first step, you and your classmates will be divided into teams of 5–7 students. You will stay in these teams for the entire course. Staying in the same group for the entire course is important because it helps you learn how to get along with your peers and to resolve, when needed, challenging interpersonal problems – one of the major skills gained from working in a team.

Step 1: Out-of-class preparation. Before each class, you will be expected to complete a series of learning tasks in the form of readings and/or video lectures. The completion of these tasks will help you master the specified material and prepare you to help your team during in-class activities. It will also render the learning within your team much more valuable.

Step 2: Readiness assurance. You will start class with a short readiness assurance test (RAT) that is designed to assess your out-of-class efforts and hold you accountable for learning the material. In most cases, you will first take the RAT as an individual (IRAT). Then you will retake the same RAT as a group (GRAT). Typically, both your IRAT and GRAT scores will count toward your final grade in the course.

Step 3: Application activities. Once the RATs are complete, you will move on to team problem-solving assignments. These tasks are done in class with all teams working in the same room on the same assignments. The assignments often take the form of clinical cases where your team will be asked to make diagnostic and treatment decisions. Solving these problems provide you with the opportunity to consolidate your learning as you discuss, deliberate, teach each other and decide on issues as teams.

You will be given time to discuss a problem in class. Then, your team must come to a single, collective answer, which you will share with the whole class. When teams disagree, each group is asked to defend its answer. (The instructors purposely write questions that generate diverse answers and stimulate class discussion.) In the process of preparing, comparing and defending team answers, you get immediate feedback about your own knowledge as well as the knowledge of your team members. You can use this feedback to continually enhance and enrich your understanding of the material and improve your ability to use this knowledge in a team setting.

Team-based learning versus problem-based learning: What is the difference?

Both team-based learning and problem-based learning involve groups of students trying to learn and apply clinical knowledge together. A critical difference between the two approaches is reflected in the difference between their names. In problem-based learning, the *problem* is the focus. The problem is designed to trigger learning issues for out-of-class study and to promote in-class discussions using this new knowledge. In team-based learning, the *team* is the focus. Students come prepared to class so they can support their team's efforts to agree on defensible answers during in-class discussions. In the process, the students not only learn how to apply material; they also learn how to work together toward a mutual goal. Other important differences between team-based learning and problem-based learning are summarized in Table 15.1.

TABLE 15.1 Differences between team-based learning and problem-based learning.

	Team-based learning	Problem-based learning
Number of faculty	Teams meet at the same time in the same room with a single instructor who walks between groups to listen in on discussions or answer questions.	Groups each have a faculty facilitator and meet in their own room.
Type of feedback	Teams receive frequent and very specific feedback about their content knowledge while completing GRAT questions in Step 2 and when comparing and defending their group answers in Step 3.	The facilitator and students verbally give each other feedback at the end of case discussions, usually focused on the group process.
Determining final course grade	IRAT, GRAT, peer assessment and individual performance on course exam.	Facilitator ratings and individual performance on course exams.

(For a more complete discussion of the problem-based learning technique, please see Chapter 13 of this handbook.)

Why is team-based learning an effective method of learning?

The development of team-based learning was informed by cognitive, motivational and social development theories. The practice of team-based learning is designed to enhance students' cognition (learning), motivation and social development.

Many of you have experienced courses where you were asked to read large amounts of information in preparation for lectures. You were then tested on the material, typically with a midterm and final exam. Unless you took the initiative to discuss what you read with others in your class, you probably had minimal opportunity to actively engage with the material. The chances are, even if you studied in groups, you were still focused on memorizing the material in order to pass the exam, not for the purpose of working with others to apply your knowledge to cases and clinical scenarios that represent the real world. This type of educational environment creates minimal opportunity to develop critical-reasoning and problem-solving skills that are essential when you enter the professional realm.

From a cognitive standpoint, team-based learning promotes active learning by engaging students to learn by "talking, listening, writing, reading, and reflecting" on the material.[3] Team-based learning creates an opportunity for you to apply your knowledge to real cases and, in this process, develop critical reasoning skills. Not only does this process help you to retain the information long term, but it provides a contextual framework that will increase comprehension of the information. You will foster the problem-solving skills that are essential in clinical professional work.

Team-based learning has also been shown to have several motivational factors that benefit learning. Team-based learning holds you accountable for out-of-class preparation so that you can serve as an effective team member. Also, the IRATs and the GRATs help you stay on track with your reading and studying so that you do not fall behind and wait until the end of the course to learn all of the material. Finally, the team-based learning focus on cases asks you to think like a real clinician, helping to remind you that the material you are learning is meaningful and serves a purpose in your preparation for your career.

Third, team-based learning has social benefits by promoting the development of teamwork skills that are essential to the professional realm. By working in teams, you will inevitably be asked to use and foster your communication and collaboration skills. In addition, you will also learn how to work effectively with your classmates, who have varying personalities, backgrounds and learning styles.

What are the potential challenges with using team-based learning in the classroom?

While there are many benefits to learning in a team environment, there are also several challenges.

A significant roadblock to the formation of a cohesive team can be conflicts in learning style. For example, how would you handle a lazy team member who never prepares for class? Or a team member that always dominates the conversation and does not allow others to talk or give input? Or how will you deal with a member who remains quiet the entire session? You should not expect that your team will work perfectly from the start. In fact, the formation of your team will go through a developmental process. Psychologist Bruce Tuckman proposed that there are four stages of team formation: forming, storming, norming, and performing.[4] Once you and your classmates are placed together in a team (forming), you will be forced to encounter everyone's unique learning styles, so conflicts may arise in the first few sessions (storming). Your team may experience a lack of balance (e.g. dominating student, quiet student) among team members that can cause you great frustration and discouragement. It often takes several sessions for these imbalances to be worked out so that all members of your team are contributing equally (norming). Once your team reaches this state, you will begin to work efficiently and effectively (performing). It is very normal for teams to evolve through these four stages; therefore, it is important that you remain aware and stay patient during this natural progression of team development.

Additionally, you may be asked to provide peer feedback. While peer feedback has been shown to be effective, students often express discomfort with the method.

You may feel you are being "judged" by your classmates and you may feel this judgment could have negative repercussions for future working relationships. However, peer feedback has many positive effects. It can improve your team's ability to work effectively by offering constructive criticism to your teammates. Any behavior issues or imbalances in the team (e.g. dominant student, lazy student) will ideally be exposed in a constructive manner, so that your team works well together.

Making team-based learning an effective learning experience: Tips for students

If you are new to team-based learning, you may feel some trepidation about how the experience will go – especially if you have had negative group learning experiences in the past. Keep the following tips in mind as you begin working in the team-based learning format:

Come prepared. Completing the out-of-class assignments in team-based learning is important for multiple reasons. First, it is necessary to perform well on the IRAT. Second – and more importantly – you want to be prepared to help your team maximize its score on the GRAT and participate fully in the in-class assignments. This does not mean that you have to understand every point: If there is a difficult concept that you are struggling with, you will be able to turn to your team for help. But you will be better prepared to ask questions of your team and your instructor if you do the preparation in advance.

Learn to challenge each other – with respect: When conflicting opinions arise, team members may err on the side of being polite. But avoiding conflict can be detrimental to team growth. When conflicts arise, consider them an opportunity to deepen the team's knowledge base. Listen actively to your teammates and state your opinions openly and clearly. As your team's cohesion strengthens, you will feel increasingly comfortable challenging each other in constructive ways.

Be patient with your team: Teams take time to evolve and grow. It is normal to feel awkward or even frustrated with your team in the early stages of formation. Remember that team-based learning is designed to teach you medical material *and* the process of team building. Just as you would not know all the material on the first day of class, you would not know how to work well together as a team on the first day either. If you are patient and open with your team, you will likely be happy with the progress you make together over time.

Beyond team-based learning: Team training for all healthcare professionals

Some medical schools have adopted team-based learning into their curriculum, while others only use a curriculum that is focused either on problem-based learning or on lectures. Medical students who do not experience courses using team-based learning should consider other ways to develop their team skills. Some examples are listed below:

- Simulation training – especially training that involves multiple disciplines (e.g. medicine, nursing, respiratory therapy, etc.) – can be a great opportunity to learn team skills. Look for opportunities to participate in mock codes or other crisis-management scenarios. Such simulations are especially valuable when they are videotaped with a review-and-feedback session. Use such sessions to observe how you work as a team member to identify your strengths and weaknesses. If your school does not typically videotape sessions, ask if they can be recorded in the future for improved feedback.
- Medical schools also sometimes offer team skills workshops without simulation. Such workshops can introduce you to teamwork concepts that are critical for a high-functioning team. Such skills can then be carried to the wards and clinics.
- Lastly, if not explicitly offered, you should solicit feedback from preceptors, faculty and peers about your teamwork skills in the classroom and on the wards. It is not always easy to ask for or receive feedback, but these are critical skills for building your teamwork skills. The earlier you start asking for feedback, the more time you will have to grow and adapt during medical school and residency.

Looking back: Key points about team skills and team-based learning

- Clinical care is moving away from an individualistic, physician-centric model and toward a team-oriented model.
- There are critical differences between a group (individuals working alongside each other with individual accountability for their work) and a team (individuals working together for a common goal with accountability as a team).
- Transforming your group into a team is a process that takes time and skill.
- Team-based learning is one way that students can learn how to work together in teams.
- Team-based learning promotes active learning, resulting in increased comprehension and problem-solving skills.
- Team-based learning involves individual advanced preparation, readiness assessment and group-assignments with frequent and specific feedback.
- Even if you do not have the opportunity to try team-based learning at your school, you can seek out other opportunities to learn inter-professional team skills through simulations, workshops, and by soliciting explicit feedback about your teamwork abilities.

References

1. Morrison G., Goldfarb S., Lanken P.N. Team training of medical students in the 21st century: Would Flexner approve? *Academic Medicine,* 1985; (2): 254.
2. Michaelsen, L.K., Knight, A.B. and Fink, L.D. *Team-Based Learning: A Transformative Use of Small Groups.* Westport, CT: Praeger, 9; 2002.
3. http://www.cat.ilstu.edu/additional/tips/newActive.php
4. Tuckman, B. Developmental sequence in small groups. *Psychology Bulletin*, 1965; 63: 384–399.

Chapter 16

Communication Skills

Geke A. Blok

Objectives

- Understand the importance of communication skills.
- Understand what effective communication is.
- Understand the importance of learning communication skills.
- Appreciate how best to learn communication skills.
- Understand how communication skills are assessed and how you can prepare.

The importance of effective communication

Communication is the basis for all human interaction and therefore is the core of medicine.

It is thus important to know what communication is, which communication skills there are, how to use them, and how these skills are assessed during medical training and in professional practice and which lifelong learning activities are needed to keep your competence at an adequate level. During medical training and in actual medical practice, it is important to be able to communicate with a wide range of people, both formally and informally, to form and maintain adequate interpersonal relationships, and to work effectively in teams.

Communication skills are also core skills for learning and employment. Other skills that are viewed as key skills are cognitive skills, problem-solving skills, interpersonal skills, teamwork skills, personal management skills, learning skills, and self-awareness. Although communication skills are listed as a separate skill, it is easy to see that you will need these for almost all of the other skills. These are all relevant, transferable skills that future employers (or colleagues) want. It makes sense to think about the type of setting where you want to be employed, to identify the relevant skills and competencies and make sure that you develop them. Organizations – healthcare organizations as well – nowadays seek graduates who are 'enthusiastic', 'self-motivated', 'have excellent communication skills', are 'self-starters with the ability to communicate', 'have excellent communication and interpersonal skills' and 'are able to get on harmoniously and productively with colleagues'.[1] (p. 209)

The above key skills are general. Why they are essential for medicine becomes clear from the fact that the many studies that are published in the international journals over the last 40 or so years show that adequate communication can significantly improve health outcomes for patients, and also for doctors (for an overview see [2]). The use of appropriate communication skills increases patient satisfaction and compliance, and helps doctors feel less frustrated and more satisfied with their work. In essence, in medical practice your success as a doctor is dependent on how well you are able to build trust; the only way through which you can earn this is through quality communication.

In medical school, and during your career as a doctor, the way you communicate and how you use communication skills will be evaluated in informal and formal ways. Informal evaluation is an ongoing process and involves peers, supervisors, patients, and colleagues. Their verbal or nonverbal feedback will give information about how effective you are. Formal evaluation (assessment) is a standard part of the curriculum in medical school, but also during residency and as part of continuous medical education.

Communication skills for study and medical practice are the same

The communication skills needed for medical training are the same skills to be used in tutorials, work groups, teamwork assignments, feedback sessions, reflecting, keeping a portfolio, and in your clerkships in order to have effective consultations with patients and satisfying collaborations in healthcare teams.

There are ample opportunities to learn and practice communication skills in working with peers, both in collaborating on a daily basis and in structured educational activities such as tutorial groups and team assignments. Also, as most medical schools have opportunities for students to practice communication skills in structured training programs, you can practice the skills in simulated or real patient contacts and by using web-based applications. After graduation there are several educational programs for residents providing opportunities to improve communication skills. Usually this is tied to specific issues, e.g. palliative care, breaking bad news, negotiations, giving and receiving feedback.

How to communicate effectively has to be addressed early in education

Recent studies have shown that if professional behavior is not sufficiently addressed in students' and residents' medical education and training, problems with professional behavior can continue to exist in their professional career. Doctors who were confronted with disciplinary measures had a higher incidence of unprofessional behavior during their medical studies.[3] The necessity for medical students to become effective communicators is evident when one considers that it is estimated that doctors perform over 200,000 consultations during their career, have ongoing collaborations with colleagues, and that the majority of (official) complaints by patients and colleagues are related to inadequate communication on the part of the doctor.[2]

The role of communicator as a professional competency

In the CanMeds framework – a framework that describes professional behavior – the competencies that belong to the role of the physician as a communicator are described as follows: Physicians enable patient-centered therapeutic communication through shared decision making and effective dynamic interactions with patients, families, caregivers, other professionals, and other important individuals. The competencies of this role are essential for establishing rapport and trust, formulating a diagnosis, delivering information, striving for mutual understanding, and facilitating a shared plan of care. Poor communication can lead to undesired outcomes, and effective communication is critical for optimal patient outcomes. The application of these communication competencies and the nature of the doctor–patient relationship vary for different specialties and forms of medical practice.[4]

In order to fulfill the role as a communicator, Frank et al.[4] identify a number of key competencies. Physicians should be able to:

- develop rapport, trust and ethical therapeutic relationships with patients and families;
- accurately elicit and synthesize relevant information and perspectives of patients and families, colleagues and other professionals;
- accurately convey relevant information and explanations to patients and families, colleagues and other professionals;
- develop a common understanding on issues, problems and plans with patients and families, colleagues and other professionals to develop a shared plan of care; and
- convey effective oral and written information about a medical encounter.

How you can develop the competencies described above is described throughout the remainder of this chapter.

Literary discussions, hard case discussions, writing about important incidents, discussion of legal issues, leadership/management skills, feedback skills, communication skills, reflection skills, development of a reflection portfolio, are all part of professionalism and should be part of the training to become a doctor.

To become a good communicator, you will need time to reflect and a safe, open atmosphere, two things that may be missing in a busy clinical workplace. Self-assessments in order to identify learning needs is not enough; you will need your peers, a mentor and a portfolio to help you to critically reflect on your performance, identify your strengths and weaknesses and develop a strategy for improvement.[5]

Effective communication and critical reflection are related

Communication and communication skills make up a significant part of the dimensions of professional behavior, either directly or indirectly. Acquisition of effective, goal-oriented communication skills requires both practicing skills and reflective thinking. Reflection is a cyclic process of perceiving and analyzing communication behavior in terms of goals and effects and designing improved actions. Early introduction of critical self-reflection facilitates the acquisition of abilities for continued lifelong learning in order to become a mindful practitioner.[6] The ability to reflect consciously upon one's professional practice is generally considered important for the development of professional expertise. However, critically reflecting on one's own behavior presumably is not a natural habit; it is a skill that has to be learned as people tend to be selective in what they consciously process.[7]

How to learn to reflect is not the topic of this chapter; some remarks, however, will be made. In order to become a reflective practitioner, it is helpful early on during your studies to develop a curiosity for feedback by other people on your communicative behavior. Very few people are natural talents in communication; the majority have to learn. Learning is easier if you actively ask people for their feedback and are also attentive to the verbal and nonverbal reactions of those you interact with. Additionally, it helps to observe others, pick your role models, evaluate what makes them effective and decide which behaviors you want to add to your own repertoire. It requires a lot of self-discipline to sit and think about how you communicate with other students, with supervisors or with patients during the day. Summarize in writing what you have done, whether you have accomplished your goals and what your strengths and weaknesses are. Constructing a personal development plan can help you to systematically learn to be an effective communicator.

Summary

- Communication is the basis for all human interaction.
- Communication is a core competence of the medical professional.
- Trustworthiness of the medical professional is dependent on the quality of communication.
- Adequate communication increases compliance and satisfaction of patients.
- Adequate communication increases satisfaction in doctors.
- Acquisition of effective, goal-oriented communication skills requires active practice and reflection.

What is communication?

Communication is a core clinical skill and an essential component of clinical competence. All your knowledge and intellectual efforts are of no use without appropriate communication skills. Being a good communicator is essential as about 70% of our professional work is communication. Moreover, sensitivity to your own nonverbal behavior and that of those you communicate with is essential, as 80% of communication is non-verbal. Communication turns theory into practice; how we communicate is just as important as what we say. It is impossible to describe what communication is in detail, many good books are available. The outline here just sums up the basics:

- **The essence of medical communication is about building trust**
  In order to be effective as a doctor you must earn the trust of the patient. Your trustworthiness solely depends on the quality of how you communicate. It is essential that you keep in mind that there is an information asymmetry between you and the patient. The patient only has a subjective idea about his or her physical condition and is depending on you for professional explanations and care. You have expert knowledge on diagnosis, treatment and prognosis. It is unreasonable to assume that the patient will reach the same understanding as you have. Therefore, cooperation between you and the patient is built on trust. It is your responsibility to manage the trust relationship: this is the very essence of medical practice. It requires continuous reflection on your professional performance; lifelong learning and practicing is just as important for you as for the concert pianist.

  Effective communication is tailor made and requires not only mastery of communication skills but also the ability to assess a situation and recognize which skills will be effective with a particular person or group at a particular time. Each person/group and situation requires a tailor-made approach, especially when you bear in mind that, for a patient, meeting with you may be a one-time event. For you this patient is one of the many. The uniqueness of the occasion dictates careful consideration: announcing the death of a patient to relatives or explaining to a patient that he is going to die or will suffer from a serious disease has to be done right the first time.

- **Empathy**
  It is through appropriate communication that you can show understanding and empathy for other people. In order to have a real relationship with patients, families and colleagues you need to understand their perspectives, take an active interest in their concerns and be able to sense their feelings. The ability to empathize with others is strongly related to our self-concept, our self-esteem, our self-awareness, and our self-control; hence the necessity for critical self-reflection. Besides learning distinctive communication skills, it is important to master a certain degree of emotional intelligence. This involves the perception, processing, regulation and management of emotions. Higher levels of emotional intelligence contribute to better doctor–patient relationships and increased empathy.[8]

- **Two levels**

  Communication involves both sending and receiving information. Every message has two levels of information: the content level and the context level. The content level refers to the verbal contents of the message. The context level guides us in interpreting the information we receive; it is the information that helps us read between the lines. Intonation, volume, choice of words (paralinguistic aspects), facial expression and body posture are the channels through which we can read the information on this second level. If both levels are in accordance, behavior is congruent. Lack of congruence erodes trustworthiness.

- **Two styles**

  There are two distinct styles of communicating with patients or families: *the doctor-centred approach* and the *patient-centred approach*. These are also respectively known as the 'directive' style and the 'explorative' style. Both styles are necessary for interaction with patients and their families, and the order in which they are used can be quite crucial.

  The main difference between the two styles is whose frame of reference is guiding the interaction. In the patient-centred or explorative style, the patient's perspective – his thoughts, emotions, attitudes and behavior – is the focus of attention. In the doctor-centred approach, the doctor gathers information to test his hypotheses, gives explanations, or provides information he thinks is important for the patient. In order to find out about the preferences, values, thoughts and feelings of patients or family members, the explorative style is more appropriate. Usually physicians find the explorative style more complicated to apply.

- **Communication skills**

  The harmonious use of all communication skills is needed to establish rapport, build trust and form effective therapeutic relationships with patients and families. However, it is not only the adequate use of distinct skills that will enable you to reach these goals. It is of crucial importance that the truth is what you convey, that you are honest, show respect and – most of all – that you yourself are authentic.

  Specific skills are needed to accurately elicit and synthesize relevant information and take into account the perspectives of all relevant stakeholders, as well as to accurately convey relevant information and explanations to them. All skills are needed to develop a common understanding on issues, problems and plans in order to develop a shared plan of care. It is important to convey effective oral and written information about a medical encounter; this is essential and often forgotten. For your own safety, and for patients and their families, your colleagues and other (health) professionals, it is important that your (electronic) notes and letters are clearly written, that you use understandable and unambiguous language, and that they are written in such a way as to reflect what has been exchanged in the encounter.

  The skills that are outlined below are attentive listening, asking questions, paraphrasing, reflecting, explaining, checking understanding, summarizing, concretizing, and structuring. Most of these skills are basic to every interaction; some are needed in specific situations to ensure that communication is effective. Many may already be familiar to you, and you may even be an expert user of them. It is of practical importance to be fully aware of what they are and how you can use them.

- *Attentive listening* is a non-selective listening skill, which means it needs to be used throughout the encounter. Attentive listening consists of verbal and nonverbal behaviors such as facial expressions, eye contact, head movements, supporting gestures, 'ahums', short attentive silences, and so-called minimal verbal encouragers (Yes...? So...? And...?). The purpose of attentive listening is to create an atmosphere in which the other person is encouraged to speak freely. The verbal and non-verbal encouragers should not be used too often or suggest restlessness, as they may distract the speaker from his/her story.
- *Eliciting information – Asking questions* is used if information gathering is the purpose. There are two kinds of questions: *open-ended* and *closed* questions. Both types of questions are necessary in communication. Open-ended questions are best used when you want to explore; closed questions can be used to acquire specific information.

    Open-ended questions can be used at various points in an interaction. At the start of an interaction they invite the other person to talk, and thus they show that you are interested in his or her point of view. Used during the conversation, they are helpful if you want to know more about a certain topic, if you do not understand what the other person just said, or if you want to introduce a new topic. Closed questions restrict the possible answers, and usually start with a verb: 'Can I', 'Will you', 'Is it', 'Do you'. They originate from the frame of reference of the person who is asking the questions. This poses the risk that they may be suggestive, and also that the person asking the questions will pay less attention to the answers because the questioner is busy thinking of follow-up questions. In order to avoid sounding like a cross-examiner, use closed questions sparingly.
- *Paraphrasing* is restating, in your own words, the most important issues in the verbal message the other person has given you. Paraphrasing has several goals: to show understanding, to check if you have correctly understood what you have been told, and to present the other person's information in a more concise manner. It is used to stimulate others to elaborate on content.
- *Concreteness* is a skill in which listening, encouraging, asking questions, reflecting feelings, and summarizing are combined. It is used to ensure that you have the personal, concrete and specific information you need for a full understanding of a situation the other person has described. The aims of concreteness are to help the other person move from global statements to specific ones, from implicit statements to explicit ones, and from general statements to statements that are personal. Possible ways to stimulate the other person to be more concrete include: asking direct questions;

being specific in your reactions; splitting up complex problems into smaller units and exploring each unit separately; and paying special attention to vague and ambiguous words. Concreteness can be used with an explorative as well as a directive style.

- *Providing information* is a skill applicable to almost every interaction. Good explanations are essential for successful communication, especially with patients and families. It is therefore helpful if you separate the topics, give information in small chunks, and clarify details. Use language that is comprehensible, avoiding medical jargon. Several techniques can be used for explaining. Signposting – announcing the next message – is often useful. Another technique is to start with the most important information, as people remember best what they are told first. You can also use visual aids, such as pictures, drawings, leaflets, and videos.

- *Dealing with emotions* – reflecting feelings is used to draw out the unspoken feelings underlying the words or behavior of another person. It is important to use your own words when reflecting feelings, and to express them in a tentative way. The intensity of your reflection should mirror the intensity of the other person's feelings. Reflections of feelings are most powerful when they relate directly to what the other person has just expressed. The aims of reflecting feelings are to communicate understanding, to invite the other person to elaborate on his/her feelings, and to show the other person that you are listening. If used too often, reflection may either be threatening or give the impression that you are employing a technique.

- *Summarizing* is used when you want to order different subjects in a logical way; essentials are separated from side issues. The purpose of summarizing is to structure what the other person has said. Summaries are characterizations of the other person's story, giving an overview of both cognitive and emotional aspects; they are to the point, formulated in your own words, and ideally communicated in a tentative mode. Summaries are indicated after you have received a bulk of (confusing) information from the other person, or when sufficient information has been gathered about a certain subject. They often mark the transition from one stage of the interview to another, or to a new subject. They can be used to list items that have been agreed upon, or at the beginning of a follow-up interview.

- *Structuring* is helpful to make interactions more productive, keep the participants focused, and guarantee that important issues are addressed. Many techniques can be used to structure interactions, such as opening and closing a meeting, providing an agenda and a timeframe, and making sure that all subjects are discussed. Most professionals know these techniques, but it is essential to apply them in a disciplined way. For example, when you ask participants to approve the agenda at the beginning of a meeting, it is easier to control deterioration by referring to this agreement. An effective way to start an interaction with patients and relatives is to summarize what has been discussed so far. An effective way to end an interaction is to summarize the plan of action or the agreements made.

Knowing 'what' to say or do is not enough, 'how' you communicate is equally important. Communication is effective when there is an interaction instead of just transmission of messages, when all parties involved understand each other and are aware of what should be the outcome. This requires planning and thinking in terms of outcome.[2]

- **Providing and receiving feedback is also communication**
  Feedback is structured information about the impact or effect of behavior. It is necessary for building relationships with other people in social life and work and it differs from criticism, which is often unprepared and hurtful. Providing quality feedback is a key factor in learning new skills, so it is important that the above-mentioned skills are also used in providing and receiving feedback. Feedback is only effective when it is given and received with respect for the other person. Feedback helps you to be aware of your strengths and weaknesses as a communicator, and you can help others by providing them with information about their performance.

Summary

- An effective doctor manages the trust relationship with patients.
- Effective medical communication is tailored to the uniqueness of the patient.
- Communication is a two-way process and involves both sending and receiving information.
- There are two distinct styles of communicating with patients or families: the *doctor-centered* approach and the *patient-centered* approach.
- Every interaction requires prudent use of communication skills.
- Providing and receiving feedback requires adequate use of communication skills.

How to improve communication

Only few people are naturally talented in communication; the majority have to learn and practice. Learning occurs not through sheer experience, or by just being told what to do, but through extensive training. Additionally, as the degree of critical self-reflection and self-awareness and emotional intelligence increases, communication improves. The combination of communication skills training with professional development training, including reflection, seems to yield the best results, as all skills that you will need as a medical student and as a medical professional are addressed. These are not only the communication skills you need for patient contacts, but also the skills that are helpful in teamwork with peers or in healthcare teams.

Formal and informal (vicarious) learning

Formal learning occurs in specified courses and training programs. In formal learning, goals and objectives are outlined, programs run along (varying degrees of) structured formats, specific educational materials are used (often developed for the educational activity at hand), and teachers generally are trained to provide this type of education, e.g. the communication skills training that you will attend. These training programs are usually assessed by formal examinations, such as a communication skills test and review of your portfolio, or a formative assessment to help you improve your skills. In the preclinical years, this formal learning primarily takes place in the medical school. In the clinical years formal learning in the teaching hospitals is tied to the particular clerkship you are doing (e.g. observed consultations with real patients, case-based presentations) and nowadays as well at the medical school where, usually, disciplines transcending educational activities are offered.

Informal or vicarious learning can occur anywhere. Vicarious (observational learning or social learning) refers to learning that occurs as a function of observing, retaining and replicating behavior observed in others.[9] People learn by copying or modelling the behavior of another person. In the medical school this is part of what is called the 'hidden curriculum'. All staff in the learning environment should preferably model the professional and communication behavior they want you to learn, although they are not always fully aware of this. This is also applicable in the teaching hospital. All facilitators, supervisors and practicing doctors observed by learners are modeling skills, behaviors and attitudes. It is a well-known fact that students also learn ineffective, unnecessary and unhelpful communication behavior from the professionals they have observed in teaching hospitals. Beware of developing the wrong habits, and try to be a critical observer.

Supportive learning climate

Students' learning is strongly influenced by the climate of their workplace. You will value a workplace for the opportunities it provides to learn skills and knowledge that are directly relevant to your daily work. You will find that if you feel safe, if you are taught by trainers with expertise in communication and if you are given positive comments and constructive feedback about how you perform as a communicator,[10] learning the 'tips and tricks' in this area is much easier and gives a lot of fun. It also enables you to show your vulnerabilities and be open about your strengths and weaknesses.

In teaching hospitals it is important that you have periods of time for practicing skills, to experience more difficult and complex work, learning 'why' as well as 'how,' and to have mistakes corrected in a constructive way by those who took it upon themselves to guide you to becoming a doctor.

Structured training programs – interactive, experiential, practice based, and authentic programs that incorporate interactive methods of teaching – are often more successful in helping individuals to acquire communication skills than more didactic methods of teaching (lectures, presentations, teacher-centred). The most effective way to acquire communication skills is in small groups, with structured feedback behavior being exercised by such means as student–(simulated) patient contacts or working as a team. This requires a systematic approach on behalf of the medical school, where attention has to be paid to knowledge (what), competence (can), performance (how) and results. Most medical schools now have communication skills training as part of their curriculum. Training of these skills should be an ongoing process during medical education, and this training should be longitudinally integrated in the curriculum and be followed up after graduation.

Essential ingredients of an experiential educational approach are:

- Systematic delineation and definition of essential skills (in writing or by video modeling).
- Formal instruction that is intentional, systematic, specific and experiential.
- Division of complex skills into smaller units.
- Observation (by peers, patients and trained facilitators).
- Well-intentioned, detailed and descriptive feedback.
- Video or audio recording and review (with peers and trained facilitators).
- Practice and rehearsal of skills.
- Active small group or one-to-one learning.

The above approach is based on the micro-training model, developed by Ivey[11] and copied by many others. In this approach, complex tasks are divided into discrete, behavioral units, based on the precise analysis of the complex task. The learning principles used stem from the behavioral theories (step-by step learning, precise didactic instruction (including modeling), behavioral practice, self-observation, immediate feedback, reinforcement).

The combination of micro-training (or its derivatives) with a cognitive approach to communication skills training has led to training programs that also pay attention to understanding the relevant and correct conceptual models that underlie the actions to be undertaken. In exercises, the real world is portrayed as much as possible – hence the term authentic – to optimize transfer to the workplace. Through observation, feedback, and rehearsal, fluency in skills can be acquired.

Educational aids that may be used in these programs are used to provide you with the necessary background information, practicalities and written instructions for role-plays with peers, written scenarios for (simulated) patient contacts, information on how to give constructive feedback, and information about how you will be assessed. So the whole package consists of a training guide, instructional videos, role-play scenarios/cases, simulated or real patients, feedback forms, and rating scales (preferably the ones that are used for assessments).

Simulated patients, real patients, virtual patients and written or video-vignettes

Simulated patients, real patients, peers, virtual patients, written or video-vignettes may help you acquire the necessary communication skills you need for your contacts with patients.

- A *simulated patient* is a person who has been trained to simulate a patient or any aspect of a patient's illness plus the psychological, emotional, historical, and physical aspects. There are a number of advantages in working with simulated patients: they are always available; they can be programmed to the specific skills that you have to practice (as simple or complicated as needed); as they are not real patients, trial and error is accepted and rehearsal is possible as often as needed. Simulated patients are trained to give feedback, so you will get direct feedback immediately after an encounter.[12] You will like working with simulated patients because you can practice in a safe situation, you do not have to worry about hurting 'the patient' and they prepare you for authentic, real working life situations.

  It is instructive, when simulated patient contacts are recorded on video, to watch them with one of your peers, with your teacher or with the whole training group. This is more helpful than watching the tape on your own, as others may observe behavior for which you have a blind spot. The advantage of this is that you may receive richer feedback, and that other students can also learn from your example. This is also the case when a simulated patient is interviewed in front of a small group and a supervisor/ trainer, where immediately afterwards feedback from the peer and supervisor is given.

- *Real patients* offer you a real-life situation. You can link the theory with a practical experience, you can learn about the perspective of real patients, you will get experience with realistic time-management (you cannot talk too long with a real patient just for the sake of exercise) and you will get an appreciation of the complexity of a real patient case. The advantage of real patients is the very fact that they are real and that you are confronted with a real-life experience. The most important thing to realize, however, is that you may hurt or exhaust the patient. It is essential for all parties that an expert facilitator is present to guide the process and make sure that feedback is adequate, not too overwhelming and does not affect the patient.

- *Peers* are perfect to practice on. You interact with each other during the day, meet each other in tutorial sessions and work groups and maybe carry out team assignments. Many medical schools now have training programs for interactive study skills (teamwork, leadership, negotiation, and presentation skills) that help students to maximize study effects. In training programs with a focus on one-to-one interactions, peers are very helpful in playing roles that are relevant for the skills to practice, for example, certain patient roles. The advantages are that peers are always available and, because they attend the same training, they know exactly what you have to practice, so they can give you focused feedback. Knowing what the training is about is also the drawback of peers. They may want to help you by making the exercise too easy, or too difficult.
- *Virtual patients* are patients that are portrayed by electronic means. The programs that use these patients offer the possibility to practice anywhere, anytime. The only prerequisite is a computer with (internet) access to the programs. In some programs different ready-made scenarios are available and what you have to do is choose the most adequate intervention by pushing a button or type the intervention of your choice. Basically, you get the opportunity to practice communication skills in these programs. The newer programs that are currently being developed are interactive and use voice recognition. With these programs you can have a real consultation with your virtual patient.[13]
- In *written or video vignettes* patient cases are portrayed. The challenges that are built into the description can be made as simple or complicated as needed. These educational aids can be used individually, where you will be asked to write down your interpretation of the case or your intervention. The result can be discussed later with peers and supervisor. It is also possible to use these aids in small groups where written and oral reactions of group members are discussed plenarily. Advantages of vignettes are that they can be used for any type of skill, on a level dependent on what you have to learn. Plenary discussion ensures that you will learn from each others' reactions.

Other ways to learn communication skills: learning in the workplace

Certain important clinical communication skills do not develop spontaneously with exposure to clinical environments, so it is important that learning these skills is facilitated. In the clinical environment there are many opportunities to learn and improve your communication skills. All day through you will have contacts with other people: patients, peers, supervisors and medical and nursing staff and other health professionals.

The types of activities you will come across in the workplace in which you will need and have opportunity to improve your patient communication skills are ward rounds, outpatient clinics and consultations with general practitioners. Other opportunities are clerking patients, formulating assessments, presenting on ward rounds, proposing management plans, writing progress notes, attending at the operating table, participating in delivery room activities or presenting in, for example, morning reports. You will learn most when you have a teacher who lets you take responsibility, introduces you to patients, gives guidance and constructive feedback and generally provides an emotionally safe learning environment. The best validated educational activity in the workplace is the 'one-minute-preceptor model', where a preceptor trained in this model uses five micro-skills to debrief a student on a clinical encounter: *get a commitment, probe for supporting evidence, teach general rules, reinforce what was done right, and correct mistakes.* Obviously, discussing the quality of communication (skills) will be part of this exercise (see [10] for an overview of workplace learning).

Reflection is a necessary condition for learning to communicate

In order to maximize your learning experiences in communication, develop insight into your strengths and weaknesses and decide for yourself what kind of doctor you want to be. It is absolutely essential to reflect on your experiences, formulate your personal goals and objectives with respect to communication, make a personal development plan and decide who and what you need to accomplish your plans. For this purpose, a reflective portfolio can be very helpful.[5]

To remain skilled is lifelong learning

Patient-centeredness, as well as the communication skills that are helpful for a patient-centred approach, has a tendency to decline during medical education. One of the explanations is that students find it difficult to keep focused on the patient while at the same time they have to deal with a growing amount of medical knowledge. In their clerkship, students may not show what they have learned once they are in the hospital environment. Possibly the role models they see may exhibit different behavior to what they have learned in order to become a member of the community they want to belong to. It is possible that, with little personal experience of working with patients, students find it difficult to integrate the abstract concept of 'patient-centeredness' with their own developing skills. Likewise, the loss of proficiency in actual performance of skills over time in medical practice is a well-recognized problem. An ongoing focus on communication skills training may help to maintain mastery of adequate patient-centred communication, and regular booster sessions during medical practice are necessary to remain skilled.

Summary

- Few people have natural talents in communication; the majority have to learn.
- Learning about communication occurs formally and informally.
- A supportive learning climate is important.
- Structured training programs that are interactive, experiential, practice-based and authentic are the best way to learn how to communicate.
- Simulated patients, real patients and virtual patients are instructive.
- Learning in the clinical setting offers many opportunities to learn and improve your communication skills.
- To remain a skilled communicator means lifelong learning.

Assessment of communication skills

Assessment means measuring performance so as to provide you with information about how well you perform against predetermined criteria. However, it is impossible to cover in assessments the wealth of occasions in which you communicate, because you can only be assessed on those aspects that can be measured and, by definition assessments are measurements at only specific moments in time and therefore cannot fully reflect day-to-day performances.

There are two types of assessment. *Formative* assessment is the identification of learning goals; this is part of ongoing teaching and learning. It has primarily a developmental goal. It gives learners insight into gaps in knowledge, skills and competencies and provides a direction for further development. An integral part of formative assessment is provision of feedback. In communication skills training formative assessment occurs all through the training process. It helps you to uncover your strengths and weaknesses. Evaluations of your portfolio may also be formative; you will get advice about the areas you have to cover in future training sessions and how to improve your reflective skills regarding communication.

Summative assessment refers to examinations (e.g. a performance test) in which you can pass or fail, or when certification or recertification is at stake. It is a way to gather information about your progress at the end of a learning process.

It is important that you know what is being assessed, how you will be assessed, which criteria are used and what the purpose of the assessment is. What will be assessed is whether you know what communication is, for what purposes different communication skills can be used and whether you are able to use the theory and the different skills in the appropriate way. Smart students, however, try to reach an understanding of what communication encompasses beyond the assessment methods and rules; merely preparing for assessments does not make you a good doctor.

Assessment methods

Methods can be either direct or indirect evaluations of performance. Direct methods concern observations of actual performance; indirect methods use other sources that retrospectively reflect the results of your performance. Assessment of written material (portfolio, patient files, progress notes) about communication provides insight into your deeper understanding of the quality of an interaction and the content matter, but also indicates whether you are able to adequately reflect on your performance.

Assessment methods are basically the same for formative and summative assessment. The main difference is that the requirements for validity and reliability for summative purposes are more stringent, they are standardized to enable fair comparisons with preset criteria and other students, and you can pass or fail with summative assessment. It is now widely accepted that a variety of methods in a wide range of situations, with many observers at many different points in time, is the best way to assess competence in communication.

For the assessment of communication skills the following methods are used:

- observed (or video- or audiotape) encounters with peers or simulated or real patients;
- written- or video vignettes;
- knowledge of skills tests (paper-and-pencil test);
- self- and peer assessments;
- appraisal of the review of the patient encounter or patient notes; and
- reflective portfolios.

Ideally, the feedback forms that are used in training situations for formative assessment are also used as checklists and rating scales for summative assessment. Obviously, the content of these structured standardized forms is dependent on the specifics that are assessed. If technical use of communication skills is the focus, you will only find the criteria for the specific skills to be assessed. If content and structure (phases in the process) of certain interactions are relevant, then criteria for these are part of the instrument, e.g. accuracy and completeness of the information and the phases in breaking bad news, respectively. Raters (you and your peers, facilitators, faculty or clinical teachers and simulated/standardized patients) are usually trained to use the forms in the appropriate way, especially because there are only 'soft gold standards'.

You will find that assessing the communication skills of peers is very difficult. Purely observing what you see without interpreting it is a hard task, as well as judging whether skills are used in the proper way. Your raters face the same difficulty. Detailed checklists do not cover all aspects of communication; if global ratings are used, certain crucial details are missed. It is inevitable that there will be a 'personal touch' to any interaction that you observe: for assessment purposes this is a complication; for real life it is a merit.

Assessment formats

- **Objective structured clinical examination: authentic performance assessments**
  The objective structured clinical examination (OSCE) is the best known summative assessment procedure in medical education. OSCEs are examples of authentic assessment in which the professional context is replicated as much as possible. An OSCE usually consists of 15–20 stations in which your competencies in different areas are assessed. Communication skills are needed in all stations, but usually they are formally assessed in only some of them; the examiners are specifically trained for proper use of rating scales and/or checklists that are used for assessment. After completion of all stations, your scores are totaled and this is your final score that indicates whether you have passed or failed the test. Sometimes you may get the scores of individual stations for meaningful feedback.
- **Written and video vignettes**
  The use of *vignettes testing formats* is a time-efficient way of testing large groups of learners. They have reasonable reliability, but only cover parts of communication processes. In video vignettes what is tested is knowledge about communication skills and about when to use which interventions. In written vignettes, additionally, cognitive use of skills can be assessed, in which you are asked to write down literally what you would say or do in the situation presented. Checklists and rating scales have been developed for this specific way of assessing communication skills. This type of assessment can be used for both formative and summative purposes.
- **Knowledge of skills test**
  Knowledge of skills tests are paper-and-pencil or electronically administered tests that assess your knowledge about communication processes, the separate communication skills and how to use them. In these tests, patient cases may be introduced in which you are asked to indicate the appropriate intervention. The association between these tests and performance is usually low or absent; presumably something else is measured. Usually these tests are used for summative purposes. Questions about communication may be part of a progress test.
- **Self- and peer assessment**
  Self- and peer assessment is generally used for formative assessment purposes. These assessments are used in communication skills training programs to evaluate ongoing progress. The reliability of self-assessment is low: people are poor self-assessors of performance, and medical students and residents are no exception. Peer assessment has a better record, presumably because it is easier to assess other people than oneself (peers and teachers often agree). A specific example of peer assessment is multi-source feedback (360 degree feedback).

  How you communicate as a team member is assessed with multi-source feedback or 360 degree feedback, which is rapidly gaining attention in medical practice. Peer teams, or members of healthcare teams in which you participate, are asked to rate your behavior on a set of competencies, including your communicative and collaborative behavior.

* **Review of the patient encounter/patient note exercise**

  Assessment of the reviews of patient encounters may take three different forms. In one option standard questions are asked about medical content, diagnosis and management plan (patient notes); in another option you may ask to review the process and the effects of your interventions combined with your appraisal of the feedback provided by peers, facilitator, and simulated patient. The third option combines the first two. In medical practice the assessment of patient notes and, for example, letters to other health professionals is part of the formative assessment of your competence as a doctor. An example such an assessment is the patient note exercise, conducted after a 15-minute interview with a standardized patient who is specifically used to assess students' ability to summarize and synthesize the data collected.

* **Reflective portfolios**

  The purpose of the reflective portfolio was described earlier in this chapter. A reflective portfolio with regard to communication skills consists of reflective commentaries, a collection of evidence (e.g. audio and/or video recordings, observer feedback and rating forms, patient evaluations, peer evaluation forms) from training sessions, simulated patients' contacts, or other activities on which performance is evaluated. Portfolios are generally used for formative assessment. With clear assessment criteria and good rater training they can also be used for summative assessment.[14,15]

Personal development plan

Now that you have reached the end of this chapter, it will be clear that you should make a personal development plan. You have already had many years of experience with communication. Evaluate your history in communication and see if you can detect where your strengths and weaknesses are. Study the curriculum of your medical school and find the opportunities to work on your communication skills and develop thorough knowledge of the assessment procedures and criteria.

Evaluate your personal history and find out whether there are personal weaknesses or personal characteristics that you may want to compensate with extra attention for certain communication skills or certain training activities. Make sure that your personal communication goals are SMART (specific, measurable, attainable, realistic and timely). Specific goals – well defined – have a greater chance of being accomplished than general goals. You can make your goals measurable if you establish concrete criteria for measuring progress, so you will know when you have achieved them. Be realistic: make sure that you take goals you are willing and able to work with. Set yourself a timeframe that makes sense and is workable. Use all the resources that are available to improve your communication skills (do not forget friends and family).

Your future as a competent communicator, who is able to communicate with a wide range of people, both formally and informally, to form and maintain adequate interpersonal relationships and to work effectively in a team, is best served when you develop from a reflective student into a reflective practitioner.

Summary

- Assessment is systematic measurement of performance in order to determine abilities and achievements using predetermined criteria.
- Assessments may be formative or summative.
- There are several instruments with which communication skills can be assessed.
- A personal development plan maximizes your chances to become a competent communicator.

References

1. Cameron S. *The Business Student's Handbook. Learning skills for study and employment.* Fourth ed. Harlow: Prentice Hall and Financial Times; 2008.
2. Kurtz S, Silverman J, Draper J. *Teaching and Learning Communication Skills in Medicine.* Abington: Radcliffe Medical Press; 1998.
3. Papadakis MA, Theherani A, Beanch MA, Kenettler TR, Rattner SL, Stern Dt et al. Disciplinary action by medical boards and prior behaviour in medical school. *N Engl J Med.* 2005;353: 2673–2682.
4. Frank JR. *The CanMEDS 2005 physician competency framework. Better standards. Better physicians. Better care.* Ottawa: The Royal College of Physicians and Surgeons of Canada; 2005.
5. Mook WNKAv. *Teaching and assessment of professional behaviour. Rhetoric and reality.* Maastricht: University of Maastricht; 2011.
6. Hulsman RL, Harmsen AB, Fabriek M. Reflective teaching of medical communication skills with DiViDU: assessing the level of student reflection on recorded consultations with simulated patients. *Patient Educ Couns.* (2008 Dec 4):2009 Feb;74(2):142–149.
7. Mamede S, Schmidt HG. The structure of reflective practice in medicine. *Med Educ.* 2004;38:1302–1308.
8. Coleman D. *Working with emotional intelligence.* New York: Bantam Books; 1998.
9. Bandura A. Self-efficacy: Toward a unifying theory of behavioral change. *Psychol Rev.* 1977;84(2):191–215.
10. Dornan T. *Experience based learning. Learning clinical medicine in workplaces.* Maastricht: University of Maastricht; 2006.
11. Ivey A. *Microcounseling: Innovations in interviewing training.* Springfield, IL: Thomas; 1971.

12. Vleuten van der CPM, Swanson DB. Assessment of clinical skills with standardized patients: State of the art. *Teaching and Learning in Medicine.* 1990;2(2):58–76.

13. Stevens A, Hernandez J, Johnsen K, Dickerson R, Raij A et al. The use of virtual patients to teach medical students history taking and communication skills. *Am J Surg.* 2006;191: 806–811.

14. Driessen EW, Tartwijk Jv, Dornan T. The self-critical doctor: Helping students become more reflective. *BMJ.* 2008;336:827–830.

15. Rees CE, Sheard CE. The reliability of assessment criteria for undergraduate medical students' communication skills portfolios: the Nottingham experience. *Med Educ.* 2004;28: 138–144.

IV
LEARNING IN THE LABORATORY

Chapter 17

Learning in the Skillslab

Robert J. Duvivier and Jan van Dalen

Objectives

After reading this chapter, the student will be able to:

- Explain the background of skills training in a designated skills training center or Skillslab.
- Describe different formats of skills training and explain their specific characteristics, advantages, and disadvantages.
- Categorize study behavior that will allow him/her to benefit maximally from skills training in a Skillslab.

Introduction

Even in today's world of technologically advanced diagnostic tools, doctors still make use of clinical skills to determine a diagnosis. History taking, physical examination and clinical judgment remain invaluable for reaching correct conclusions. The Scottish Clinical Skills Network defines clinical skills as follows:

> ... any action performed by staff involved in direct patient care, which impacts on clinical outcome in a measurable way. These include cognitive or 'thinking' skills (such as reasoning and decision making); non-technical skills (such as teamworking and communication), and technical skills (such as clinical examination and invasive procedures).[14]

Box 1: Types of skills training in a Skillslab

Blood pressure measurement is a common clinical skill used in practice. Training in the Skillslab will focus on several aspects of these skills in consequent steps. First, students will learn how to use a stethoscope. Then they will be introduced to a sphygmomanometer (blood pressure meter) and use it to take another student's blood pressure. Now students will decide when blood pressure should be taken in a specific case presented by a simulated patient. The final step involves interpretation of the blood pressure of a patient with hypertension and a discussion on the implications for clinical management.

Historically, students acquired those skills during their time in hospital wards by observing and imitating experienced physicians. However, it was not always ethically appropriate to first practice a procedure such as venapuncture on a patient.

Moreover, the rapid turnover of patients in hospital made skills training in this way too dependent on the accidental population of patients in the ward.

Additionally, emerging insights in medical education showed that learning by role modeling was not the most efficient way to acquire new skills. Skills training would benefit from another, more gradual approach.

These insights led to the establishment of clinical skills training centers or Skillslabs. The aim of these educational facilities is to provide training in a systematic and safe environment where mistakes do not yet have grave consequences. Skillslabs use effective educational methods which can be tailored to the level of experience of the students.

In this chapter we address various aspects of student learning in the Skillslab, based on scientific literature and our personal experience as student, teacher, and educational researchers.

What is a Skillslab?

The best description of a Skillslab is: a teaching and learning facility for acquisition of clinical skills (physical examination, procedural, laboratory, and communication skills) for future doctors or other health professionals. Training in a Skillslab is not intended as a substitute for teaching with patients but rather as a *preparation* for teaching with patients, and is thus complementary.

Skillslabs are characterized by a 'safe' environment, where students have the opportunity to be observed and receive feedback while they learn to perform their skills. Depending on their individual level and progress, skills training in a Skillslab gradually increases in complexity and realism. (See Box 1, for an example.)

Skills' training is set up in such a way that the teacher plays an important and influential role in the beginning. By demonstrating skills, observing students' performances and providing constructive feedback, the teacher helps students to acquire appropriate skills performance. Additionally, the students become aware of their limitations and develop appropriate self-confidence. Consequently, the teacher becomes less important towards the end of the skills training program, giving way to maximum student responsibility and lifelong learning.

Scientific evidence shows that training students in clinical skills will help them to benefit from their clerkships.[2,13,11,16,15] Well structured training in a longitudinal format is especially helpful in preparing students for the hospital.[13,15]

Different methods of skills training can be found in health professionals' educational institutions around the world. Most of them have a few common characteristics, justified by evidence from studies in medical education:

- Training is better than no training.
- Longitudinal skills training is better remembered than concentrated training.

- Skills training should include practice, observation and feedback.
- Training should include the opportunity to practice again after feedback.

Are there different ways of training?

Four objectives can be distinguished in skills training:

- The technique of a skill should be performed correctly.
- The skill should be performed in interaction with a patient; communication is part of all procedures.
- Knowledge and skills are integrated.
- Findings have to be correctly interpreted.

Different ways of training are indicated for these different objectives. Most skills training require thorough *preparation* before actual practice. Using *models* and *manikins* can create a safe and standardized context, which is particularly useful when learning the technique of a skill. Subsequent steps of training can involve practicing on **fellow students** (under supervision) to allow feedback to be incorporated. Also, students become familiar with the broad spectrum of normal findings, including different characteristics, when practicing on real persons. Practicing with **simulated patients** has the additional benefit of integrating knowledge and skills in a realistic doctor–patient encounter. Using **real** *patients* will help students to understand the physical examination and interpret their findings.

Throughout these various stages students should have maximum opportunities to maintain their mastery of skills by training outside scheduled and programed training sessions in *teacher-independent training*.

Finally, most students train their skills outside the school with whomever they can find. As one student mentioned in our focus group study: *"I sometimes go to my grandmother. She is very old and that makes such a difference. She thinks it is great. She is 90 years old, so when you listen to her lungs you hear almost nothing because it is all much muted. Or my friend's grandmother. They all have lungs. Everybody has to know what I am studying."*[4]

How can one benefit most from training at the Skillslab?

Research has indicated some conditions that help Skillslab training to be most efficient. Usually training is better appreciated when teachers help students to *discover* the guidelines for a skill, rather than *model* it. Students need the opportunity to practice, be observed, and receive personal feedback in order to develop their skills. Moreover, in optimal training conditions students can freely ask questions and receive answers to these questions.

So, practice, observation and feedback are crucial components of clinical skills training. A constructive teaching and learning climate, including the opportunity to practice again after feedback, is also important.

Our studies have revealed specific guidelines for benefitting optimally from every phase of skills training:[7,3]

- *Preparation.* Students *may* benefit from skills training without having prepared. They can pick up much from the context to participate and focus on acquiring the 'tricks': *how* to perform. However, when compared to training with preparation they benefit much less. Thorough preparation can also help students to understand the principles of physical examination: the *why* of a skill. Through preparation, students may be able to begin to focus on possible pathology that they may detect in the examination. They may begin to generalize beyond this one occasion and discuss possible alternative findings, such as "what would you expect if this patient was a 70-year-old carpenter?"[1]
- *Training with manikins* has the drawback of limited realism. Advantages are the ample opportunity to focus on technique and systematics of examinations. Models are obviously very patient and they feel no pain. They provide the opportunity to practice the technique and systematics of a skill that cannot be simulated in another way, or which would provoke much anxiety (initial venapuncture, bladder catheterization, gynecological examination, resuscitation). Practicing with models requires students' willingness to overcome the unrealistic aspect of a rubber or leather model.
- *Training with each other (peer physical examination)* is somewhat more realistic than with models; at least the performance involves a 'live' counterpart. The focus in this practicing stage is obviously also on the correct procedure, but in this type of training students can pay attention to the emotional wellbeing of the other, including asking for (informed) consent and adequately addressing undressing. Here the training is most beneficial when students give each other honest and constructive feedback. Moreover, the teacher should be available for questions the students have while they attempt to perform the skill. If most students have a similar question the teacher should ask for attention and address this issue plenarily.
- *Training with simulated patients.* Simulated patients are healthy people who have been trained to portray an illness scenario and to give feedback

---

Box 2: Rules for giving feedback

- Describe behavior ("you did ..."); do not judge ("you are ...").
- Describe the effect the behavior had on you; speak on your behalf.
- Relate feedback to what the receiver asked.
- Give alternatives.
- Ask for a reaction.[10]

to students. Simulated patients preferably come from different age and social groups than students, in order to complement peer physical examination training. Moreover, students can practice whole consultations with simulated patients: from clarification of this patient's reason to visit the doctor, via history taking and physical examination, to discussing and agreeing on further management of the patient's problem. A hybrid use of simulated patients in combination with models has been described by Kneebone,[6] allowing students to integrate communication skills with procedural skills such as inserting an IV drip or performing minor surgery.

Training with simulated patients works best when the student acts as much as possible as a (future) doctor. Some schools have the opportunity to record simulated patient encounters. This is always embarrassing and confrontational, but at the same time very instructive. Students benefit most from simulated patient encounters when they can see their own performance and receive feedback about the effects of their behavior. The most challenging aspect of learning from simulated patient encounters is to see them as a practicing situation rather than an exam situation.

When asking for feedback, students must make sure of asking specific questions. When giving feedback, be sure to formulate comments according to specific feedback rules. See Box 2 for these rules.

- *Training with patients* is excellent when pathology is introduced. It can very well be organized in a Skillslab, involving patients with stable dysfunctions who have been properly introduced and have consented. At the end of a series of training with healthy counterparts, students can now search for and recognize pathology. Patients' involvement in training can help the transition from training of skills to training clinical reasoning.
- Practicing outside the Skillslab's scheduled sessions encompasses both theory and practice. Early in the course, students focus on precise guidelines for each skill, provided by the school where available, or on checklists of previous skills tests, as well as on notes taken during training. Later, students focus on *principles* of physical examination and find back-up for these principles in handbooks (of physiology or internal medicine, for example).

How to prepare for skills assessment: the OSCE?

Skills are most often assessed by means of a multiple station test, the Objective Structured Clinical Examination or OSCE.[5] Rudland et al.[12] identified practice behavior for medical students in preparation for the OSCE. Strategies used to identify topics for the OSCE included a list of examinable problems, past OSCE papers and talking to peers. Preparation undertaken for the OSCE included both theoretical and practical preparation, as indicated above. Theoretical preparation referred to consulting textbooks and reviewing the physical examination handbook.

Practical preparation consisted of practice with fellow students, either individually or in groups, (simulated) patient contacts or practice OSCE runs ('mock exams').

Strategies to avoid when studying for the OSCE include getting too detailed, and focusing on rare diseases. Also, students are not advised to leave practice to the last moment.

The most important guideline for preparing for the OSCE is: practice, practice and practice.[1] Students who volunteered as subjects to be examined in an OSCE reported this to be very helpful in preparation for their own, future OSCEs. Senior students are also consulted by those in doubt about what to expect in an OSCE. When studying, it is helpful to also focus on the theoretical background of skills (for example: anatomy and neurology when preparing for an exam on locomotor examination).

Epilogue

Skillslabs have seen increased recognition in medical education, and are now inherent aspects of medical training. Students can contribute to their clinical skill teaching by accepting their responsibility for their professional training.

References

1. Boshuizen HPA. Does practice make perfect? In: Boshuizen HPA, Bromme R, Gruber H (Eds): *Professional Learning: Gaps and transitions on the way from novice to expert* (pp. 73–95). Dordrecht: Kluwer, 2004.
2. Busari JO, Scherpbier AJJA, Boshuizen HPA. Comparative study of medical education as perceived by students at three Dutch Universities. *Advances in Health Sciences Education,* 1997;1:141–151.
3. Duvivier RJ, van Dalen J, van der Vleuten CPM, Scherpbier AJJA. Teacher perceptions of desired qualities, competencies and strategies for clinical skills teachers. *Medical Teacher,* 2009;31(7):634–641.
4. Duvivier RJ, van Geel K, van Dalen J, Scherpbier AJJA, van der Vleuten CPM. Learning physical examination skills outside timetabled training sessions: What happens and why? *Advances in Health Sciences Education, Theory Practice,* published 28 June 2011.
5. Harden RM, Gleeson F. Assessment of clinical competence using an objective structured clinical examination. *Medical Education,* 1979;13:41–54.
6. Kneebone R. Simulation in surgical training: Educational issues and practical implications. *Medical Education,* 2003;37:267–277.
7. Martens MJC, Duvivier RJ, van Dalen J, Verwijnen GM, Scherpbier AJJA, van der Vleuten CPM. Student views on the effective teaching of physical examination skills: a qualitative study. *Medical Education,* 2009;43(2):184–191.
8. Pendleton D, Schofield T, Tate P, Havelock R. *The consultation: an approach to learning and teaching.* Oxford: Oxford University Press, 1984.
9. Remmen R, Derese A, Scherpbier A, Denekens J, Hermann I, van der Vleuten C, van Royen P, Bossaert L. Can medical schools rely on clerkships to train students in basic clinical skills? *Medical Education* 1999;33:600–605.

10. Rudland J. Wilkinson T, Smith-Han K, Thompson-Fawcett M. "You can do it late at night or in the morning. You can do it at home, I did it with my flatmate." The educational impact of an OSCE. *Medical Teacher*, 2008;30(2):206–211.

11. Scherpbier AJJA. Kwaliteit van vaardigheidsonderwijs gemeten. [Measuring quality of skills training.] (Dissertation) Maastricht: University Press, 1997.

12. Scottish Clinical Skills Network. http://www.scsn.scot.nhs.uk/, accessed 28 November, 2010.

13. van Dalen J, Bartholomeus P, Kerkhofs E, Lulofs R, van Thiel J, Rethans J-J, Scherpbier AJJA, van der Vleuten CPM. Teaching and assessing communication skills in Maastricht: the first twenty years. *Medical Teacher,* 2001;23:245–251.

14. van Dalen J. Communication skills: teaching, testing and learning. (Dissertation) Maastricht: University Press, 2001.

V
LEARNING IN THE HOSPITAL

Chapter 18

Clinical Reasoning

Silvia Mamede

Objectives

- To provide a synthesis of research on clinical reasoning relevant to medical students.
- To understand clinical reasoning and its development throughout medical education and professional practice.
- To know how medical students become experts in the course of their education.
- To help medical students reflect on how to make use of their learning opportunities in the course of their undergraduate education.
- To know how to benefit from research on clinical reasoning.

A 23-year-old married woman presented with moderate intensity abdominal pain that had commenced 48 hours earlier. At first, the pain was in the upper abdomen, but later it became localized in the right lower quadrant. The pain started abruptly and was accompanied by anorexia and nausea. She had no important morbid antecedents. She reported amenorrhea for 2 months and irregular menstruation since menarche. Physical examination showed an oriented, moderately pale patient. Her pulse was 100/min, respiration 20/min and temperature 37.8°C. Examination of her heart and lungs was unremarkable. The abdomen was quite painful on palpation in the right hemiabdomen and especially in the right iliac fossa, with rebound tenderness. Peristaltic sounds were audible but normal.

What is the most likely diagnosis for this patient? Addressing this question is not a straightforward task. A physician would need to consider the findings obtained through history taking and a physical examination, as well as distinguishing between what is relevant and what is irrelevant to the current problem. He would need to evaluate the relationship of the several pieces of information – generating hypotheses, verifying how the findings relate to each hypothesis, exploring alternative plausible diagnoses and, finally, making decisions for instance on whether diagnostic tests should be ordered to confirm or refute his hypotheses. While thinking through the problem, the physician would be engaged in clinical reasoning: *the largely unseen set of mental processes through which physicians solve clinical problems.*

Clinical reasoning critically defines the performance of physicians in any clinical setting. Although several other aspects play a role in a good clinical performance, the accomplishments of most physicians have roots in appropriate clinical reasoning and decision making. Consider the breadth and complexity of medical knowledge, the myriad of known diseases and the almost endless ways in which they manifest themselves in real life. It is intriguing how physicians think through clinical problems and arrive at what in most cases is a successful diagnosis. How is it possible that a young student entering medical school develops, in the course of a few years, the ability to solve such complex problems?

Not surprisingly, researchers have been attracted by the challenge of understanding clinical reasoning and its development throughout medical education and professional practice. Over the last decades, a small but very productive group of researchers in several countries have directed their efforts into clarifying these issues. As a result, we now know more about the mental processes through which physicians make diagnosis, how a young student becomes an expert, and what can go wrong in clinical reasoning.

Throughout their years of undergraduate education, efforts are concentrated on providing the students with opportunities to acquire knowledge about normal and abnormal functioning of the body, the processes underlying diseases, the signs and symptoms that characterize disease, and diagnosis and treatment. It is assumed that by acquiring this large amount of complex knowledge, students will "naturally" be able to "apply" this knowledge to solving clinical problems when they start to encounter patients. Not so much attention is directed to making explicit what is usually an implicitly large unconscious process: how expert doctors reason while solving clinical problems. This chapter addresses this issue by providing a synthesis of research findings on clinical reasoning that are more relevant to medical students.

First, we summarize how medical students become experts in the course of their education. Subsequently, we present the different modes through which physicians think through problems and discuss how they affect clinical performance. Finally, some implications for medical students are drawn from this overview. Our intention is to help you to reflect on how you can make the best use of the learning opportunities you have in the course of your undergraduate education.

How students become experts: Transitory stages towards expertise

Early researchers on expertise development assumed it was largely a process of expansion of knowledge about a domain. Throughout their years of education, students would acquire more and more relevant concepts and construct meaningful relationships between them. By gradually extending their knowledge base, beginners would become experts. Modern theories on medical expertise, however, advocate a different view: shifts in the way knowledge is organized in the memory and used occur throughout the years of medical education. Becoming an expert, therefore, involves not only acquiring more knowledge, but also progressing through different stages in a process of knowledge restructuring.[1,2] A detailed description of this process is beyond the scope of this book (if you are curious, the references cited in this section will provide you with further explanation), and these distinct stages or "phases" are only briefly outlined in the following:

- **Stage 1:** During the first years of their training, students rapidly develop rich, elaborate causal networks that explain the causes and consequences of diseases in terms of general, underlying biological or pathophysiological processes. At this stage, students do not yet recognize patterns of symptoms that fit together, and therefore they try to make sense of clinical cases presented to them by analyzing isolated signs and symptoms and relating them to the pathophysiological mechanisms they have learned.[1,2,3]
- **Stage 2:** As students extensively and repeatedly apply the knowledge that they have acquired and are exposed to patients' problems, a first change in their knowledge structure takes place. The networks of detailed, causal and pathophysiological knowledge become encapsulated into diagnostic labels or high-level, simplified, causal models, explaining signs and symptoms.[3,4] The concept of encapsulation came about from studies in which students and experienced doctors were asked to explain patients' symptoms in clinical cases, such as the one we presented to you. An advanced medical student would probably say:

> *This patient probably has an obstruction of the appendix lumen by a fecalith or enlarged lymph nodes. This raises the intra-luminal pressure and leads to distension of the wall of the appendix and a reduction in blood supply. The appendix gets little or no nutrition or oxygen. The supply of white cells and other natural fighters of infection are also reduced. Bacteria normally found in the bowel overgrow and invade the appendiceal tissue. White blood cells are recruited to fight the bacterial invasion, releasing pus from dead white cells, bacteria, and dead tissue. Pain occurs due to the distension of the appendix wall and when the augmented, inflamed appendix rubs on the inner wall of the abdomen…*

An expert doctor, however, would explain the symptoms in a much more concise way by saying:

> *This patient has appendicitis, with pain that is caused primarily by distension of the appendix and later on by infection and inflammation…*

Concepts such as appendicitis and inflammation "encapsulate" the detailed student's explanation of pathophysiological processes. Experts have many of these encapsulated concepts available, describing simplified, causal mechanisms or syndromes, and they tend to use this so-called clinical knowledge while reasoning through cases.[5,6]

- **Stage 3:** When students enter the clinical years and start to practice extensively with patients, another transition occurs. The different ways in which diseases manifest with signs and symptoms merge with pathophysiological mechanisms, and students start to pay attention to the contextual conditions within which diseases emerge. Instead of causal mechanisms, the clinical manifestations of a disease become the anchor points of their thinking. Gradually, their encapsulated knowledge reorganizes into *illness scripts* for different diseases.[1,4] Illness scripts are mental structures, containing relatively little knowledge about pathophysiological mechanisms but a wealth of clinically relevant information about the disease.[7,8] An illness script of a disease

TABLE 18.1 Example of an illness script for appendicitis.

Enabling conditions	Fault	Consequences
Factors that generally make the occurrence of a certain disease or family of diseases more likely.	Malfunction that explains the consequences, which may consist of diagnostic labels or a simplified description of pathophysiological mechanisms.	Complaints, signs and symptoms that arise from the fault.
Boundary conditions: Age: more common in the teens and 20s; Gender: more common in males.	Obstruction of the appendiceal lumen, with bacterial overgrowth, ischemia and inflammation. If untreated, necrosis, gangrene and perforation occur.	Pain initially in the epigastrium or in the periumbilical region, shifting after a few hours to the right lower quadrant. Pain increases with cough and motion. Brief nausea, vomiting and anorexia. Diarrhea or constipation may be present. Low-grade fever. Classic signs in physical examination: Right lower quadrant – direct and rebound tenderness located at McBurney's point, Rovsing sign, psoas sign, and obturator sign. Classic findings appear in less than 50% of the patients. Many variations of signs and symptoms occur.

contains *enabling conditions, faults* and *consequences*. Table 18.1 defines these elements and presents an example of a possible illness script for appendicitis.

- **Stage 4:** When a physician encounters a patient like the one we have described, he would search for an appropriate illness script in memory, and after selecting one (or a few) would verify the script by matching its elements to the information provided by the patient. During this process of script verification, an interpretation of that instance of the script takes place; the script then becomes "exemplified" or *instantiated*.[1, 4] These "instantiated scripts" remain in memory as traces of previous patients and may be used in the diagnosis of similar, future problems. Storing these different representations constitutes another transition – a fourth stage in the course of expertise development. Illness scripts therefore exist in different forms, from representation of disease categories to representations of individual patients previously seen.[1,8] They play a crucial role in experienced doctors' reasoning, as we will see in the next section.

Summary

In the course of their education, medical students progress towards expertise in transitory stages, characterized by different ways in which knowledge is organized in their memory and utilized:

- development of *elaborate networks of knowledge,* explaining the causes and consequences of diseases in general terms underlying pathophysiological processes;
- gradual *encapsulation* of these networks of knowledge into smaller numbers of diagnostic labels, syndromes, or high-level simplified causal models, explaining signs and symptoms;
- reorganization of encapsulated knowledge into *illness scripts,* structures that contain mostly clinical, relevant information – signs and symptoms and contextual factors about a disease; and
- storage of *examples of patients* actually seen, as instances of illness scripts of particular diseases.

How experienced doctors reason while solving clinical cases

Suppose that an experienced physician sees the patient whose description opened our chapter. In the first minutes of the clinical encounter, the hypotheses of appendicitis would probably come to mind. He would perhaps also consider the alternative possibility of a ruptured, ectopic pregnancy. The physician would not have arrived at the plausible diagnosis by analyzing, one-by-one, the patient's symptoms and trying to figure out the pathophysiological mechanisms that could explain them. You can imagine that such reasoning processes would take much more time than the very few minutes an expert doctor would need before the hypothesis of appendicitis suddenly "appears" in his thoughts. In fact, this is a better description of what most frequently occurs: the diagnosis just pops into the physician's mind. How would this happen?

The key to answering this question is "pattern recognition." The physician quickly recognizes similarities between the patient at hand and illness scripts, such as in Table 18.1, or examples of patients with appendicitis previously seen, which are stored in his memory throughout the years of clinical practice. Such scripts, or examples, are activated and retrieved from the physician's memory very early in a clinical encounter by cues in the patient's appearance or clinical findings. This allows experienced physicians to quickly generate diagnostic hypotheses.[1,9] In fact, illness scripts and instances of patients already seen have a crucial role, not only in generating hypotheses but also in that they guide physicians while they search for additional data through history taking, or physical examination and interpretation of findings, thereby refining their hypotheses and verifying their diagnosis.[10]

This mode of reasoning based on pattern recognition is fast, largely beyond conscious control[5,6] and explains how hypotheses seem just to rapidly and effortlessly appear in physicians' minds without requiring them to analyze individual signs and symptoms or explain their causal mechanisms. Research has shown that this so-called "non-analytical reasoning" develops with practice, and experienced physicians tend to rely mostly on this reasoning mode for making diagnosis in routine situations.[1,11] However, non-analytical reasoning is better conceived as one pole of the clinical reasoning spectrum. At the opposite pole of the spectrum, the so-called "analytical" or "reflective" reasoning involves an effort and conscious analysis of findings for a patient's problem before diagnostic decisions are made.[11,12] Physicians may adopt different reasoning strategies, depending on the situation. The non-analytical reasoning typically encountered in common problems may be replaced by reflective approaches when physicians are faced with complex, unfamiliar cases.[13,14] Clinical reasoning tends to be so flexible because the several knowledge structures – causal networks of pathophysiological mechanisms, encapsulated concepts, illness scripts and examples of patients – acquired throughout education and practice, apparently remain as layers in the memory. When matching the current case to illness scripts or the experience of previous patients is not possible (that means, pattern recognition fails), a physician may turn to his pathophysiological knowledge to try to make sense of a patient's clinical manifestations. This has been shown to happen,[1,14,15] but this shift between the different reasoning strategies is not straightforward, as we will see.

As you might have already noticed, expert physicians solve most of the problems encountered in their professional practice successfully (for the good of the patients!). This means that the non-analytical mode of reasoning works quite well in most situations. However, there is also another side to the coin. Relying excessively on non-analytical reasoning may introduce bias in diagnostic reasoning, thereby provoking errors.[16,17] Such errors have attracted public and professional attention in the last few years, especially after the Institute of Medicine's well known report *To Err is Human*,[18] which estimated that medical errors result in 44,000 to 98,000 unnecessary deaths and around one million injuries each year in the United States alone. Similar problems have been reported by studies in other countries and have nurtured the efforts to understand the origins of medical mistakes. Of course, not all medical errors can be attributed to failures in physicians' reasoning, but the reality is that faulty reasoning has been shown to play an important role, especially in diagnostic failures. What then can go wrong with physicians' reasoning?

We like to conceive medical decisions as the result of objective and rational applications of well-established knowledge to a patient problem. This, however, is not entirely true. Uncertainty is inherent in medical practice. The ways in which diseases present range from typical to very atypical manifestations which sometimes are hardly recognizable. Clinical judgment involves perception and interpretation of findings within the context of each particular patient and is subject to multiple, usually unperceived influences.[19,20,21] Research has shown that physicians' experience, beliefs and perspectives influence their perception and interpretation of features in a patient.[22,23] Findings that corroborate a certain perspective may be recognized and emphasized, whereas another line of reasoning may not receive appropriate attention. In our case, for instance, a physician who initially generated the hypothesis of a ruptured, ectopic pregnancy, triggered by the report of amenorrhea, may persist in this line of thought without appropriately considering the whole configuration of the clinical manifestations. Indeed, difficulties in restructuring the initial reasoning have been pointed to as an important cause of diagnostic failure among experienced physicians.[24] Studies have shown that a suggested diagnosis for a patient influences not only physicians' diagnostic decisions but also recognition and interpretation of clinical signs.[23] Physicians have been shown to change their reasoning mode, make better diagnoses and judge the same clinical cases differently, only because they were told that other doctors had incorrectly diagnosed the cases before.[25] Misperceptions and misinterpretation of evidence are therefore not unusual in clinical problem-solving. They may happen at any stage – hypothesis generation, hypothesis refinement and diagnosis verification – and may compel physicians toward incorrect judgments and decisions. More than 30 types of bias which potentially distort physicians' reasoning and lead to diagnostic errors have been identified.[16] The question of how such errors can be prevented is not easy to answer, but has raised the debate about reflection in medical practice.

Reflective practice has been conceptualized as to doctors' ability to critically reflect on their own reasoning and decisions.[27] A reflective physician tends to recognize difficulties in solving a problem and accepts uncertainty while further exploring the problem, instead of searching for a quick solution. This thoughtful approach is not expected in routine problems, but would be triggered by troublesome situations, when a reflective physician would switch from the usual non-analytical to a more reflective mode of reasoning.[27] When engaged in reflection, a physician would not only carefully consider the findings in a case but would also critically examine his own reasoning. Patients' problems would, therefore, be explored more thoroughly; alternative hypotheses would be more easily considered and extensively verified. Clinical judgments would improve and errors could be minimized.[27,28]

Although apparently reasonable, these statements have only recently been supported by empirical studies. Experimental studies with internal medicine residents have explored the effects of the two main modes of reasoning – non-analytical and reflective – on quality of diagnoses. Residents were asked to diagnose simple and complex cases by using either a non-analytical or a reflective approach. Reflective reasoning was shown to improve accuracy of diagnoses in complex clinical cases, whereas it made no difference in the diagnoses of simple, routine cases.[29] In a subsequent study with internal medical residents, the positive effect of reflective reasoning on the diagnosis of difficult, ambiguous clinical cases was reaffirmed.[25]

Should we advocate, then, that reflective reasoning is the best approach to diagnosing patients' problems? Unfortunately, things are not so simple. As we said, non-analytical reasoning allows a physician to make diagnoses timely and efficiently in most situations. What seems clear, is that minimization of avoidable diagnostic errors depends on the physician's ability to adjust reasoning strategies appropriately and with flexibility to the problem at hand, and to combine non-analytical and reflective reasoning.[11] While the usual pattern-recognition, non-analytical approach makes it possible for a physician to efficiently solve familiar problems, diagnoses of complex or unusual problems would benefit from reflection.

Summary

- Experienced physicians diagnose mostly routine, simple problems through non-analytical reasoning. This is based on fast, largely unconscious recognition of similarities between the problem at hand and illness scripts or examples of previously seen patients.
- Physicians may shift from the usual non-analytical to a more reflective reasoning when they encounter complex, unusual problems.
- When diagnosing a case through reflective reasoning, physicians tend to engage in conscious, elaborate consideration of case findings and scrutinize their own reasoning.
- Non-analytical reasoning allows physicians to solve most of the routine problems efficiently but may lead to distortion in clinical reasoning, thereby provoking diagnostic errors.
- Empirical studies have indicated that reflective reasoning leads to higher diagnostic accuracy for solving complex, unusual problems, whereas it makes no difference in the diagnoses of simple cases.

How can you benefit from research on clinical reasoning?

Many questions still require further exploration. Research over the last few decades has produced a substantial amount of evidence about how medical expertise develops and how doctors reason while solving clinical problems. Some implications may be drawn for medical education. As a conclusion to this chapter, we highlight a few key suggestions that may help you make the best use of your learning experiences:

- Keep in mind that an extensive, multi-dimensional knowledge base is the primary requisite for good clinical performance. You should not expect to acquire "reasoning skills" simply, because there is no such thing as general reasoning skills that can be developed and applied to solve any problem, independent of domain knowledge.[11] Knowledge of clinical reasoning, different reasoning modes and the potential sources of errors may help, but only if you have stored in your memory relevant knowledge of the basic biomedical sciences and a wealth of illness scripts and examples of patients.
- Learning from patients' problems has many advantages. The more patients you encounter, the more you will accumulate a larger mental set of examples upon which non-analytical reasoning processes can rely. These examples will represent a wide spectrum of diseases and the vast range of ways in which specific conditions present. You should see not only many patients with a diverse range of problems, but many examples of how the same disease may present itself. Learning around examples also makes it possible to integrate basic biomedical and clinical sciences and allows you to continuously restructure and enrich both your biomedical knowledge and your clinical knowledge throughout the years of undergraduate education.
- Use your experience with patients to expand and restructure your knowledge base. This requires you to take time to think about the patients you encounter with the purpose of recognizing contextual information, underlying mechanisms and clinical presentation of diseases. Try to make comparisons with the problems you see: identify the similarities and differences between new problems and those previously seen; differentiate between superficial characteristics that may make a problem seem different and structural, underlying concepts or principles, and relate such principles back to similar principles in past examples. Simply working with many patients, without consciously reflecting on the problems you are faced with, is not enough to develop a rich and multiple knowledge structure that will allow you the flexibility to solve patients' problems.
- Engage in reflection on your experience with patients; reflect not only on the patient's problem but also on yourself. Learn to critically question your own reasoning; check the grounds for your conclusions and verify whether alternative lines of reasoning exist, and whether other plausible hypotheses could

explain the patient's symptoms. Try to become aware of feelings, perspectives and concerns that influence your reasoning when you are dealing with clinical problems. Physicians' previous experience influences the way they interact with new problems, and self-awareness, therefore, has been considered a crucial attribute for a good clinical performance.

References

1. Schmidt HG, Boshuizen HPA. On acquiring expertise in medicine. *Educ Psychol Rev* 1993; 5: 1–17.
2. Schmidt HG, Norman GR, Boshuizen HPA. A cognitive perspective on medical expertise – Theory and implications. *Acad Med* 1990; 65(10): 611–21.
3. Rikers RMJP, Schmidt HG, Boshuizen HPA. Knowledge encapsulation and the intermediate effect. *Contemp Educ Psychol* 2000; 25(2): 150–66.
4. Schmidt HG, Rikers RMJP. How expertise develops in medicine: knowledge encapsulation and illness script formation. *Med Educ* 2007; 41: 1133–39.
5. Boshuizen HPA, Schmidt HG. On the role of biomedical knowledge in clinical reasoning by experts, intermediates and novices. *Cogn Sci* 1992; 16(2): 153–84.
6. McLaughlin KJ. The contribution of analytic information processing to diagnostic performance in medicine. Rotterdam: Erasmus University, 2007.
7. Feltovich PJ, Barrows HS. Issues of generality in medical problem solving. In: Schmidt HG, De Volder ML, editors. *Tutorials in problem-based learning*. Assen/Maastricht, the Netherlands: Van Gorcum, 1984.
8. Charlin B, Boshuizen HPA, Custers EJ, Feltovich PJ. Scripts and clinical reasoning. *Med Educ* 2007; 41: 1178–84.
9. Norman GR, Brooks LR. The non-analytical basis of clinical reasoning. *Adv Health Sci Educ Theory Pract* 1997; 2: 173–84.
10. Charlin B, Tardif J, Boshuizen HPA. Scripts and medical diagnostic knowledge: theory and applications for clinical reasoning instruction and research. *Acad Med* 2000; 75: 182–90.
11. Norman G. Research in clinical reasoning: past history and current trends. *Med Educ* 2005; 39: 418–27.
12. Croskerry P. The theory and practice of clinical decision-making. *Can J Anesth* 2005; 52(6): R1–R8.
13. Mamede S, Schmidt HG. The structure of reflective practice in medicine. *Med Educ* 2004; 38: 1302–08.
14. Elstein AS, Shulman LS, Sprafka SA. *Medical problem solving: an analysis of clinical reasoning*. Cambridge, MA: Harvard University Press, 1978.
15. Rikers RMJP, Schmidt HG, Boshuizen HPA. On the constraints of encapsulated knowledge: Clinical case representations by medical experts and subexperts. *Cogn Instruct* 2002; 20(1): 27–45.
16. Croskerry P. The importance of cognitive errors in diagnosis and strategies to minimize them. *Acad Med* 2003; 78: 775–80.
17. Bornstein BH, Emler CA. Rationality in medical decision making: a review of the literature on doctors' decision-making biases. *J Eval Clin Pract* 2001; 7(2): 97–107.
18. Institute of Medicine. *To Err is Human: Building a safer health system*. Washington, DC: National Academy Press, 1999.

19. Maudsley G, Strivens J. "Science", "critical thinking" and "competence" for tomorrow's doctors. A review of terms and concepts. *Med Educ* 2000; 34: 53–60.
20. Tonelli MR. The philosophical limits of evidence-based medicine. *Acad Med* 1998; 73: 1234–40.
21. Hall KH. Reviewing intuitive decision-making and uncertainty: the implications for medical education. *Med Educ* 2002; 36: 216–24.
22. Malterud K. Reflexivity and metapositions: strategies for appraisal of clinical evidence. *J Eval Clin Pract* 2002; 8(2): 121–26.
23. Leblanc VR, Brooks LR, Norman GR. Believing is seeing: The influence of a diagnostic hypothesis on the interpretation of clinical features. *Acad Med* 2002; 77 (10 Suppl October): S67–S69.
24. Eva KW. The aging physician: Changes in cognitive processing and their impact on medical practice. *Acad Med* 2002; 77 (10 Suppl), S1–S6.
25. Mamede S, Schmidt HG, Rikers RMJP, Penaforte JP, Coelho-Filho JM. Influence of perceived difficulty of cases on physicians' diagnostic reasoning. *Acad Med* 2008; 83: 000–000.
26. Graber M., Gordon R., Franklin N. Reducing diagnostic errors in medicine: What's the goal? *Acad Med* 2002; 77: 981–92.
27. Mamede S, Schmidt HG. The structure of reflective practice in medicine. *Med Educ* 2004; 38: 1302–08.
28. Epstein RM. Mindful practice. *JAMA* 1999; 282: 833–39.
29. Mamede S, Schmidt HG, Penaforte JC. Effects of reflective practice on the accuracy of medical diagnoses. *Med Educ* 2008; 42: 468–75.

Chapter 19

Learning and Teaching around the Bed

Hossam Hamdy

Objectives

After reading this chapter, you will be able to:
- Know the challenges of learning in a clinical environment.
- Learn the outcomes in clinical teaching.
- Learn the strategies for effective learning in a clinical context.
- Learn how to evaluate a clinical teaching and the behavior of an effective clinical teacher.
- Understand the theoretical perspective of learning in relation to clinical teaching.

While in a meeting with the Dean of the College of Dentistry I received a call from Prof Magzoub. He asked me if I could contribute to a book by writing a chapter entitled "Learning and teaching around the bed." I accepted this invitation. As I looked at my dental colleague, I thought perhaps the title should also include the "dental chair." A few hours later, I had a meeting with the clinical nutritionists who showed me their wonderful new lab. It had a beautiful kitchen; so I came up with an idea for the title – "Learning around the kitchen table." A few days later, I was dining with a well known French scientist and I mentioned the title of the chapter to him. He immediately reacted exclaiming, "this is very important – I always tell my daughter not to study in bed!!

Introduction

Learning around the bed, or "bedside teaching," describes a common learning and teaching practice applicable and entrenched in the culture of many health professionals' education. It describes a learning situation and an environment in which a triad of interaction takes place between the clinical teacher, the student and the patient. At the center of the interaction is the patient's problem; all this takes place in a healthcare environment where service to the patient and other patients is provided. This is what is commonly described as the "clinical learning environment."

It not only differs from a classroom or laboratory but it is influenced by many factors related to the context of the healthcare delivery system. It can be difficult to control and requires attention to detail.

The challenges of learning in a clinical environment

The clinical learning environment encompasses many settings, i.e. hospital inpatients, outpatient clinics, operating rooms, emergency departments, day care surgery, and primary healthcare centers. The modern practice of medicine has led to a change in the clinical context and a shift from teaching in the hospital to teaching in an ambulatory care setting. At present, hospitals are populated with critically ill patients, short-stay patients and newly diagnosed patients with little or no physical signs. Teaching and learning close to the patient bed continues to be an important medical education activity and, if properly conducted, is highly valued by students.

The quality of learning in the hospital environment, particularly in the wards, has been called into question.[1-7] Concerns have been raised in relation to inadequate supervision,[6-14] poor induction,[11] insufficient time available for the clinician to teach[9,10] and inadequate systems of structured educational appraisal[8]. Students need guidance, clear goals, and objectives. It is important to view students in the clerkship phase of the undergraduate medical curriculum as apprentices, shadowing the role of an intern or foundation doctor.

Learning outcomes in clinical teaching

Learning around the "bed" or on the "ward" is one of the strategies which should help the medical student to acquire competencies related to patient care and decision making, core of knowledge, evidence-based medicine, interpersonal and communication skills, ethics and professionalism, and cost-effective practice.

It is important that clinical teachers ensure that the students have acquired through bedside teaching the following competencies and skills:

- good communication and data gathering;
- history taking and physical examination;
- clinical reasoning;
- decision making – investigation and treatment;
- ethics and professionalism; and
- patient safety.

Theoretical perspective of learning in a clinical setting

It is not the purpose of this chapter to discuss in detail different learning theories. Several learning theories have influenced learning and teaching in a clinical setting.

It is important to highlight the main features of contemporary learning theories and how they translate into action in relation to clinical teaching.

1. **Behavioral theories**[15]
   These theories emphasize:
   1.1. learning by action;
   1.2. frequent practice in varied contexts;
   1.3. reinforcement as a prime motivator; and
   1.4. clear behavioral objectives that are communicated to the student.

2. **Cognitive theories**[16]
   "Learning through knowing" emphasizes what goes in the student's head. It emphasizes the reasoning process, whether analytical or pattern recognition, generating schemata and mental images. It makes the clinical teacher thinking, visible.[17]
   In the cognitive school, "focus is on the internal world of the student." Acquisition of knowledge and skills take place through a process of transmission from the teacher or through engagement with one's own experiences (Piaget constructivism). Related to the cognitive schools are concepts of andragogy or adult learning principles,[18] experimental learning,[19] and reflection.[20, 21]

3. **Social theories of learning (Bandura)**[22]
   Several theoretical and psychological stands have been proposed and have applications to the clinical environment. In health professional education, learning and practice take place within a context and in communities which have their specific social, cultural, and behavioral norms and practices, e.g. the "tribe" of surgeons.
   3.1. *Social cognitive theory* proposes a module of learning which captures the dynamic interplay between the student, doctors, nurses, patients etc. It also captures cognitive knowledge and skills, the environment, ward, clinic, operating rooms, etc., all of which combine and determine an individual's behavior. It is considered by many educators as a relevant model for work-based learning in medicine.[23–25]
   3.2. *Social constructivism theory* (Vygotsky)[26] – this theory emphasizes social engagement, and how students can make sense of new ideas and information by engaging with teachers, fellows, patients, and nurses so that learning is "with others" and "from others." It also entails identifying the students' needs, their prior knowledge and level of competency, and provides them with guided assistance as well as support and coaching, which will enable them to move forward successfully.
   3.3. *Socio-cultural learning theories*[27,28] – these theories show no distinction between learning and practice and are part and parcel of everyday experience and practice. They show, for example, clerkships or attachment to a department as "time spent in communities of practice."

Learning takes place by student engagement in real, work-based activities. Teachers and students should identify, and use, the learning resources embedded in this day-to-day activity.[29]

Strategies for effective learning in a clinical context

Learning theories and research on workplace learning have guided learning and teaching strategies, which may increase its effectiveness. A *set-dialogue* and *closure approach* can constitute an organizational framework for improving clinical teaching in general and bedside teaching in particular. This approach integrates and organizes many educational principles into three phases – the *planning phase, patient encounter phase, and closure phase*. The timeframe of the three phases can vary from a few minutes to hours, or even weeks, for a session or a whole clerkship rotation.

Set "Planning phase" – Pre-round

1. Workplace environment and culture. Ward routine practices should be explained to the students. They should be introduced to the nurses, and facilitate their integration into the Ward daily work. Students should be seen as a help and not a burden. The clinical environment should be considered as a "community of practice and learning." The clinical teacher needs to explain to the students the culture and expectations in terms of dress code, the way to address team members and patients, proposed ways of practice and participation and professional behavior.[30] All this should take place on the first day of joining the department.
2. Clinical teachers need to be familiar with the clinical curriculum and outcome competencies at the end of the training period. Realistic expectations need to be planned, taking into consideration the time allocated for training and availability of patients.
3. Students should be exposed to multiple learning experiences. A balance needs to develop between short periods of training in different subspecialties and longer periods of training in clinical departments. This ensures a deeper understanding of the workplace culture. A training period of less than two weeks is not effective. It is not recommended to rotate the students in too many silos, e.g. surgical subspecialities: colorectal, cardiac, pediatric, plastic, etc., There are so many sub-specializations that it is impossible to cover them all.
4. It is important to make a differentiation between a *service ward round* and an *educational ward round*. In a service ward round the students join the team and observe how senior clinicians and the service team make decisions and communicate with each other. The student's role on a service round is usually limited. On the other hand, an educational ward round or "bedside teaching session" is characterized by being a student's protected time, a two-hour session with interaction between the teacher, students, and patients.

5. Orientate the students on the objectives of each bedside teaching session and together negotiate their needs and expectations. Goals should be appropriate to the setting, i.e. patient problems, student level, and "prior knowledge and skills."

6. The clinical teacher should demonstrate professional behavior by introducing himself, being available on time, appropriately dressed, knowing the names of his students and asking permission from patients to ensure their comfort, respect, and dignity.

7. Select patients who would be appropriate for bedside teaching, and involve the students in this process. Communication skills, physical examination skills and professionalism are best taught around the bed.

8. Explain the main theme of the session, the timeframe and the roles of the student and teacher, i.e. history taking, examination of the abdomen, etc.

Dialogue: "The patient encounter"

1. The clinical teacher should be close to the patient and student; corridor teaching should be avoided.

2. Observe the student with the patient and avoid taking over the interaction.[31]

3. Train the students to take a detailed history and examination, i.e. hypothesis driven history and physical examination. Encourage early generation of probabilities and working diagnosis.

Clinical reasoning is key to the practice of medicine. For bedside teaching, it is essential in driving the process by taking a detailed history and examination, and for decision making.

A combination of non-analytical reasoning, "pattern recognition" and analytical reasoning are used for clinical diagnosis. Students should be trained on early generation of diagnostic hypothesis from the cues in the chief complaint and its duration. This guides the generation of relevant history questions. Each question should be considered as a diagnostic test with variable degrees of sensitivity and specificity. The answer, or result, will have an impact on supporting, modifying, or rejecting the early diagnostic hypothesis. The clinical teacher should guide the students in modeling professional thinking and decision making, so that "the implicit becomes explicit." The same applies to physical examination, which should be guided by a diagnostic hypothesis. It is important that the student should not ask questions or do physical examinations in a mechanical way.

The teacher should:

1. Review with the students the diagnostic probabilities and rationale for investigation and treatment decision.

2. Probe the student's clinical reasoning skills and use questioning techniques to challenge the student – this should be done without humiliating the student and by using gentle correction when needed.
3. Keep students engaged and avoid lecturing at the bedside.
4. Capture "unique" moments which may arise[32] during the patient encounter. These could be positive or negative incidents, e.g. superb humanistic skills by a trainee, or missed clues in the history or physical examination. Teachers should grab these moments, applaud good work and correct mistakes. There is no need to wait until the end of a session to give feedback. "Feedback is like fish – you need to eat it fresh!"

The *"one minute preceptorship"* model, described by Furney et al.,[33] is widely used for clinical faculty training in order to improve teaching with patients. It describes five micro-skills[34] which will help the teacher on how to guide the teaching interaction. The five micro-skills are:

1. *Commitment:* i.e. ask the student to articulate his/her own diagnosis or plan.
2. *Probe* for supporting evidence: evaluate the student's knowledge or reasoning.
3. *Teach general rules:* teach the student common "take home points" that can be used in future cases and are preferably aimed at the student's area of weakness.
4. *Reinforce* what was done well and offer feedback.
5. *Correct errors:* feedback with recommendations for improvement.

Closure

"Reinforce with the students what they have been taught." Prior to leaving the patient, the teacher needs to summarize what was taught and learnt during the encounter. It is important to explain to the patient what was discussed or found in relation to their illness and management.

Further discussion about the patient's problem and management needs to take place away from the patient. Students have the opportunity to ask more questions and clarify any confusion.

Feedback and reflection are interrelated, and need to take place at the end of the session. This should be short, focused, and constructive. Strengths and weaknesses "areas that need improvement" should be described: "What went well, and what needs improvement?" Students' and Teacher's reflection are important components of any clinical teaching episode. It should be kept in mind by the teacher during and after the teaching episode, and be evident in the teacher's "actions." A good practice for the teacher is to write down his/her own thoughts, including strengths, ideas for improvement and how things could be done differently the next time.

Students should also be encouraged to reflect on their experiences. It is advisable to ask them to write down their thoughts as part of a reflective portfolio. This can have a positive effect on learning.[35] Bedside Teaching provides opportunities to practice evidence based medicine. Being close to the patient allows the students to identify, describe and discuss ethical and professionalism incidents.

Evaluation of clinical teaching

Evaluation of the clerkship, the clinical learning environment and the effectiveness of the clinical teachers is essential. Several factors in the literature have been shown to influence the effectiveness of student learning in a clinical environment, e.g. the number and mix of patients encountered by students, the number of students, organizational quality of the training and the supervision they receive.[36]

Good supervision appears to be the key to clinical training success.[37] Checklists recording the clinical teacher's effective behavior have been described, including how to summarize the student's responses and how best to present them, using what has been described as "visual indicators of teaching and learning success" or "VITALS."[38]

Effective clinical teacher behavior

1. To be available as scheduled.
2. To give orientation and clarified clerkship objectives at the beginning of a rotation.
3. To arrange training opportunities that meet student learning needs.
4. To facilitate student access to patients and to integrate students with the team providing care.
5. To effectively communicate knowledge and train students to master new skills.
6. To encourage students to use clinical reasoning and critical appraisal in patient problem-solving.
7. To test student progress and to give continuous feedback.
8. To motivate student learning and stimulate self-directed learning.
9. To function as a good, professional role model in one's relationships with patients, team members and students.
10. To demonstrate respect and sensitivity to the needs of the students.
11. To demonstrate overall effectiveness as a clinical tutor.

Ward-based teaching and "teaching around the bed" offer a unique opportunity for student learning in the clerkship phase. It was found by students to be the most valuable method of clinical teaching. To attain maximum benefit, patients, students and tutors must each be prepared. Clinical faculty development and training are essential in order to ensure quality education in the clinical environment. Most importantly, to be an effective clinical teacher is to be willing to teach and be enthusiastic about it.

References

1. Bourne M and Paterson-Brown S (1999) Calman and the new deal – compromising doctor training and patient care. *Scottish Medical Journal.* 44:147–8.
2. Bruch G, Bahrami J and MacDonald R (1997) Training the SHO grade: how good is it? *British Journal of Hospital Medicine.* 57:565–8.
3. Cooke L and Hurlock S (1999) Education and training in the SHO grade: a cohort study. *Medical Education.* 33:418–23.
4. Davis J, Tan K and Jenkins H (2000) The current status of SHO postgraduate education in a single region. *Medical Education.* 34:367–70.
5. Field A, Baker M and Williams J (2001) Formal education programmes for SHOs: comparison of experience in three hospital specialties. *Postgraduate Medical Journal.* 77:650–3.
6. Paice E (1998) Is the new deal compatible with good training? A survey of SHOs. *Hospital Medicine.* 59:72–4.
7. Pease R, Mitra A and Heymann T (1999) What the SHO really does. *Journal of the Royal College of Physicians of London.* 33:553–6.
8. Murphy D and Kelly M (2003) SHO formative assessment: an observational study. *Education for Primary Care.* 14:158–65.
9. Leverton T (2000) A method of assessment of hospital posts accredited for GP training. *Education for General Practice.* 11:405–11.
10. Rickenback M, Dunleavy J, Little P and Mullee N (1997) Impact of existing peer review visits needs to be increased. *British Medical Journal.* 314: 1828–30.
11. Hand H (2000) Evaluation satisfaction with hospital training for general practice: a comparison of two surveys in East Anglia for the JCPTGP. *Education for General Practice.* 11: 385–90.
12. Hand H and Adams M (1998) The development and reliability of the RCGP questionnaire for measuring SHO satisfaction with their hospital training. *British Journal of General Practice.* 48:1399–1403.
13. Hand H, Shepstone L and Dawson H (2003) Judging the quality of SHO training: the work of the HRC of RCGP in England and Northern Ireland. *Education for Primary Care.* 14:18–24.
14. Grant J, Marsden P and King R (1989) SHOs and their training: Personal characteristics and professional circumstances and perception of service and training. *British Medical Journal.* 299:1263–8.
15. Hartley J (1998) *Learning and Studying. A Research Perspective.* Routledge, London.
16. Wooley N and Jarvis Y (2007) Situated cognition and cognitive apprenticeship: a model for teaching and learning clinical skills in a technologically rich and authentic learning environment. *Nurse Education Today.* 27:73–9.
17. Collins A, Brown J and Newman S (1989) Cognitive apprenticeship: teaching the crafts of reading, writing and mathematics. In: Resnick L (ed.) *Knowing, Learning and Instruction: essays in honour of Robert Glaser,* pp. 453–94. Lawrence Erlbaum Associates, Hillsdale, NJ.
18. Knowles M (1973) *The Adult Learner. A Neglected Species.* Gulf Publishing, Houston, TX.
19. Kolb D (1984) *Experiential Learning.* Prentice Hall, Englewood Cliffs, NJ.
20. Schon D (1983) *The Reflective Practitioner: how professionals think in action.* Basic Books, New York.
21. Schon D (1987) *Educating the Reflective Practitioner: towards a new design for teaching and learning in the professions.* Jossey-Bass, San Fransisco, CA.
22. Bandura A. Social Learning Theory, New York: General Learning Press; 1977.
23. Bleakley A (2006) Broadening conceptions of learning in medical education: the message from teamworking. *Medical Education.* 40:150–57.

24. Swanwick T (2005) Informal learning in postgraduate medical education: from cognitivism to 'culturism'. *Medical Education.* 39:859–65.
25. Bleakley A (2002) Pre-registration house offi cers and ward-based learning: a 'new apprenticeship' model. *Medical Education.* 36:9–15.
26. Vygotsky, L.S. (1978), Mind in Society. Cambridge, MA: Harvard University Press.
27. Lave J and Wenger E (1991) *Situated Learning: legitimate peripheral participation.* Cambridge University Press, Cambridge.
28. Wenger E (1999) *Communities of Practice, Learning, Meaning and Identity.* Cambridge University Press, Cambridge.
29. Morris C (2005) *Moving beyond See One, Do One, Teach One: developing pedagogy for doctors as teachers.* Institute of Education, University of London, London.
30. Cave J, Goldacre M, Lambert T et al. (2007) Newly qualifi ed doctors' views about whether their medical school had trained them well: questionnaire surveys. *BMC Medical Education.* 7:38.
31. Kroenke K. (2001) Attending rounds revisited (President's Column). *Society of General Internal Medicine Forum,* 24(1):8–9.
32. Ramani S, Orlander JD, Strunin L and Barber TW (2003) Whither bedside teaching: a focus group study of clinical teachers. *Academic Medicine.* 78:1–7.
33. Furney Scott, Orsini Alex, Orsetti Kym et al (2001) Teaching the One-minute Preceptor – A randomized controlled trial. *Journal of General Internal Medicine.* 16:620–24.
34. Neher JO, Gordon KC, Meyer B and Stevens N (!992) A fi ve-step "microskills" model of clinical teaching. *Clinical Teacher.* 5:419–24.
35. Irby D and Bowen JL (2004) Time-effi cient strategies for learning and performance. *The Clinical Teacher.* 1(1):23–28.
36. Dolmans DHJM, Wolfhagen IHAP et al. (2008) Factors adversely affecting student learning in the clinical learning environment: a student perspective. *Education for Health.* 20(3).
37. Durak HI, Vatansever K et al. Factors determining students' global satisfaction with clerkships: an analysis of a two year students' rating data base. *Advances in Health Sciences Education.* 13(4):495–502.
38. Hamdy et al. (2001). Application of "VITALS" Visual Indicators of Teaching and Learning Success in reporting student evaluations of clinical teachers. *Education for Health.* 14(2): 267–76.

VI
LEARNING IN THE COMMUNITY

Chapter 20

Community-based Education: What? Why? How?

Bashir Hamad

Objectives

On completing the chapter, you will be able to:
- Define the meanings of community-based and community-oriented medical education.
- Explain the rationale/justification for community-based education (CBE).
- List six criteria for effective implementation of CBE, giving practical examples of programs for such implementation.
- Describe your role as a student in critiquing and improving CBE programs in your college.

Introduction and rationale – Why this chapter?

You must have realized from reading Chapter 3 (Current Trends in Medical Education) and other chapters in this handbook that studying medicine within the walls of a university campus and a university/tertiary hospital is far from being adequate or relevant. As students, if we are to be trained properly, we should receive what we call a *balanced training in all three levels of health care (primary, secondary, and tertiary) as well as training within our community*. The purpose of this chapter is to explain to you this kind of training, what it is for, and how best it should be done. This should help you exercise your positive role in it as a student and prepare for graduating as a competent doctor who is better *able and willing* to serve patients, their families, and the community at large.

What is community-based education?

Community-based education is defined as:

All learning activities that take place within the community, in a rural, suburban or urban setting (i.e. a setting other than that within a tertiary hospital), where students, faculty and community members are involved.[1] Examples of these learning activities are: attachment to a family, attachment or assignment to a primary healthcare (PHC) centre, general practice, rural hospital or community-based national program or research project, etc.

These activities which make up community-based education represent the means by which a community-oriented medical education (COME) program is put into practice.

What is COME?

For a full definition of COME and major misconceptions about it, please refer to Hamad (1991).[2]

In general, COME may be defined as an education that is *relevant* to the needs of the society within which it is operated. Its aim is to produce community-oriented health professionals, irrespective of their future specialty. The term, therefore, is used to describe the *approach* and basic characteristics of the health training institution's program as a whole.

To be called community-oriented, the program should display the following characteristics:

1) Learning objectives which are based on, and responsive to, community needs and priority health problems.
2) Comprehensive curriculum addressing the biological, psychological, and social aspects of individual patients, their families, and community; with its focus being not only on disease and cure but also on health and prevention.
3) Balanced practical training in the three levels of healthcare (primary, secondary, and tertiary), starting early in the curriculum and continuing throughout.
4) Use of available community resources, and appropriate technology for teaching/learning and research.
5) Partnership or optimum working relationship with the health system of the country (no ivory-tower isolation) to create a *teaching health system* and a *serving educational institution*.
6) Product/graduate with the following desirable attributes and abilities:

   - Community-oriented;
   - Problem-solver and lifelong learner;
   - Humane, caring and discreet in dealing with patients, their relations and his/her own colleagues;
   - Manager;
   - Communicator; etc.

On implementing CBE to achieve the above-mentioned requisites of COME, we need to make sure that the criteria for the success of a CBE program are met (see Box 1).

Box 1: Criteria for effective CBE[3]

CBE should:

1) Have clearly stated objectives, and be well planned, organized, supervised, and evaluated (with emphasis on learning objectives and effective supervision);
2) Be student-centered and geared toward active learning (not passive or touristic);
3) Enjoy total faculty commitment (not dependent on one department);
4) Involve community, faculty, students, and related sectors together (including program evaluation and development);
5) Benefit (not "use") the community; and
6) Have available the required resources.

Why community-based education?

Having defined what it means, let us think of the reasons why we should use CBE. Is it of any benefit to any of those involved in the education program as a whole (what we call the stakeholders)?

After considering some basic reasons or justifications, we will proceed to describe the benefits of CBE and highlight the evidence from research results to-date for these benefits.

Accountability to society (Social Contract)

It is a basic requirement of societies that their health professionals should be accountable to them for addressing priority health needs. As stated clearly by the World Health Organization,[4] health professionals must attend to "the priority health concerns of the nation they have a mandate to serve". This cannot be achieved through practices restricted only within hospitals, and "... substantial change in the orientation of medical education towards greater relevance to the needs of society is necessary, unavoidable and urgent."[5]

Drawbacks and shortcomings of traditional systems of medical education in light of changes in education and healthcare

In spite of the emergence of strong forces for change and new trends in the field of medical education and healthcare (see Box 2), the movement in traditional systems of education is still rather slow. Rote learning through lectures and other, out-dated methods of teaching/learning and student assessment are predominant.

Clinical training is largely limited to bedside teaching within the walls of hospitals. "A steady diet of lecturing leads to intellectual anaemia."[6]

An academic who only presents facts is not a teacher, a teacher is one who nurtures the learning process and thereby modifies behavior and patterns of thinking for a lifetime.[7]

Box 2: Forces for change and changing healthcare needs

Forces for change (summarized in five environmental trends):
1. Increased clinical productivity
2. Multidisciplinary culture
3. New learning science and information technology (IT)
4. Changing health care needs
5. Demands for accountability[8]

Changing healthcare needs
1. Curative to health promotion
2. Episodic to continuous and comprehensive care
3. Individual physician to team care
4. Centralized to decentralized primary health care (PHC) system
5. Care of individual to community care
6. In-patient to home, day and intermediate care[9]

If medical education is to respond to these changes, as it must, then CBE has a lot to offer in this regard as it tends to provide, among other things, authentic, real-life environments for teaching and learning.

Targeting excellence and relevance

The relevance issue has been discussed in the sections above, but cannot be over-emphasized. We cannot, by any means, claim to be producing competent doctors for a society when we limit their training to tertiary-care hospitals receiving at best only 10% of the patient population in that society. Graduates should also be well grounded in the context of their society and the milieu of medical practice in its broadest sense.

Obviously, the aim of change is not just for the sake of change, but for change for the better, and curricula should not be stagnant and static but constantly evolving. They should be updated on a regular basis in keeping with new developments in health profession education and healthcare.[10]

Cost-effectiveness
According to the experience of the author as a founding dean of two medical schools, CBE is cost-effective, but literature support for this is still hazy except for one earlier study from New Mexico.[11] As yet there are not many studies in this area.

Benefits to stakeholders
The main stakeholders in this connection are the students, the faculty and other health personnel (mentors, preceptors), the training institution, and the community.

Students
In community-based settings, students are expected to understand the community and its culture and the prevailing knowledge, attitudes, and practices related to health and disease. They will be more acquainted with the different roles of health-related personnel, and be exposed to role models in health practice. It is also expected that they will develop the desired skills and right attitudes in effective communication, empathy, teamwork and leadership. In addition, applying their knowledge in real-life situations and diverse settings should enhance their motivation to learn. But what is the evidence from the literature? Some examples are quoted below.

A study from Australia[12] found that students in a full-year community-based clinical placement expressed marked ownership of their education, had more direct personal involvement with patients, felt more autonomous and self-directed, and had more collegial relationship with faculty than their counterparts placed in tertiary hospital practice.

The program evaluation of three medical schools in the United States (Dartmouth, New York and Virginia)[13] revealed that students performed as well or better than their peers in hospital wards and that CBE experiences contributed positively to student education, critical thinking and problem-solving skills.

Fifth-year students in a CBE placement at the University of Western Australia[14] did as well as urban-placed students, were more embedded in daily care provision, were more involved in interdisciplinary projects and teamwork, and enjoyed a richer experience.

In the nursing field, service-learning students (1999) reported benefits of personal satisfaction, professional growth, critical thinking skills, and preparation for nursing practice in a diversity of settings.

Faculty and other health personnel

According to the author's experience, many faculties in classical schools have never reached out to the community and many do volunteer to report it as their first experience. CBE paves the way for a faculty to have a closer relationship with its society and for students to shoulder some responsibilities for community development. It also opens venues for them to take responsibility for leadership or training of field staff and to make their education and training more relevant to the needs of their society. These outcomes are unlikely to be achieved without the full involvement of the whole faculty in CBE activities. As an example, the coordination of CBE courses in Gezira Faculty of Medicine, Sudan (Research Training and Rural Development, Rural Residency, Family Attachment and PHC Centre Practice), has been the total responsibility of faculties of other disciplines than community medicine (Surgery, Pathology, Medicine, Pediatrics and Obstetrics and Gynecology, respectively).

The process of evaluation of the integrated PHC clerkship[15] has provided the faculty with innovative evaluation methods, and the results have shown that there were enhanced recruitment, retention and development of CBE in the faculty and more local and PHC leaders engaged in scholarly activities.

Similar results were reported from the family medicine clerkship in Georgia. The most important factor in dealing with part-time or field staff (clinical instructors, mentors, preceptors, etc.) is to use a participative leadership style and treat them "as respected partners, receiving constant support in implementation."[16]

Community

Community benefit was stated earlier as one of the criteria of effective CBE programs (Box 1). Through these programs the community becomes more health aware and is enabled to identify its problems and seek feasible solutions with the help of students and faculty. The facilities and resources of the health system in the locality are likewise improved. In the process, sustainable development of the community can be realized, in addition to empowerment, leadership, and self-reliance.

The option of graduates to practice in a rural community is another advantage. This has recently been supported by a report on five studies in 2005: "It is now well established that students from rural backgrounds are more likely than urban students to opt to practice in a rural community" and this is "greatly enhanced by greater exposure to rural health issues."[17]

Institution

CBE activities provide the institution with more detailed and up-to date information on the local community or country and its health problems. The information can then be utilized to improve the relevance of the education and research programs of the institution and streamline its curriculum accordingly.

We would like to conclude this section on the reasons for CBE by quoting the results of a Best Evidence Medical Education (BEME) systematic review on "How can early experience in clinical and community settings contribute to basic medical education?"[12] covering the period 1992–2001:

- "Early experience fostered medical students' self-awareness and empathetic attitudes towards ill people;
- Boosted their confidence, motivated them, gave them satisfaction, and helped them develop their professional identities;
- It made entering clerkships a less stressful experience by developing interpersonal skills;
- Early experience taught students about professional roles and responsibilities, healthcare system and population health needs;
- It gave biomedical, behavioral and social sciences relevance and made them easier to learn;
- It motivated and rewarded teachers and patients and enriched curricula;
- In some countries junior medical students were a source of preventive healthcare for underserved populations; and
- Early experience increased recruitment to primary care/rural medical practice in the USA."

The reader must have realized by now that these results have provided literature support for many of the areas we have been discussing.

How about community-based education?

The purpose of this section is to make you familiar with some methods and examples of CBE programs. We should remind ourselves, though, that these programs or learning activities should satisfy the effectiveness criteria for CBE outlined above in Box 1.

Community-based learning activities are described under four main categories[1]

- "Training in PHC facilities;
- Community surveys and related projects;
- Family care programs; and
- Work in a defined community for community development."

For detailed information on these, with examples, see also Feletti et al. (2000)[18] Examples of CBE courses initiated by the author and his colleagues at the Gezira Faculty of Medicine in Sudan are summarized in Table 20.1 (a synopsis of these courses appears in Magzoub and Hamad (1995)[19]).

The proportion of time allotted for community-based education programs out of the total curriculum time varies among different medical schools within a range of 20–70%. For example, it is about 20% in Gezira, Sudan (established 1978);

TABLE 20.1 Community-based experiences and activities for medical students at Gezira, Sudan (from Magzoub and Hamad, 1995, in Education for Health[19]).

Course	Duration/ semester	Site	Main activities
Introduction to Medicine and the Study of Medicine	Two weeks in Semester 1	Villages, factories, urban slums	Collection of data, identification of community problems
Interdisciplinary Field Training, Research and Rural Development Program	Four weeks in each of Semesters 4, 6, and 8	Villages	Community diagnosis, health interventions, community development, and evaluation
Primary Health Care (PHC), Centre Practice, and Family Health	Longitudinal: one day every week through Semesters 4–8	Families and PHC units	Family visits, clinical attachment to PHC units
Doctor and Society	Three weeks in Semester 4	Different community sites and hospitals	Students conduct interviews with patients and community members
Rural Attachment	Four weeks following Semester 7	Single-doctor rural hospitals and surrounding villages	Clinical attachment and community diagnosis
Primary Health Care Clerkship	Four weeks in Semester 8	Villages and PHC units	Orientation to managerial aspects of PHC and exposure to health teams, leadership

New Castle, New South Wales, Australia (1978); Suez Canal, Egypt (early 1980s); Arab Gulf, Bahrain (1980s); more than that in Manchester, UK (1994) and even more (70%) in Florida State, USA (2000).

It has to be realized that the planning and implementation of CBE programs are by no means easy and the challenges are many. Since these are beyond the scope of this chapter, the reader is recommended to read the relevant papers.[19,20,21]

Your role as a student

In this system of education the role of students is never passive. Students have the responsibility to participate in the management of courses or blocks as student coordinators, and in critiquing and giving constructive feedback in program evaluation. Questionnaires and open discussion are often used in this regard to obtain your opinions for purposes of improving and developing the educational programs.

Questionnaires are usually anonymous to allow you free expression of your opinion without fear of any personal incrimination. In addition to the open discussion by faculty during or at the end of each block, there may be regular (e.g. monthly) meetings, preferably chaired by the dean, to discuss with you a variety of college matters and plans according to his discretion. You should therefore make it a point of being actively and fully involved in these and other activities for your own benefit and for the benefit of your colleagues and the college as a whole. In addition, you should be proactive and come up with initiatives for change. For example, one of the students of the Faculty of Medicine, University of Gezira, Sudan, suggested the introduction of a new block in the curriculum, to which the faculty and leaders agreed. The block thereby carried the name of the student: 'Imam.'

References

1. World Health Organization. Community-based Education of Health Personnel. *Technical report Series No. 746*. Geneva: WHO, 1987.
2. Hamad B. Community-oriented medical education: What is it? *Medical Education* 1991; 25: 16–22.
3. Hamad B. What is community-based education? Evolution, definition and rationale. Chapter 1 in: Schmidt H, Magzoub M, Feletti G, Nooman Z. and Vluggen P (eds) *Handbook of Community-Based Education: Theory and Practices*. Maastricht, the Netherlands: Network: TUFH Publications, 2000.
4. World Health Organization.
5. Towle A (1998) quoted by Gwee MCE medical education: Issues, Trends, Challenges and Opportunities. *SMA News* 2003; 35 (2): 5–9.
6. Myers and Jones (1993). Ibid.
7. Woosly (1997). Ibid.
8. Irby DM, Wilkerson LA. Educational Innovations in Academic Medicine and Environmental Trends. *Journal of General Internal Medicine* 2003; 18, 5: 370–376.
9. Jones R, Higgs R, de Angelis C and Prideaux D. The changing face of medical curricula. *The Lancet*. 2001; 357: 699.
10. World Federation for Medical Education. *Global Standards for Quality Improvement*. Copenhagen: WFME, 2003.
11. Mennin SP and Martinez-Burrola N. The cost of problem-based versus traditional medical education. *Medical Education* 1987; 20: 187–194.
12. Dornan T, Littlewood S, Margolis SA, Scherpbier A, Spencer J and Ypinazar V. How can early experience in clinical and community settings contribute to basic medical education? BBEME, 2006 at: *http//www.bemecollaboration.org/topics.htm* Accessed July 2009.

13. Carney PA, Bar-on ME, Grayson MS, Klein M, Cochran N, Eliassen MS, Gambert SR, Gupta KL, Labrecque MC, Munson PJ, Nierenberg DW, O'Donnell JF, Whitehurst-cook M, Willett RM. The Impact of Early Clinical Training in Medical Education: A Multi-Institutional Assessment. *Academic Medicine* 1999; 74: S59-S66.

14. Denz-Penhey H, Shannon S, Murdoch J, et al. Do benefits accrue from longer rotations for students in Rural Clinical Schools? *Rural and Remote Health* 2005; 5. (Article No. 414).

15. Pipas CF, Peltier DA, Fall LH, Olson AL, Mahoney JF, Skochelak SE, Gjerde CL. Collaborating to Integrate Curriculum in Primary Care Medical Education: Successes and Challenges From Three US Medical Schools. *Family Medicine* 2004;36(1):S126–S132.).

16. Australian Learning and Teaching Council. Influence of student placements on practice location upon/after graduation from other disciplines? In: Delivering optometric graduates ready for practice beyond the cities and ready to service an ageing population The University of Auckland and Queensland University of Technology 2011 p 26.

17. Tesson G, Curran V, Pong R, Strasser R. Advances in Rural Medical Education in Three Countries: Canada, the United States and Australia. *Education for Health* 2005; 18, 3: 405–415.

18. Feletti G, Ja'afar R, Joseph A, Magzoub M, McHarney-Brown C, Omonisi K, Rifaat A, Wachs J and Schmidt H. Implementation of community-based curricula. In: Schmidt H, Magzoub M, Feletti G, Nooman Z and Vluggen P (eds) *Handbook of Community-Based Education: Theory and Practices.* Maastricht, The Netherlands: Network: TUFH Publications, 2000, p. 147 (Chapter 10).

19. Magzoub M and Hamad B. The struggle for relevance in medical education. *Education for Health* 1995.

20. Hamad B. Milestones of leadership strategies for planning and implementation of community oriented medical education (COME). *Newsletter of Network of Community-oriented Educational Institutions for Health Sciences* 1992; Maastricht, The Netherlands; 6–8.

21. Murray E, Moddel M. Community-based teaching: the challenges. *British Journal of General Practice* 1999; 49: 395–398.

Chapter 21

Primary and Ambulatory Care Education

Samuel Scott Obenshain

Objectives

By the end of this chapter, you will be able to:
- Know the definition of primary care.
- Know the definition of ambulatory care.
- Know the advantage of learning in a primary care environment.
- Be able to list the learning opportunities in primary care.
- Be able to compare and contrast learning in a primary versus a tertiary care environment.
- Know the importance of asking for a critique of your performance in primary care.
- Be able to know how to develop one'syour own learning issues from patients oneyou sees.
- Be able to recognize the importance of the opportunities to enhance your clinical skills in the primary care setting.
- Know why "Communication is the prime clinical skill" of the clinician.
- Know the importance of physical examination in the care of patients.
- Know the importance of getting feedback from your patients.
- Be able to explain the role of intermediate-level practitioners in the provision of primary care.
- Know how you can continue your education in primary care.

What is primary care?

Primary care is first-line care that is delivered by physicians or intermediate care providers. The vast majority of all patient care is provided in this setting, not in the hospital where most medical student education takes place. It is generally provided in the care provider's own office, clinic or even in the home of the patient. It includes well-care visits, screening and the care of illnesses that can be treated in that particular setting. It is also provided outside of a hospital, although, the site of care may be in an outpatient or clinic facility that may actually be in a hospital. The providers are family physicians, general pediatricians, general internal medicine physicians or, at times, obstetrician/gynecologists who may be providing the primary care of their female patients.

How are primary and ambulatory care related?

Ambulatory care means the care of patients who are able to come to the care provider's facility, an office, a clinic, or may be seen in the patient's own home. Primary care is delivered in an ambulatory facility, so these terms are often used interchangeably. At times the patients may be referred to as the "walking ill," that is, patients who are sick but whose care can be managed outside of the hospital. With the more recent changes in the medical care environment more and more patients are having their care managed outside of the hospital, which is referred to as a secondary care environment. As the care becomes more and more specialized it may be referred to as tertiary or even quaternary care.

Why learn in an ambulatory primary care setting?

This setting provides the best opportunity for you, as a novice physician or medical student, to enhance your clinical skills, i.e. communication, critical reasoning and physical examinations skills. In addition, this also provides the best chance for you to see the natural history of a particular disease from the beginning on through its entire course. Also, you can see patients as they first present with a complaint and will have to think through the patient's diagnosis by yourself. Too often the patients you see in the hospital environment already have a diagnosis before they are admitted and you just follow what the others who have seen the patient before have thought.

The other major reason for learning in the ambulatory-primary care environment is that you are working side-by-side with an experienced care provider and will see how such an individual organizes his or her life. Both of the latest books on improving medical education[1, 2] deal with the development of identity of the physician in training and comment that this can best be developed in the primary care location.

What are the major opportunities for learning in a primary care setting?

Some of the opportunities and advantages of learning in the primary care setting are listed below:

- First-line care provides you with the opportunity of being the first to see the patient.
- The patient presents his or her problem first-hand to you, providing the opportunity to think through the patient's problem and come up with your own diagnosis.
- It presents the opportunity of learning the natural history of a disease since you may see the patient from the outset of their problem.

- Most care of patients with a chronic disease is provided in the ambulatory setting, not in the hospital. What you see in the hospital are acute exacerbations of the chronic disease.
- The patient is able to tell his or her own story.
- You are able to listen to the patient's story in the patient's own words.
- You are able to develop and test your own hypotheses.

How is primary care setting different from the tertiary care setting?

As noted above, the primary care setting is first-line care in which the patient first presents to the care provider with an illness or other health concern. This provides the learning opportunity of seeing the course of a disease from the beginning to the end, whereas in the secondary or tertiary care environment the hospital sees patients with acute episodes of chronic disease and/or very acute illnesses. The latter environment puts the learner in a subsidiary role, dealing with a patient whose diagnosis has already been made or someone who is so sick that they are unable to communicate with the learner.[3]

In my role as an ambulatory educator I once had a student who was almost through his third year in medical school, most of which had been spent in the hospital environment he told me, when he was seeing an 8-month-old child, "This is the first patient I have seen all year who could sit up by himself" – meaning that all his patients had been so sick they could not even sit up without any help.

As has been noted in the two books mentioned earlier,[1,2] more of our student's learning should be in the environment where the majority of care of patients is provided, i.e. the primary-ambulatory care environment, and this should begin earlier in the learner's experience in medical school. This would and should turn medical education, as we know it today, upside down.[4] The learner should begin to encounter patients in a setting where he or she can actually learn from them.

Why should I ask for constructive criticism?

To enhance your learning, you must have a constructive critique that will help improve your performance. Teachers find giving critique one of the most difficult things they have to do, and to overcome this difficulty you must request and expect to receive critique. Just saying "you are doing a good job" is not constructive critique. The term critique is partly why the job is so difficult, since critique implies criticism in most minds. This is understandable, but at the outset of a clinical rotation ground rules should be set and one component of this, besides being on time, etc., should include constructive critique. To accomplish this, you must be observed in carrying out the task expected of you and then receiving comment on how you might improve your performance. Being a learner means learning from your experiences, but without comments on how you may do it better you will find it hard to improve.

How do I learn from my own patients?

Learning from your own patients is the most important learning you can do. To do this you must be honest about what you know and then work to build upon this knowledge base. Asking for feedback from your patients is one step, although, as noted above, when teachers have trouble giving feedback one can expect patients to have the same problem.

The second way to learn from your patients is to develop learning issues from the patients' problems. What do I know about this problem and what more do I need to know to be able to provide for them the best care possible? Asking questions of one's preceptor (teacher) about why they are using this or that drug? How they came to their decision about what the patient's problem was? Or why they decided to follow this regimen or refer the patient for a second opinion? All of these will help you better understand not only the role of the physician but also his/her thinking.

Once you have done this, you must read about your patients in order to expand your knowledge about their problems. Even if you think "I have seen this many times," there is always something more one can learn. Then you should discuss what you have learned with your teacher, thereby making the information more yours. As they say, "To teach is to learn."

Can primary care learning expand my worldview of medicine?

The answer to this question is YES! As noted above, most of the current medical education occurs in the hospital, which is a tertiary care setting and limits the experience a student could have. Getting into a primary-ambulatory care setting will give you a view of medical care as seen in first-line care, that of a patient's and physician's first experience with a patient's problem. This view will certainly help you to understand the entire spectrum of the health care system.

What learning may be unique to the ambulatory or primary care setting?

The greatest advantage of a primary-ambulatory care setting is that it provides time for the learner to interact with patients and to have the opportunity of being the first care provider to speak with the patient before a diagnosis may have been made. This provides you with the opportunity to expand your abilities in interacting with patients and receiving feedback on how you carry out these tasks. In addition, you may be observed doing those tasks and receive feedback as to how they were performed.

- The patient is able to communicate about his or her own problems.
- The patient's diagnosis has not already been established.
- The learner may try different techniques in obtaining information from the patient:
  - open-ended questions

- focused listening
- overcome tendency to be thinking of the next question instead of listening to the patient's answers
- being able to ask the patient what he or she thinks the problem may be
- learn to re-cap what the patient has said to be sure you have the story correct
- practice patient-centered care
- learn to set the agenda for the encounter rather than delve into the depth of the first problem suggested.

Why is communication considered the prime clinical skill of the physician?

Seventy percent of diagnoses come from the patient's history. Learning to take a complete history from the patient and allowing them to tell their own story can greatly enhance your ability to come to the correct diagnosis. The primary care setting is the best place to learn to enhance your skills in communicating with the patient.[5] It was for these reasons that the Chair of Medicine at the University of New Mexico stated "Communication is the prime clinical skill of the physician."

What is the role of the physical examination?

A physical examination can confirm what has been learned from the patient's history.

It is also an important clinical skill. However, it should be used primarily to confirm the conclusions you have reached from taking a complete history from the patient. Expanding your skills with physical examination is an opportunity provided by the primary-ambulatory care setting.

What is the role of the primary care physician in caring for patients with chronic disease?

The vast majority of care for patients with chronic disease is provided in the primary-ambulatory care setting. Having experience in this setting will give you a much better understanding of the long-term care of the patient with a chronic disease. While you will see acute exacerbations of chronic disease in an in-patient hospital experience, the best place to get the total understanding of the physician's role in care for chronic disease is in the ambulatory setting. There you can observe how the disease is managed, from an educational perspective, to drug management, to understand how one can follow the course of the patient's disease. Whether following an asthmatic's pulmonary function tests, or a diabetic's management of their blood glucose levels, or monitoring the progression of the complications of their disease, such as foot care, these are the opportunities provided in the primary-ambulatory care setting, whereas in the hospital the care providers are mainly interested in stabilizing the patient's condition so they can discharge the patient back to the care of their primary care physician.

What role is played by intermediate-level practitioners in the provision of primary care?

Intermediate-level practitioners, such as physician assistants and nurse practitioners, play a major role in providing primary care to patients in all settings. They are most valuable in areas of low population density where the population may be too low to support a physician. While these individuals may also work in secondary or tertiary care settings, many education programs have been developed to educate primary and intermediate care practitioners. These people can be very helpful for a student who is learning in a primary-ambulatory care setting by assisting in the supervision and education of the student, since they may have more time available to spend with the learner.

How may I continue my education in primary care after medical school?

In the United States you can opt for a primary care residency training position in several disciplines. Family medicine is primarily an ambulatory training program with more limited time in the hospital or tertiary care setting. The amount of time spent in primary care in a family medicine residency increases as one moves through the residency. There are also primary care internal medicine residencies. These programs have their learners spending increasing amounts of time in an ambulatory setting compared to the more tertiary intense regular internal medicine residency. Pediatric residencies also allot more time in the ambulatory setting since they have recognized for many years that most pediatric care is provided by pediatricians in the primary-ambulatory care setting.

These disciplines are supported by their own journals and societies.

Take home questions

1. Explain the difference between your education in a primary care and a tertiary care setting.
2. List those skills you are able to expand or enhance while participating in a primary-ambulatory care setting.
3. How are the patients you see in a primary-ambulatory care setting different from those seen in the tertiary care setting?
4. How might you continue your education in primary care?

References

1. Cooke, M, Irby, DM and O'Brien, BC (2010) *Educating Physicians: A Call for Reform in Medical School and Residency*. San Francisco: Jossey-Bass/Carnegie Foundation for the Advancement of Teaching.
2. Bleakley, A, Bligh, J and Brown, J (2011) *Medical Education for the Future: Identity, Power and Location (Advances in Medical Education)*. Springer Dordrecht Heidelberg London New York.
3. Steward, DE (1993) Moving medical education out of the hospital. *Teaching and Learning in Medicine*, 5(4), 214–216.
4. Kriel, JR, Hewson, MG, Zietsman, AI and Coles, C (1988) Teaching medicine upside down: Some educational implications of the theory of cognitive structures. *SA Family Practice*, February, 42–49.
5. Murray, E, Jolly, B and Modell, M (1999) A comparison of the educational opportunities on junior medical attachments in general practice and in a teaching hospital: a questionnaire survey. *Medical Education*, 33, 170–176.

Chapter 22

Leadership in Medicine

John Bligh and Julie Browne

Objectives

- The objective of this chapter is to introduce medical students and junior doctors to the concept of medical leadership and to encourage them to reflect on and develop their own leadership styles and roles.
- The authors discuss the importance of medical leadership in improving the care of patients, outline the differences between leadership and management, examine medical leadership in terms of values, skills, personality traits and leadership styles, and show how effective medical leaders must take account of the organizational structures and cultures within which they work.

Introduction

Medical students are tomorrow's doctors. In accordance with Good Medical Practice, graduates will make the care of patients their first concern, applying their knowledge and skills in a competent and ethical manner and using their ability to provide leadership and to analyze complex and uncertain situations.[1]

Throughout your medical training and subsequent career, there will be regular occasions when you are challenged to provide effective leadership. Leadership is part of a doctor's professional life, and is as fundamental to the practice of medicine as the roles of scholar, scientist and clinician.[1]

But what is medical leadership? It is not always about being 'in charge' or giving orders; it usually involves a significant amount of teamwork and collaboration. Consider the following scenarios:

- A family doctor is concerned that some diabetic patients are not attending routine appointments with the practice nurse.

- A psychiatrist wants to set up a specialist alcohol liaison team within a general hospital.
- Two medical students decide they need to know more about global health issues.
- During a consultation, it becomes clear to a pediatrician that a child's injuries were not accidental.
- A vascular surgeon has an idea for a new approach to the treatment of varicose veins.
- A junior doctor is, for the first time, faced with the challenge of telling a patient's family that she has died.
- A medical student becomes concerned that a fellow student is taking illegal drugs.

Although these scenarios differ from each other in many ways, they all involve some of the basic leadership challenges faced by doctors and medical students in everyday practice.

Medical leadership requires the doctor or medical student to have an understanding or vision about what clinical and professional practice should be, and to recognize that action is needed; it requires him/her to initiate the decision making and planning process that will identify a pathway for bringing about change, and to work with other people to pursue and eventually achieve that change. So if leadership is about anything, it is about initiating, managing, guiding and achieving change.[2, p. 35] Adair[3] splits this process of leading change into five key stages, where the leader has a fundamental responsibility for making things happen:

1. *Setting objectives* – The leader defines or identifies the purpose, aims and objectives that are to be achieved as part of an overall vision for change and improvement. He or she may work as part of a group to do this, and in these circumstances his or her role is to synthesize and summarize the group's objectives.
2. *Planning* – The leader ensures that there is a plan in place to achieve the objectives that have been set.
3. *Communicating* – The leader explains the vision, objectives and the plan so that everyone involved knows why it is necessary, what will be done and how it will be achieved.
4. *Organizing* – The leader ensures that everyone is briefed, supported and adequately equipped to play their part, and if necessary organizes the training and resources to do it. The leader supervises and monitors the work and keeps it all on track. This team-building work is vital to keep the project or organization moving forward effectively.
5. *Monitoring and evaluating* – The leader reviews and evaluates performance, and gives accurate and timely feedback to individuals and groups so that progress can be monitored and improvements made.

What is the difference between management and leadership?

> 1. You would expect a leader to set objectives, plan a course of action, communicate a vision, lead a team, keep it on track and monitor progress. Would a manager do this?

The stem of the word 'management' comes from the Latin word *manus*, meaning *hand*. It still has that connotation: managers 'handle things' such as planning, organizing, staff and controlling. Although there is a considerable overlap between management and leadership, a leader requires qualities over and above those of a good manager. If management is about planning, organizing and solving problems, then leadership is about the production of change and requires a different, if overlapping, set of skills and attributes.[2] As Ramsden[4] says: "Management is about 'doing things right' ... Leadership is about 'doing the right thing'."

> 2. Look again at the leadership scenarios on page [218–219]. How many of the people in these scenarios would you describe as managers?

Managers are generally appointed to their position, but leaders emerge. Leaders are not necessarily the most senior members of the team and, depending on the situation, the role of the leader may shift from person to person within the team. Sometimes, even the most junior member of the team may become the leader, perhaps because certain innate qualities make him or her the best qualified to lead at this time, or because he or she possesses the skills and experience that the situation requires, or is able to adopt the right approach to guiding the team. Clearly, leaders have something extra about them that make them more than managers.

> 3. Think of a leader who has inspired you. What are the special qualities that set him or her apart? Make a list of these qualities.

In your response to the question in box 3 you may have come up with a list that contains a mixture of personality traits, skills, leadership styles, and values that, to you, typify a great leader.

Values: These are the fundamental principles which underpin a leader's actions and which define who they are as people, such as respect for others, honesty and a sense of fair play.

Skills and abilities: It is sometimes argued that few people are truly 'born leaders', and that leadership consists of a set of learnable skills. These include things like abilities in conflict resolution, problem solving or experience of the task in hand.

Personality traits: These are the innate characteristics that great leaders are said to possess. They may include qualities such as decisiveness, persistence or confidence.

Leadership styles: These depend in part on the context and situation, and may be defined by adjectives such as autocratic, motivational, nurturing, etc.

The need for medical leadership

The most important area for developing new concepts, methods and practices will be in the management of society's knowledge resources – specifically in the areas of education and healthcare, both of which are today over administered and undermanaged.[5, p. xii]

We live in a rapidly changing environment and the medical profession and medical practitioners have to respond to modern times with effective leadership. It has been recognized for a long time that doctors as a group have traditionally found leadership difficult and need more specific training for leadership roles. Smith,[6] in an essay in the *BMJ*, offered various explanations for this: doctors, he argued, traditionally do not like being led; they have tended in the past to think about individual patients rather than about organizations and systems; they frequently find working in teams problematic since they usually want to be in control; their education does not provide enough training for leadership, particularly in the fields of economics, finance, policy and strategy development; and doctors have historically resisted compromise and negotiation. His essay was, in some ways, prophetic. In 2007, a major failure of the UK system for recruitment into specialist training, Modernizing Medical Careers, precipitated a national inquiry into the crisis. The Inquiry's report[7] concluded: "There has been a dearth of medical professional leadership over this period".[p. 105] It was clearly the Inquiry's view that doctors had failed as a profession in their duty to lead change and improvement in health service delivery. This may be hard to accept: harder still is the recognition that absence of good leadership may also compromise patient care.[8]

Medical schools, postgraduate training departments and doctors' organizations everywhere are, to their credit, responding to the challenge of improving medical leadership. Leadership training and experience is increasingly appearing as an outcome requirement in various competency frameworks and curricula at all levels from undergraduate, postgraduate, specialty training and continuing medical education in countries throughout the world – particularly the Netherlands, Denmark, Canada and the UK – and opportunities for medical students to develop their leadership skills are increasing all the time.[1, 9–11]

Leaders in medicine

Leadership is the most personal thing in the world, since it is just plain you.[3, p. 47]

As a doctor you have a responsibility to lead, so it is important to think about how you will discharge your duties, reflect on your leadership skills and consider what type of leader you will be.

---

4. Try sub-dividing the list you made in your response to question 3 into columns headed (a) personality traits, (b) skills, (c) leadership styles and (d) values. To what extent do these characteristics reflect the kind of leader you would like to be?

In this section we will discuss in more detail what characterizes a leader in medicine. Where possible we will use evidence to back up our views, but it is important to stress that leadership is not an exact science and that everyone has a unique view of what makes a good leader, since every good leader is unique.

Values

Medicine is a value-led profession and everything a doctor does should be driven by a clear set of values. You cannot make ethical decisions unless you know what the fundamental issues are and have resolved your basic principles and values.

In order to lead a team in a particular direction you need to know where you are going. But even as you are deciding where you are going, you need to have in mind the question of why you want to go there, and the driver for this will be your values.

Some medical students, at graduation, take part in a 'Hippocratic Oath' ceremony where they make a public declaration of their values. Here is the oath taken by the students of Imperial College, London:[12]

Box 1: Imperial College School of Medicine's Declaration of a new doctor [12]

Now, as a new doctor, I solemnly promise that I will to the best of my ability serve humanity – caring for the sick, promoting good health, and alleviating pain and suffering.

I recognize that the practice of medicine is a privilege with which comes considerable responsibility and I will not abuse my position.

I will practise medicine with integrity, humility, honesty, and compassion – working with my fellow doctors and other colleagues to meet the needs of my patients.

I shall never intentionally do or administer anything to the overall harm of my patients.

I will not permit considerations of gender, race, religion, political affiliation, sexual orientation, nationality, or social standing to influence my duty of care.

> **Box 1: Imperial College School of Medicine's Declaration of a new doctor[12] (*Continued*)**
>
> I will oppose policies in breach of human rights and will not participate in them. I will strive to change laws that are contrary to my profession's ethics and will work towards a fairer distribution of health resources.
>
> I will assist my patients to make informed decisions that coincide with their own values and beliefs and will uphold patient confidentiality.
>
> I will recognize the limits of my knowledge and seek to maintain and increase my understanding and skills throughout my professional life. I will acknowledge and try to remedy my own mistakes and honestly assess and respond to those of others.
>
> I will seek to promote the advancement of medical knowledge through teaching and research.
>
> I make this declaration solemnly, freely, and upon my honour.

---

5. Note how many of these undertakings are 'active' rather than passive. They commit the oath taker to initiate and lead improvements rather than merely not to do wrong.
6. If your medical school does not have a graduation oath, why not try writing your own?

Obviously, as a member of a profession, you will share some fundamental values with all members of that profession and your actions will be measured against those values. Documents such as *Good Medical Practice*[13] and *Management for Doctors*[14] by the UK's General Medical Council show in more detail how professional values should underpin the actions of every doctor, while the *Professional Standards* of the Academy of Medical Educators define underpinning values for medical teachers.[15]

Skills

---

7. What skills does a leader in medicine need? Think of a good leader in your university, medical school or hospital. Apart from their medical and academic qualifications, what else can they do that qualifies them to lead?

Schwartz and Pogge[16] propose the following skills "as a minimum":

- Strategic and tactical planning
- Persuasive communication
- Negotiation
- Financial decision-making
- Team building
- Conflict resolution
- Interviewing

Bordage et al.[17] add to these: searching for information, developing and training staff, abiding by and applying regulations, preparing papers and visits, and teaching and supervising.

> 8. All of these skills can be learned, and can be improved with practice. What skills do you need to become a better leader? What can you do to acquire these skills?

Personality traits

The following have been proposed as attributes of medical education leaders:[17]

- Dedicated
- Enthusiastic
- Sense of humor
- Assertiveness, confidence
- Charismatic
- Energetic
- Willing to learn
- Motivator
- Optimist
- Visionary
- Imaginative, creative, resourceful, insightful

These are indeed a wonderful set of natural gifts, but few possess all of these all the time! There is no doubt that some rare individuals are 'born leaders' who seem to have a natural talent, not so much for getting things done, but for inspiring others to *want* to get things done. This is such a powerful personal attribute that it is even known by its Greek name "charisma," literally meaning a divine gift. Defining leadership as a natural gift may, however, be discouraging for those who do not feel themselves to be natural leaders.

We would argue that there is more to leadership than simple force of personality. Even where leadership does not come naturally, leadership skills can be improved where there is:

- a genuine desire to work with a team to bring about change;

- an ability to understand and reflect on one's own strengths and weaknesses with honesty and humility; and
- a desire for continuous improvement.

Although some people find leadership easier than others, there is no one perfect personality type that qualifies someone for leadership at all times and in all circumstances. There are only individuals with the best skills, experience and attributes to fit the particular circumstances and the task; such individuals are made, not born.

Box 2: Principles for public servants

The Nolan Committee on Standards in Public Life sets out seven principles for the conduct of holders of public office.[18] These are:

- Selflessness;
- Integrity;
- Objectivity;
- Accountability;
- Openness;
- Honesty; and finally
- Leadership.

Holders of public office should promote and support the first six principles by leadership and example.

---

9. Look at the Nolan Committee's seven principles[18] (Box 2). Are they inborn personality traits? Are they beliefs and values? Or are they a mixture of both?

Leadership styles

Leadership style is intimately linked to a leader's vision and values, and personality and skills will affect the way in which these are played out in practice. For example, a military leader may find that an authoritarian, directive approach works effectively on the battlefield during times of conflict but is unsuccessful in the office during peacetime. Highly effective leaders adapt to the demands of the team, the task and the context, which are in constant change. Variable organizational factors include:[19, p. 117]

- the power or position of the leader;
- the relationships within his or her group;
- organizational norms;

- structure and technology; and
- variety of subordinates.

Handy describes[19, chapter 7] four different organizational cultures and the role of the leader within them (see Figure 22.1).

10. As you read the following four descriptions think of an organization in which you are part of a team. Which description best describes the culture of that organization?

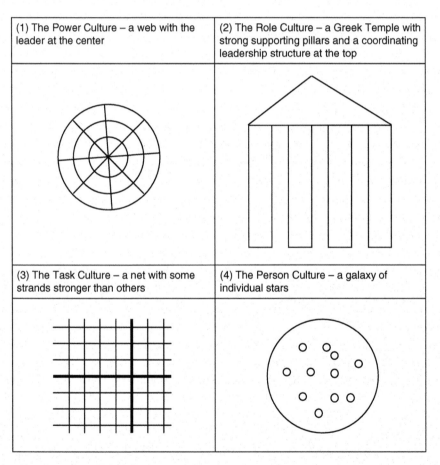

FIGURE 22.1   Handy's four organizational cultures

(1) The Power culture

The power culture is like a spider's web, with Zeus – the all powerful leader – as its patron god. The organization depends on a central authoritative figure. Influence comes only from proximity to the center. Family businesses are often power cultures. Organizations with power cultures are often built on trust, shared values and beliefs. They can react quickly and efficiently to threats, and bureaucracy is minimal. However, they may have difficulties if they grow in size because they are strongly dependent on one dominant leader, and they struggle if that leader is lost. Democracy and equity are not a priority in this type of organizational culture. Power cultures offer a highly traditional view of the role of the leader and are becoming increasingly rare in clinical practice, where teamwork is now seen as essential to effective patient care.

(2) The Role culture

Handy pictures the role culture as a Greek temple with Apollo – the god of reason – as its patron. The role organization rests on its strong pillars (Finance, Purchasing, Production departments, etc.), coordinated at the top by a narrow band of senior management, the pediment. Roles are often more important than individuals. Communication, systems and procedures are formal, with strict standards and outcome measures. Hospitals, universities and healthcare systems tend particularly towards this type of culture, as do the finance and public sectors, since it is usually found where economy of scale is more important than product innovation.

Such organizations thrive when doing routine, stable, unchanging tasks, and they offer security and reliability to the individual as long as nothing changes. But they can be threatened when the environment changes and are sometimes slow to respond to emergencies, leading to catastrophic collapse – such as during the recent banking crisis. For some talented, innovative and ambitious doctors a role culture can be frustrating, since role cultures place little emphasis on an individual's capacities.

(3) The Task culture

Handy pictures the task culture as a net, with some strands stronger than others. Its patron deity is Athena, the warrior and champion of achievements. The whole emphasis is on getting the job done. This culture seeks to bring together the right individuals in the right teams, ensure they have the appropriate resources and then let them get on with the job. Research teams, surgical 'firms' and product development groups often develop a task culture.

A strong team ethos means that leadership within the group is based on expert power rather than age or status, and as a consequence staff satisfaction is usually high. Such teams are quick to respond to change. However, organizations built around task cultures find it hard to produce economies of scale and can founder when resources become scarce. Because there is a relatively flat hierarchy, task cultures are inherently unstable and difficult to control, and they are prone to shift towards role or power culture when the organization finds itself challenged.

(4) The Person culture

The person culture is pictured by Handy as a galaxy of individual stars, with Dionysus – god of the self-oriented individual – as its patron. In a person culture, the individual comes first; the organization is subordinate to the individual and depends on the individual for its existence. Influence is shared and any power base is expert. Doctors' private practices, along with architects and law firms, are frequently person cultures, since success depends on the talents of the individual practitioners. Since these individuals may view the culture simply as a place to do their own thing, conflict is a constant risk, and the organization may lack strength and a sense of team spirit.

---

11. In which organizational culture would you be most comfortable as an employee?
12. In which organizational culture would you be most comfortable as a leader?

Conclusion

In recent times, there has been increasing emphasis on the values of democracy, inclusivity and transparency in decision making. This reflects a cultural change in the West towards less hierarchical structures throughout society. Consequently, the leader's role is increasingly viewed as being much more to do with motivating others to achieve the group's aims, and, instead of remaining aloof from the rest of the team, the leader is pivotal in developing a cultural environment where change can be achieved.

To some extent, this style of leadership should come naturally to doctors, since working with others is a key part of their role. Doctors, unlike managing directors of national companies, meet and talk daily with the end users of their services – patients – and they already know that real and lasting improvements depend on good teamwork. It is therefore right and natural that doctors should embrace the challenge of medical leadership, and a doctor's career in leadership starts right at the beginning of medical studies.

References

1. GMC. *Tomorrow's Doctors*. London: General Medical Council, 2009.
2. Kotter JP. *A Force for Change: How Leadership Differs from Management*. New York: Macmillan, 1990.
3. Adair J. *Not Bosses But Leaders: How to Lead the Way to Success* (3rd edn). London: Kogan Page, 2004.
4. Ramsden P. *Learning to Lead in Higher Education*. London: Routledge, 1998.
5. Drucker PF. *On the Profession of Management*. Boston: Harvard Business Review, 2003.

6. Smith R. What doctors and managers can learn from each other. *BMJ* 2003; 326: 610–611.

7. Tooke J. *Aspiring to Excellence: A Report of the Independent Inquiry into Modernising Medical Careers.* London: MMC Inquiry, 2008.

8. Allard J, Bleakley A, Hobbs A, Vinnell T. 'Who's on the team today?' The status of briefing amongst operating theatre practitioners in one UK hospital. *Journal of Interprofessional Care* 2007; 21(2): 189–206.

9. Frank JR (editor). *The CanMEDS 2005 Physician Competency Framework. Better Standards. Better Physicians. Better Care.* Ottawa: The Royal College of Physicians and Surgeons of Canada, 2005.

10. NHS Institute for Innovation and Improvement and Academy of Medical Royal Colleges. *Medical Leadership Competency Framework.* London: NHS Institute for Innovation and Improvement, 2009.

11. Ham C, Dickinson H. *Engaging doctors in leadership: What can we learn from international experience and research evidence?* Coventry: NHS Institute for Innovation and Improvement/Health Services Management Centre. 2008.

12. Sritharan K, Russell G, Fritz Z, Wong D, Rollin M, Dunning J et al. Medical oaths and declarations. *BMJ* 2001; 323: 1440–1441.

13. GMC. *Good Medical Practice.* London: General Medical Council, 2006.

14. GMC. *Management for Doctors.* London: General Medical Council, 2006.

15. Academy of Medical Educators. *Professional Standards.* London: Academy of Medical Educators, 2012.

16. Schwartz RW, Pogge C. Physician leadership: essential skills in a changing environment. *American Journal of Surgery* 2000; 180: 187–192.

17. Bordage G, Foley R, Goldyn S. Skills and attributes of directors of educational programmes. *Medical Education* 2000; 34: 206–210.

18. The Nolan Committee on Standards in Public Life (http://www.public-standards.gov.uk/ Accessed 2 April 2010).

19. Handy, C. *Understanding Organizations.* London: Penguin, 1993.

VII

GETTING THE MOST OUT OF
ASSESSMENT AND EVALUATION

Chapter 23

An Introduction to Assessment

Mohi Eldin Magzoub, Hanan Al Kadri, Ahmed Al Rumayyan, and Cess van der Vleuten

Objectives

The objective of this chapter is to answer the following questions:
- As a student, why should you bother about assessment?
- What is assessment, and how are the common terms used in assessment language defined?
- How is assessment conducted?
- What are the common assessment instruments?
- What are the features of good assessment practice?
- What are the general guidelines for performing well in a test?

Introduction

Assessment is one of the most important activities in education. It comes second to teaching as a role of medical teachers and it comes almost first as a concern for students. Assessment provides evidence and important information on student progress and learning on attaining the required objectives of a course as well as achieving the competencies and outcome of the program. Assessment is always a matter of sampling across a large pool of contents and performance indicators, using certain instruments to gather information. Therefore subjectivity and bias are always introduced. Minimizing bias and making a compromise between what is ideal and feasible is a real challenge for medical educators. Assessment is not only used to make decisions regarding students and provide feedback to them, it is also one important indicator for the whole quality of the educational program. This might be used to improve the curriculum and the ways teachers are teaching as well as the ways students are learning. For this reason, teachers and curriculum planners should start to think about assessment at the early stages of curriculum design when they decide on assessment strategies, principles and instruments.

As a student, why you should bother about assessment?

Assessment will provide an excellent feedback to you and identify gaps and weaknesses in your learning, as well as strengths, which help you make the necessary plans and interventions for improvement.

Assessment is a major drive for learning. The student's goal is to survive the educational program and this can only be achieved through passing tests. This is clear when, for example, the student asks "Will this content be part of the exam?" On the other hand, students become more attentive when the teacher mentions. "This is a very important and essential content." Furthermore, most students do not care when the teacher says "Read this piece of information for your own knowledge and not for your assessment." Teachers are now becoming more aware of these facts and are trying to match the desired learning objectives with assessment. Therefore, knowing how exams are constructed and designed is more likely to assist you in preparing well for the exam.

Assessment is one of the indicators of the quality of a course or program. The results of your exams will be used by program designers to improve your learning as well as the way you are assessed. Having a well-constructed exam based on a review of previous tests will contribute to its being a high-quality exam. This in turn will help in preventing errors and flaws that affect your performance in the test.

In the near future, following your graduation, you will be expected to contribute to the education and training of other health professionals. This contribution may include teaching, supervision and mentoring. You may be also involved in assessment. Acquiring skills and knowledge in assessment during your study is of utmost importance in performing this role. In fact, even during your school life you may participate in assessing your peers and yourself. Furthermore, many schools have introduced medical education as an integral part of their curriculum, which includes assessment.

Assessment is expected to measure changes and progress in gaining knowledge, acquiring skills and modifying attitude. Different instruments are designed to serve this purpose, including a progress test. Continuous and regular assessment of student progress is expected to assist in identifying areas of problems to be averted as well as points of strength to be reinforced.

Fair assessment causes students to have motivation, encouragement and interest in their subject matter. Assessment discriminates between good students with high performance and poor students. On the other hand, if assessment is unfair this will negatively reflect on your commitment and enthusiasm.

Why are students valuable sources for improving any assessment system?

As one of the main stakeholders in your educational program you are also responsible for improving the assessment system through regular feedback. This will be gathered through a questionnaire at the end of the exam and, on some occasions, through qualitative research. Your feedback is of utmost importance in determining the acceptability, feasibility, quality and relevance of your assessment.

Many accreditation bodies are including assessment as one of the most important standards of the educational program. During self-evaluation and external visits of accreditation, your views and opinions about assessment serve as important evidence for the quality of the assessment.

Without your participation, educational research targeting assessment would not be possible. Educational research will provide evidence for improvement.

Summary

Summary of reasons why you should bother about assessment and why you are considered as a valuable source:

1. Assessment is a major drive for learning.
2. Assessment is a source of feedback to students.
3. Understanding the way you are assessed helps you in preparing well for the exam.
4. In the near future, you will be involved as an assessor of health professionals.
5. During your study you may take a role as assessor of yourself as well as your peers.
6. As one of the stakeholders in your educational program, you are involved in evaluating your assessment system through giving direct and indirect feedback.
7. Improving assessment will be reflected in the improvement of the learning process.

What is assessment, and what is the definition of common terms used in assessment language?

In this section of the chapter you will be provided with basic definitions of the common terms used in assessment. Understanding these terms will help you to familiarize yourself with the language of assessment and may improve your feedback about assessment in your school.

- **Assessment**
  Educational assessment is the process of documenting, usually in measurable terms, knowledge, skills, attitudes and beliefs. Assessment can focus on the individual learner, the learning community (class, workshop, or other organized group of learners), the institution, or the educational system as a whole.

- **Reliability**

  Reliability relates to the consistency of an assessment. A reliable assessment is one that consistently achieves the same results with the same (or similar) cohort of students. Various factors affect reliability – including ambiguous questions, too many options within a question paper, vague marking instructions and poorly trained markers.

- **Validity**

  A valid assessment is one that measures what it is intended to measure. For example, it would not be valid to assess surgical skills through a written test alone. Teachers frequently complain that some examinations do not properly assess the curriculum upon which the examination is based; they are, effectively, questioning the validity of the exam.

- **Acceptability**

  A test may be *acceptable* to some of those dealing with it and not to others.[7] The beliefs and attitudes of both examiners and examinees towards assessment may not always be in line with the research and empirical evidence. Therefore, certain assessments may not be acceptable to all.[12] Provision of necessary information and willingness to compromise may increase the commitment of both examiners and examinees.[4] However, if the beliefs, opinions and attitudes of both examiners and examinees are not considered in choosing and designing assessments, the survival of the assessment procedure is threatened.[12]

- **Educational impact**

  The educationally desirable direction that teachers expect the students to follow, conveyed to the student by the assessment, is referred to as *educational impact*. Citing many authors, van der Vleuten points out that the "assessment program has tremendous impact on learners and students to do whatever they are tested on and are not likely to do what they are not tested on."[12] It is true that high validity, reliability and positive educational impact enhance the rigor of an assessment. However, the psychometric properties and educational impact of an assessment should be balanced with the practicability and the cost-effectiveness of using an assessment instrument in a given context, and with its acceptability to people involved in the assessment process.[12]

- **Formative assessment**

  Formative assessment is a reflective process that intends to promote student attainment. It is defined as the bi-directional process between teacher and student to enhance, recognize and respond to the learning.[3] Black and Wiliam[1] consider an assessment 'formative' when the feedback from learning activities is actually used to adapt the teaching to meet the learner's needs.

- **Summative assessment**

  Summative assessment refers to the assessment of the learning and summarizes the development of learners at a particular time. The test aims to summarize learning up to that point. Summative assessment is commonly used to refer to assessment of the educational faculty by its respective supervisor. It is imposed onto the faculty member, and uniformly applied, with the object of measuring all teachers on the same criteria to determine the level of their performance. It is meant to meet the school's or district's needs for teacher accountability and looks to provide remediation for sub-standard performance and also provides grounds for dismissal if necessary.

* Standard settings
  Standard setting refers to the process of establishing one or more cut scores on a test. In some conditions (e.g., licensure and certification testing programs) only a single cut score may be required to create categories such as pass/fail, or allow/deny a license, while in other contexts multiple cut scores on a single test may be required in order to create more than two categories of performance.

Assessment instruments

* Classification of instruments:
  * First, according to what is assessed. Bloom pyramid of level of competencies.
  * Second, according to when it is assessed, such as curricular phases, for instance basic science, clinical assessment, etc., or theoretical, practical and clinical.
  * Third, according to who assesses, for instance, teacher-based, student-based. The classification we use here is according to where it is conducted, and as it is used in previous sections.
* Class-based
  * *Multiple choice questions* (MCQs) make up a test that offers several answers from which the correct one is to be chosen and marked by a tick or cross in a given space. It can normally be handled by computer.
  * *Extended matching items/questions* (EMIs or EMQs) are a written examination format similar to multiple choice questions but with one key difference: it tests knowledge in a far more applied, in depth, sense. It is often used in medical education and other healthcare subject areas to test diagnostic reasoning. Students sitting in to this test have a greater chance of answering incorrectly if they cannot synthesize and apply their knowledge.
  * *MEQs.* An essay is a piece of writing that is often written from an author's *personal* point of view. Essays can consist of a number of elements, including: literary criticism, political manifestos, learned arguments, observations of daily life, recollections, and reflections of the author. The definition of an essay is vague, overlapping with those of an article and a short story. The modified essay question (MEQ) attempts to test problem solving and decision making on the basis of an ongoing family saga, using seven or eight questions to be answered in 90 minutes.
  * *SAQs.* A teacher's primary purpose in giving a short-answer test is to test whether students have a foundation of knowing the material, usually factual.

- Short-answer exam questions (SAQs) generally require the student to remember and reproduce knowledge: for example, it may also require demonstration of understanding of knowledge in questions such as "discuss the role of . . .". Understanding what type of response the examiner wants requires that the student read and analyze the questions carefully. This analysis and accurate interpretation requires a good knowledge of the meaning of *direction words*.
- Hospital-based
  - *Mini-CEX.* Effective workplace assessment practices can provide valuable feedback to trainees at all stages of training, building on strengths and helping to overcome deficiencies. They can allow early identification of those trainees who should be encouraged to consider other career options. The mini Clinical Evaluation Exercise (mini-CEX) was developed to provide reliable and valid assessment of workplace performance for junior doctors in their first years of clinical practice. It has been extensively evaluated in the context of internal medicine and found to be a reliable assessment tool.[9]
  - During a mini-CEX assessment, a trainee is observed performing a defined clinical task during his/her normal working day, assessed against a structure rating form and given feedback. In the original design, 15 minutes of observation was followed by 5 minutes of feedback. Published studies indicate six assessments by a range of supervisors, providing reliable results for a junior doctor.
  - *DOCEE.* Direct observation of medical trainees with actual patients is important for assessment of performance-based clinical skills. Multiple tools for direct observation are available. Direct observation clinical encounter examination (DOCEE), faculty observation of residents while students' are performing clinical skills, is a relatively reliable and valid evaluation of trainees. It is a new multi-faceted approach to faculty development that leads to meaningful changes in rating behaviors and in faculty comfort with its evaluation of clinical skills.
  - *Long case.* In the traditional format, candidates are given ample, uninterrupted and unobserved time to interview and examine a real patient untrained for examinations. Candidates present their findings to the examiner(s) as in an unstructured oral assessment. Although the long case examination is purported to test the integrated interaction between doctor (student) and patient, it is being gradually replaced in undergraduate assessments by more structured examinations, i.e. by objective structured clinical examinations (OSCEs).[5]
  - *Short case.* During a short case test, each candidate spends approximately five minutes with the patient to perform the proper process of a focused task and related signs, then a further approximately 3–5 minutes to formulate a clinical or differential diagnosis. Either one or two examiners observe the encounter and mark the student on a basis of either global rating or a scale of structured marking. The process differs from mini-CEX,

being designed for summative assessment, and it does not include formative feedback.

- Skills lab-based
  - *DOPS.* Performance-based methods such as direct observation of proce-
    dural skills (DOPS) are ideal in the assessment of diagnostic and interven-
    tional procedures.[6] Virtual reality simulator models can help in training
    and assessment of the core curriculum skills and reduce the time required
    for achieving and maintaining competence.
- *Simulation and computer-based simulation.* From its shy beginnings in the 1960s,
  simulation for learning developed through the 1980s and 1990s.[2] Simulation
  has changed the face of medical education and is today widely used for learning and assessment. Simulation-based medical assessment offers medical
  students and healthcare professionals the opportunity to learn from errors
  and thus boost patient safety.[13] With standardized 'patients' and high-fidelity simulators, virtual patient simulation (VPS) systems are fairly recent additions to the spectrum of simulation. VPS can be defined as "an interactive
  computer simulation of real-life clinical scenarios for the purpose of healthcare and medical training, education or assessment,"[8] and as "computer
  programs that simulate real-life clinical scenarios in which the learner acts as
  a healthcare professional, obtaining a history and a physical exam and making
  diagnostic and therapeutic decisions."

  Learning with VPS could lead to better assessment results with different
  examination formats and ultimately provide a transferable skill. We
  believe that transfer of the knowledge and skills to live patients is the ultimate goal of simulation-based medical education, and that it could be
  achieved not just by procedural simulation,[10] but also with VPS learning
  and assessment.
- Community-based
  - *Supervisory visit.* When students are posted in community settings, special
    instruments are required due to the different nature of community-based
    education compared to classroom- or hospital-based learning. Different
    instruments are suggested in the literature, including supervisory visits
    and community members' feedback.

Clinical supervision is considered one of the vital support systems for effective
high-quality health services. The quality of the relationship between supervisor
and provider is the single most important factor for effective supervision. A framework for effective supervision for education and assessment, published in the
AMEE guideline, indicated the following provisions:

(1) effective supervision should be offered in context; supervisors must
    be aware of local postgraduate training bodies' and institutions'
    requirements;
(2) direct supervision, with trainee and supervisor working together and
    observing one another, positively affects patient outcome and trainee
    development;

(3) constructive feedback is essential and should be frequent;

(4) supervision should be structured and there should be regular timetabled meetings. The content of supervision meetings should be agreed and learning objectives determined at the beginning of the supervisory relationship. Supervision contracts can be useful tools and should include detail regarding frequency, duration and content of supervision; appraisal and assessment; learning objectives and any specific requirements;

(5) supervision should include clinical management; teaching and research; management and administration; pastoral care; interpersonal skills; personal development; reflection;

(6) the quality of the supervisory relationship strongly affects the effectiveness of supervision. Specific aspects include continuity over time in the supervisory relationship, that the supervisor controls the product of supervision (there is some suggestion that supervision is only effective when this is the case) and that there is some reflection by both participants. The relationship is partly influenced by the supervisor's commitment to teaching as well as both the attitudes and commitment of supervisor and trainee; and

(7) training for supervisors needs to include some of the following: **understanding teaching, assessment, counseling skills, appraisal, feedback, careers advice, and interpersonal skills.**

- *Community-members feedback.* Interpersonal feedback occurs when one group member shares his or her perceptions of and reactions to another's behavior with that other person. This type of interpersonal exchange provides an opportunity to compare expected with actual behavioral consequences. Thus, group members can, to a great extent, come to see themselves as others do, making possible a kind of independent reality check that is difficult to make alone. Personal growth and therapy groups would appear to provide the ideal setting for the productive exchange of feedback. The interactional nature of the group tends to elicit members' conscious and unconscious behavioral patterns in a manner reflective of behavior outside the group.[11] The elicited behaviors then provide the basis for a meaningful and accurate interpersonal feedback.

Comprehensive assessment

- *Portfolio* was originally used in the domain of business. It was defined as a collection *of* investments all owned by the same individual *or* organization. These investments often include stocks, which are investments in individual businesses; bonds, which are investments in debt that are designed to earn interest; and mutual funds, which are essentially pools *of* money invested by professionals or according to indices. Learning portfolios have been considered as a valuable and effective assessment tool, especially in the fields of education. Learning portfolios comprehensively document learning processes and outcomes and serve as a multi-dimensional assessment.

Features of good assessment practice

1. Comprehensive assessment utilizing a cocktail of assessment tools.
2. Admit subjectivity is inevitable.
3. Regular follow-ups and review of the assessment system.
4. Aligning assessment with learning objectives and educational outcomes.
5. Active involvement of students through regular feedback.
6. Caring about utility rather than the individual psychometric property of each instrument.
7. Regular monitoring and update of the assessment system.
8. Ensure summative assessments are also formative assessments.
9. Use appropriate methods that test meta-cognitive skills.

How to perform well in a test

The following points are just guidelines that may help you in preparing well for your exam. In the following chapters in this book you will find more and specific guidelines on how to perform well in specific instruments such as OSCE, MCQs and other written tests:

1. First, you should review your objectives.
2. Review the learning and assessment strategies of your school.
3. Preparation should match the nature and focus of the instrument.
4. Preparation should be continuous and not at the end of the course.
5. Review previous exams and the feedback you have received from them.
6. Know how your teachers prepare and conduct exams and make positive use of their mistakes in doing so (test-wise student).

References

1. Black, P., and Wiliam, D. (1998). Assessment and classroom learning. *Assess Educ, 5*, 7–74.
2. Bradley, P. (2006). The history of simulation in medical education and possible future directions. *Med Educ, 40*(3), 254–262.
3. Cowie, B., and Bell, B. (1999). A model of formative assessment in science education. *Assess Educ, 6*, 101–116.
4. Crossley, J., Humphris, G., and Jolly, B. (2002). Assessing health professionals. *Med Educ* (36), 800–804.
5. Harden, R.M., and Gleeson, F.A. (1979). Assessment of clinical competence using an objective structured clinical examination (OSCE). *Med Educ, 13*(1), 41–54.
6. Johnson, S., Healey, A., Evans, J., Murphy, M., Crawshaw, M., and Gould, D. (2006). Physical and cognitive task analysis in interventional radiology. *Clin Radiol, 61*, 97–103.
7. Lowry, S. (1993). Trends in health care and their effects on medical education. *BMJ, 306*, 255–258.

8. Masters, K., and Ellaway, R. (2008). e-Learning in medical education. Guide 32, Part 2: Technology, management and design. *Med Teach, 30*(5), 474–489.

9. Norcini, J.J., Blank, L.L., Duffy, F.D., and Fortna, G.S. (2003). The mini-CEX: a method for assessing clinical skills. *Ann Intern Med, 138*(6), 476–481.

10. Park, J., MacRae, H., Musselman, L.J., Rossos, P., Hamstra, S.J., Wolman, S., et al. (2007). Randomized controlled trial of virtual reality simulator training: Transfer to live patients. *Am J Surg, 194*(2), 205–211.

11. Stoller, F.H. (1972). New perspectives on encounter groups. In: L.N. Solomon and B. Berzon (Eds.), *Use of Videotape Feedback* (pp. 233–244). San Francisco: Jossey-Bass.

12. van der Vleuten, C.P. (1996). The assessment of professional competence: Development, research and practical implication. *Adv Health Sci, 1*(1), 41–67.

13. Ziv, A., Ben-David, S., and Ziv, M. (2005). Simulation based medical education: an opportunity to learn from errors. *Med Teach, 27*(3), 193–199.

Chapter 24

Student Guidelines for a Written Test

Andleeb Arshad

Objectives

By the end of this chapter, students will be able to:
• Plan effectively, write appropriately, and revise properly as they attempt a written exam.

Introduction

Different forms of written exam questions include long essays, short essays, modified essays, etc. This chapter will introduce briefly the different types of written exam questions and will then discuss general guidelines that are applicable to all of these different forms in detail. An understanding of written exam questions, and guidelines on attempting to answer them, will surely improve exam performance.

Forms of written exam questions

• *Long essay questions* usually ask for a response of 200 to 1000 words. They mostly require higher levels of cognitive activity such as critiquing, designing, evaluating, exemplifying, solving, comparing, and contrasting. Middle-level cognitive activities such as explaining, describing, narrating, and commenting, however, are also often required in long essay questions. These questions intend to assess the depth of understanding of a topic. Assignments constitute an even longer version of essays, and students get at least a couple of weeks to write them. Assignments usually require a literature review and a bibliography.
• *Short essay questions* usually ask for a response of less than 150 words. They mostly require middle and lower levels of cognitive activity such as describing, analyzing, listing, commenting, and defining. These questions intend to assess the breadth of a student's knowledge base.

- *Modified essay questions* are a series of seven to ten questions that are linked to a case or scenario which is progressively released. These questions usually require only a couple of words or sentences as a response. A trigger is released and a couple of questions follow. More questions are posed with the release of new pieces of information. Modified essay questions are a very effective tool to assess problem-solving.

General guidelines

The skill of writing is to create a context in which other people can think. (Edwin Schlossberg)

Writing for an exam is not only about writing; it is about reading, thinking, organizing, writing and then revising. Here are some guidelines that are applicable to any form of written exam question:

A. *Reading the question*
   First of all, read the question carefully at least twice before trying to answer it. Identify what the question is asking for. It is a good idea to underline or highlight important keywords in the question. A minor misinterpretation of the question can lead to a very false answer, even though you may work very hard on answering it. A question may ask you to list a few facts, to provide a definition, an explanation, an example, a solution, a critique or a synthesis. The words what, why, where, when and how in a question provide you with important directions. Clearly demarcate the requirements of the question. After reading the question you should know what is required and, more importantly, what is not required. Many exams notify the total achievable scores associated with the question, which helps you allocate appropriate time to spend on that question.[1] If you find a question difficult, it is advisable to leave it for the end of the exam, though you also have to ensure that you save sufficient time for it.

B. *Thinking and organizing*
   Most of the questions are not fact-seeking. Many questions require your own synthesis. Your thinking capabilities matter more than your ability to reproduce from memory. Your ability to express yourself in written form matters much.

   Secondly, think with concentration and organize your thoughts before attempting to write an answer. Use, if possible and if time permits you, the spider-web, the fish-bone or any other technique that you may know to brainstorm on the question and then to streamline your thoughts.[2] As a result of your brainstorming you should also be able to get to the keywords and key phrases that you would be using in your answer. Generally there is extra space available on your answer sheet. Use enough of it for draft scribbling.

While prioritizing and organizing your thoughts, keep the requirements of the question always in your mind. If you include things that are not required in the question, you can easily end up irritating the assessor. Examiners scan quickly through answers.[3] Initiatory and closing sentences, as well as keywords in the text, are hence very important. Setting a context for your answer is important but it should have an appropriate relative length. Assessors usually praise direct and bold attempts in an answer.[1,4] Make sure that you answer the question directly, at least by the second line of your answer. A long introduction can bore the assessor and have an adverse effect on the quality of your answer.

For example, if a question asks you to provide an example related to a phenomenon, do not spend time on defining or critiquing on the phenomenon. Your definition may be excellent or your critique on the phenomenon very intellectual, but they do not serve the requirements. Start directly with providing an example of the phenomenon, while ensuring that the example is an appropriate representation of it. After giving the example, you can use a couple of sentences to discuss how your given example represents the phenomenon.

C. *Writing the response*

When it comes to writing, try using short sentences. The sentences should connect and there should be a smooth flow of ideas.[3] Avoid spelling and grammatical mistakes. Be very clear and to the point. Your handwriting should be legible. Writing short but clear sentences is far more important than writing long but vague ones. Using bullets in your answer increases its effectiveness. Synthesis-level questions, however, may not be suited for the bullets format. Provide suitable headings if required. For example, if a question requires pros and cons of an idea, provide a heading for the pros as you write them and similarly a heading for the cons. Highlighting keywords in your answer may increase its readability. As a part of your preparation, writing skills can be improved by answering exam practice questions.

The intellectual richness of your answer is, of course, very important. It can only be attained by your understanding of the subject.[5] The choice of right words at right places provides an insight into your knowledge of the content. Let your knowledge be boldly visible in your answer. Your assessor will most probably be an expert on the subject. Therefore, do not shy away from using technical words of the subject if you are comfortable with them. For example, words like *assimilation, anabolism* and *catabolism* are very familiar to physiologists and they will never be considered as complex words in writings related to physiology.

D. *Revising*

Your job is not over just when you complete writing your answer. You need to revise it at least once. You must be able to identify spelling mistakes and also see if you can improve the text of your answer. It is advisable that you take a small break before revising your question. This break may allow you to bring the entire text of your answer to mind and help you to effectively critique your answer as you revise it. An effective revision will surely purge your answer of its shortcomings and help you gain better results.

> A scrupulous writer, in every sentence that he writes, will ask himself at least four questions, thus: 1. What am I trying to say? 2. What words will express it? 3. What image or idiom will make it clearer? 4. Is this image fresh enough to have an effect? (George Orwell)

Summary

Re-emphasizing what was stated earlier, writing for an exam is not only about writing – it is about reading, thinking, organizing, writing, and then revising. Read the question carefully, spare time to think and organize your writing. Write in small connected sentences and ensure that spellings and grammar are correct. Provide a small break and then revise your writing. Practicing writing in similar situations will lead to improvement.

References

1. Dernbach JC. *Writing Essay Exams to Succeed (Not Just to Survive)*, 2nd edition. Aspen, 2006.
2. Kaye S. *Writing under Pressure: The Quick Writing Process.* Oxford University Press, 1990.
3. The Writing Center, University of North Carolina at Chapel Hill (updated 2007). Available from: http://www.unc.edu/depts/wcweb/handouts/essay-exams.html
4. Center for Teaching Excellence, University of Wisconsin. Available from: http://www.uwec.edu/geography/ivogeler/essay.html
5. Coles M, White C, Brown P. *Learning to Learn: Student activities for developing work, study, and exam-writing skills.* Pembroke, 2003.

Chapter 25

Strategies for Performing Well in Multiple-choice Question Tests

Susan Case

Objectives

By the end of this chapter, you will be able to:
- Understand the structure of well-constructed multiple-choice questions.
- Understand the importance of the purpose of the exam, and of reading any published material about the exam, including sample test questions.
- Appreciate the tricks to use in guessing when you do not know the correct answer, but understand that tricks will not help in answering well-constructed questions.
- Know the approaches for use in answering well-constructed questions.
- Recognize that careful, consistent studying is the best way to prepare for a test.

Introduction

Many question formats are used to assess students' knowledge and their ability to apply that knowledge, but none is more commonly used than the multiple-choice format.

Multiple-choice questions (MCQs) are sometimes viewed as testing only memorization of isolated facts and as being less realistic in their relationship to the actual practice of medicine than other forms of assessment such as direct observation of patient interactions or even standardized patient examinations. However, research in the field of study concerned with the science of educational testing, known as psychometrics, has shown that multiple-choice questions have many advantages over other examination formats. Where the goal is to measure knowledge, or ability to apply that knowledge to a variety of scenarios or cases, the multiple-choice format is unsurpassed in content coverage as well as in grading accuracy and consistency. For large-scale standardized testing programs, multiple-choice tests produce equated scores that retain their meaning over time and across test administration dates, regardless of fluctuations in test difficulty or examinee proficiency; for example, an equated score of 200 indicates the same level of performance across time, regardless of what particular set of questions

were in the test or whether the particular group of examinees performed especially well or poorly.

Regardless of the testing format, poorly written questions may test only knowledge of isolated facts; they may contain ambiguous language; they may contain
unrealistic scenarios. These flaws, which are seen across testing formats, are
construction-related flaws rather than inherent drawbacks associated uniquely
with multiple-choice questions. Poorly crafted exam questions, whether they are
multiple-choice questions, essays, or oral interview questions, fail to assess what is
intended and fail to encourage the learning that is desired. In other words, the particular question format is not as important as the skill and sophistication with which
the questions are crafted and the exam as a whole is assembled and graded.

This chapter begins with some background information about the structure of
multiple-choice questions as well as a description of well-formatted and poorly
formatted questions. It then provides advice on how to answer these questions.

Summary

To measure knowledge or ability to apply that knowledge to a variety of scenarios or cases, the multiple-choice format has several distinct advantages over other testing formats, most notably in content
coverage, grading accuracy and grading consistency. Poor quality
questions are seen across testing formats; they are construction-related flaws rather than inherent drawbacks associated uniquely with
multiple-choice questions.

Structure of multiple-choice questions

High-quality multiple-choice questions contain three components:

- the stem (a scenario or vignette setting up the question);
- the lead-in (the question); and
- the options (answer choices, typically labeled A, B, C etc.).

The stem or vignette

The stem of a well-constructed question is written in concise, standard language.
While the well-constructed stem may include some superfluous information, it
avoids introducing facts intended to trick examinees. Multiple-choice stems should
set up straightforward, understandable problems; the challenge for examinees
should be in determining the correct answer, not in trying to understand the scenario. As discussed more fully below, the difficulty of a multiple-choice question
is best determined by the sophistication and plausibility of the options, not by the
complexity of the stem.

The stems used for patient vignettes often follow the structure outlined below
in the order indicated. This example is drawn from the National Board of Medical

Examiners website publication, available for download at no cost from www. nbme.org.[1]

1. Age, gender (e.g., A 45 year-old man)
2. Site of care (e.g., comes to the emergency department)
3. Presenting complaint (e.g., with a headache)
4. Duration (that has continued for 2 days.)
5. Patient history with family history if relevant
6. Physical findings

Depending on the question, the above elements could be followed by additional facts such as the results of diagnostic studies, initial treatment, and subsequent findings.

The lead-in

The lead-in is the component of the MCQ that frames the examinees' task. Well-constructed questions include a focused lead-in that poses a single, specific task and that naturally flows into a set of homogeneous options.
Consider the following lead-ins:

• Poor example: Given the above facts, which of the following statements is true?
• Good example: Given the above facts, what is the most likely diagnosis?

The lead-in of the poor example is not focused. It might easily lead to a set of heterogeneous options that are impossible to rank-order, making it impossible to decide which the best response is. In contrast, the second lead-in is so specific that a knowledgeable examinee could generate an answer without even looking at the options. The good example demonstrates the level of specificity that is required for a well-crafted question.

Each well-constructed lead-in controls the task demanded of the examinees in answering that question, and requires the examinee to demonstrate a particular skill that is deemed important (e.g., determining the most likely diagnosis; determining the underlying cause of the problem). Note that the examinee should be able to pose an answer to the question without looking at the options. In medicine, particularly in the clinical sciences, the tasks often are grouped into categories similar to those used by the United States Medical Licensing Examination (USMLE) Step 2: Health and Health Maintenance; Mechanisms of Disease; Diagnosis; and Treatment. Sample lead-ins include:
[For the patient described above]

• What is most likely to have prevented this condition?
• What is the most likely explanation of these findings?
• What is the most likely diagnosis?
• What is the most appropriate pharmacotherapy?

The options

Options are the answer choices. The correct option is called the *answer key*, while the incorrect options are called *distractors*. There is no rule restricting the number of options: a larger number of options reduces the success of random guessing.

Well-constructed option lists adhere to the following guidelines:

1. Options should be short, single words or very short phrases, and should not be long or complicated.
2. Options should not include vague frequency terms such as rarely and usually.
3. Options should not include absolute terms such as always and never.
4. Options should be parallel in terms of language.
5. Options should be of similar length and complexity.
6. Options should be listed in a logical order, or in alphabetical order.
7. Options should not include the phrases "none of the above" or "all of the above."
8. Options should not present any additional facts or conditions beyond what was included in the vignette (e.g., "Yes, if the patient also has a headache . . .")

The options are the question writer's main tool in controlling the difficulty of a multiple-choice question. As an illustration, consider the difference in difficulty between the two sets of options proposed below.

Comparison of option sets that control the difficulty of the test questions

Which of the following countries has the largest population?

Easy option set:
(A) Argentina
(B) Greenland
(C) Netherlands
(D) Saudi Arabia
(E) United States

Difficult option set:
(A) Bangladesh
(B) Brazil
(C) Indonesia
(D) Pakistan
(E) United States

Summary

Well-constructed multiple-choice questions include a well-written stem that clearly and concisely establishes the facts necessary to answer the question; a lead-in that presents a single focused task; and a set of options that are single words or very short phrases.

How to answer multiple-choice questions

Some of you may have encountered numerous multiple-choice questions in your classes; for others, this is a new testing format. For poorly constructed multiple-choice questions that fail to follow the guidelines shown above, there are certain tricks that may increase your chances of guessing the correct answer. Please note that these tricks do not work on well-constructed questions, including questions developed for high-stakes examinations by professional test development agencies, but they may help you a bit with some other tests.

With poorly constructed questions, if you have no idea which answer is correct, you can try the following tricks. Before guessing among all the options that are listed, first eliminate any you know are incorrect. Also, be sure there is no scoring penalty for guessing wrongly – scoring penalties for guessing are rarely used in the US, but are sometimes used elsewhere.

When you do not know the correct answer and have to guess, consider trying one of these tricks:

Tricks for use in answering poorly constructed questions

1. Choose the option with general frequency terms (e.g. often, usually) rather than the option with absolute terms (e.g. always, never).
2. Choose "all of the above," especially if you know two of the choices are correct.
3. Choose B or C, rather than A or D; if the options are numerical values, select the middle value.
4. Do not choose "none of the above," because this option is often added by teachers who cannot think of another choice.
5. Do not choose the funny option; instructors sometimes throw in funny options just to make you feel at ease.
6. Choose an option that follows logically and grammatically from the lead-in. If the lead-in asks for the most appropriate laboratory test, do not select an option that is not a laboratory test. If one of the options does not follow grammatically from the lead-in, do not choose that option. When creating exams, teachers pay more attention to the correct answer than to the incorrect ones, and are less likely to make a mistake with the correct answer.
7. Choose the longest option if one option stands out as being significantly longer than the others, because the instructor tends to include more careful language and more qualifying terms in the correct answer to ensure that it is absolutely correct.
8. Choose the option that repeats key words from the stem.
9. Choose the more general option rather than the more specific one.
10. If the option list includes a pair of opposites, one of them is probably correct.
11. If a subset of the options includes all the logical possibilities, one of these is likely to be correct. For example, if A, B and C are "increases," "decreases" and "remains the same," any additional unrelated options are unlikely to be correct.

For well-constructed questions, there are no tricks that will provide you with any advantage. For tests including well-constructed questions, there is no substitute for studying the material and learning it thoroughly. Please note that well-constructed questions are not designed to trick the knowledgeable examinee. They are typically written and reviewed several times by groups of content experts and test development experts to ensure that they are focused on important issues, and that the structure of the question is developed to ensure that those who have the appropriate knowledge will answer the question correctly.

Approaches for use in answering well-constructed questions

1. Read the vignette or stem carefully; assume all the information is there for a reason.
2. The more common diagnoses, the more common laboratory tests, the less invasive treatments and the more critically important issues are more likely to be correct than the infrequent, less important, more esoteric choices. Choose the simple interpretation: do not make the question more complex than it really is.
3. If you are deciding between two possible answers, ask yourself how the two answers differ. Then look at the question again and decide how that difference is important for the question.
4. Do not hesitate to reconsider your answer choice; first answers are not always the best choice.
5. Do not worry about the sequence of letters that you put down as correct answers. These tests are often constructed with questions in random order, without consideration of which option is correct (for example, there might be a series of questions where the correct answer to each of them is 'A'). Across the entire test, the number of questions with each letter possibility as the correct answer is likely to be nearly equal, but for any short sequence of questions, anything is possible.

For all tests, consider the following guidelines:

1. Begin studying early and often. Begin by studying in one direction and then studying again from a different perspective (e.g., first by organ system, then by presenting complaint, such as headache, abdominal pain).
2. Allow time for repeated reviews; focus on key concepts. Look for similarities and differences among similar entities such as diseases presenting in a similar fashion, or among underlying causes of disease, or among pharmacological options.
3. Be prepared physically and mentally (e.g., get enough rest, eat well, dress in layers to avoid being too hot or too cold).
4. Determine how much time you have per question; pace yourself by answering a specific number of questions every 15 minutes, every 30 minutes, every hour. Do not spend too much time on any one question.

5. Answer every question; do not skip a question unless you are sure you will be able to return to it.
6. Do not let one question influence the next. Consider each question in isolation.
7. Maintain your concentration.

Before sitting for a standardized test such as USMLE:

1. Read the website carefully to become familiar with the test material as well as the rules and regulations.
2. Think about the purpose of the test and the implication of that purpose. The purpose statement is typically provided to question writers and is used to determine whether a question should be included in the test. For example, tests used for general licensure purposes are generally focused on the knowledge and skills required for the initial practice of medicine, not those that might be expected of senior practitioners or specialists. On the other hand, if the purpose of the test is to assess knowledge of material from a particular course, the questions are likely to be more narrow in scope and more focused on what was taught in that course.
3. Review sample questions provided by the testing program in advance. There are several strategies that might make the test easier for you; try these in advance with the sample questions and decide which is best. First, try to cover up the options for each question and generate an answer in your mind before you look at the options. An alternative approach is to read the lead-in and the options before reading the vignette. Some test takers find that one of these two approaches works better for them.

Conclusion
There are many strategies for maximizing your success in multiple-choice exams. Of course, the best way to improve your chances is to study carefully before the exam. There is no good substitute for knowing the right answer. The right tricks offered are unlikely to be useful with well-constructed test questions, and should in no way be considered as substitutes for learning the material.

Reference
1. Case SM, Swanson DB. *Constructing Written Test Questions for the Basic and Clinical Sciences*, 3rd edition. Philadelphia, PA: National Board of Medical Examiners; 2001.

Chapter 26

Preparing for OSCE

James Ware

Objectives

- To familiarize students with the importance of OSCE and how it will contribute to their success during their undergraduate training.
- To disseminate the many positive attributes of OSCE to medical students.
- To prepare medical students for this type of examination format.

Introduction

OSCE is the acronym for Objective Structure Clinical Examination, first described in 1975 by Ronald Harden, an eminent medical educator from Dundee, UK. The OSCE is widely used at all stages in many modern medical programs, and so familiarity with this examining process is important and will contribute to students' success during their undergraduate training. Today, there are books available describing the skills and competencies needed and at the end of this chapter there is a short bibliography. This examination has been developed because of the dissatisfaction with the traditional long case, although much has been changed for this examination. The OSCE has many positive attributes, of which those that are of interest to a medical student are given below:

- All candidates take the same examination.
- The same criteria are rigorously applied to test the same competency or skill for all candidates.
- Many different skills, competencies and procedures are tested in one OSCE.
- The OSCE performs better psychometrically.[1]

Furthermore, from the perspective of a medical student faced with the prospect of being examined in an OSCE, there is a certain predictability which can be used

---

[1] Psychometrics is the field of study concerned with the theory and technique of educational and psychological measurement.

to provide better preparation for this examination format, and this is the focus for this chapter. Briefly, these student-friendly criteria can be listed as follows:

- The skills, competencies and procedures are known in advance.
- Often special clinical teaching is based on the OSCE format[2] and delivered in a skills lab.
- Students can practice in small groups in the specific areas they need to do so.
- Tasks required from candidates are specific and circumscribed, leaving less room for error or misunderstanding.
- The division of marks is usually given along with clear written instructions at every station.
- Many schools deliver a formative OSCE for exam familiarization and as part of the assessment program.
- The component sequence of specific skills is standardized.
- The variety of tasks is finite and to some extent predictable.

Many tasks are performed with simulated patients. A simulated patient (SP) is someone who has received training appropriate for their role – for example, at a station examining the visual fields, the SP may say he cannot see in some part of the normal visual field, thereby simulating a specific lesion which can then be diagnosed and explained. A so-called non-standardized patient, who is a *real patient*, could also be used for this particular examination, but they might have difficulty coping with more than 15–20 candidates carrying out the same examination. Examples of what a non-standardized patient cannot be used for might be *the physical examination skills to detect and confirm ascites or perform CPR*. Alternatively, mannequins can be used for many forms of physical examination, skills and procedures. In other words, simulations are frequently used in an OSCE.

Finally, the OSCE employs fixed time intervals for every station, usually well known in your own medical school. Remember that the more tasks to be tested, the shorter will be the timeframe – usually not less than five minutes. The time constraint for each station limits the nature of any given task, making most tasks more predictable; for example, history taking is usually focused and physical examinations are limited to one system. Despite this, you may be surprised, but if you remember what the OSCE is being used for, say a graduating examination before continuing to be an intern, those tasks will still be predictable. Below are some examples of stations that may not have been introduced in your school, but might be in the future:

- Information given over the telephone about a patient to a relative, in this case the examiner.
- Filling in forms correctly.
- Putting together equipment, for example to measure the central venous pressure.

---

2 Braceau C et al., Acad Med. 2002, Sep; 77(9): 932.

- Taking an ECG or measuring lung function, both of which could be with a non-standardized patient.
- Performing a local anesthesia using simulated skin.
- Suturing simulated skin held in a jig.
- Writing a referral letter.
- Examining multiple silicon breast simulations.

Any intern will tell you that these are some of the tasks that they do on a regular basis. Clearly there is a network that will provide all the information you need about those stations and tasks that have already been used in your school. Bear in mind that it takes time to develop new stations, so it is unlikely that you would be confronted with more than one or two that seem unfamiliar in any OSCE that you have prepared for. Below is an example of a duplex station – station A followed by station B:

A. At this five-minute station, a focused history is taken from an SP; the station is not observed and your efforts will receive no marks.
B. The following station instructions say that you must now write a referral letter to the appropriate hospital specialist, named Professor Smith. The candidate's letter would now receive marks for the station.

It now appears that any skills or competencies may be asked of you. A little common sense and local knowledge will serve you well. Most intimate examinations will not be carried out with either an SP or a non-standardized patient. However, you may be asked to use a mannequin. If your skills lab does not have these models you might reasonably exclude that task.

Do not forget those small tasks that are performed so many times that you might not pay any attention to the actual skills required, or indeed have any knowledge of the details, such as which fluids are used. Below is a list of some commonly performed tasks that are seldom examined:

- Hand washing.
- Putting on a theater gown and mask.
- Inserting a naso-gastric tube onto a mannequin.
- Giving instructions concerning IV fluid administration and monitoring to a nurse, who will be the examiner.
- Writing a prescription on a prescription pad.
- Opening a sterile pack.
- Weighing a patient in their hospital bed; this requires such a bed to be available.

Do not forget to wash your hands or use spirit wipes after examining a patient, even if you wore gloves for the physical examination. Forgetting this simple task may lose you marks.

Generic station skills

Except for unmanned stations, usually reserved for X-ray interpretation, or any other skill that may be tested without being observed or requires an SP, the candidate will require a set of well-practiced skills, particularly so as not to waste time at the station. These can be summarized as follows:

- Introduce yourself to the examiner, SP, or non-standardized patient, if used.
- Explain to the SP what you are about to do and how they will assist you in the examination; delivering details in layman's language needs practice.
- Deliver a commentary about what you are doing, and why, if asked to do so.
- Avoid fishing for prompts, which will almost inevitably lose you marks.
- Show empathy towards patients, simulated or otherwise, and thank your patient when you have finished.
- Equip yourself with essential equipment; this will be a plus if used correctly – for example, measuring chest expansion with your tape measure. Although such equipment is usually provided at the station, it will leave a positive impression if you have your own.

Pediatrics, obstetrics, gynecology, psychiatry and emergency medicine

Originally, OSCE was most commonly used in medicine, spreading rapidly to surgery, and today it is used in all clinical disciplines. For each, there is a set of special skills that a graduating doctor should master. Clearly, there are overlapping skills and competencies *per se*, but with a specialist's detail. Usually, these specialties issue comprehensive lists that should be carefully studied and today many of these departments hold skills lab sessions of their own. The same preparation is required for each individually and should include the following:

- Obtain a list of tasks from previous editions of the specialty OSCEs.
- Compare the known OSCE tasks with the list provided by the specialty.
- Prepare with a small group of colleagues who will rate the demonstrations and give invaluable feedback.
- Ensure that you are familiar with any special equipment which should be held in the skills lab store and available for practice.

Practice in small groups

The resources provided at different medical schools will vary, such as well-equipped skills labs that are open all the time, even when teaching is not scheduled or OSCEs are not taking place. This is the best place to practice. However, some schools using OSCEs in their assessments do not have a dedicated skills lab or may have one that is not fully equipped. Nevertheless, whatever facility your school has to offer, the best way to prepare for an OSCE is to form your own small group and practice together. Everyone will need to do a little homework.

- Each member constructs his/her one station against an agreed blueprint.[3]
- For each station, a set of marking criteria is worked out – keep it simple.
- Check the station against the relevant teaching or study resources.
- If the equipment is available, everyone does their own theoretical preparation, exam sequences, history-taking headings and/or details of procedural tasks.

Set aside one afternoon for this exercise and take turns to be first at a station. One male will usually need to volunteer as the SP, if required, in rotation. Each student will demonstrate his/her skills while the others mark according to the schema used. The station time is strictly adhered to, say five to seven minutes. If a checklist approach has been used, very soon the true method of marking will become apparent. An example of a physical examination, indicating peripheral arterial disease, is given below as:

- Introductions, 1 or zero
- Explanations, 1 or zero
- Inspection for hair distribution, 1 or zero
- Inspection for skin color, 1 or zero
- Testing for skin temperature, 1 or zero
- Others, 1 or zero

It will soon become apparent that this approach for marking cannot discriminate between something done well in a credible way and a demonstration done with little credibility. Indeed, there are reports in the literature showing that students can perform as well as specialist residents when the tick-box approach to marking is used.[4] Instead, what is called a global rating scale gives better discrimination, as shown below:

Instructions and explanation prior to the physical examination (2 marks)

2.0/2.0	Polite introduction and accurate explanations with all details.
1.5/2.0	Minor deficiencies, forgetting to ask the patient to let the candidate know if the patient experiences discomfort or pain.
1.0/2.0	Errors or omissions, such as forgetting to mention a comparison between left and right side.
0.5/2.0	Despite significant prompting, is unable to give a credible demonstration.
0.0/2.0	Unable to carry out this task.

---

[3] Examiners use test blueprints to ensure that all the necessary tasks are included in the examination according to a pre-determined representative sampling scheme.
[4] Petrusa ER et al., *Am J Med*. 1987, Jul; 83(1): 34–42.

Immediately after this method of marking is used it will force the participants to increase the care and skills demonstrated. This is the method used at most OSCE stations with observer-examiners. For example, percussion which is neither spaced nor placed correctly or gives a reasonably resonating note is rated downwards. In other words, the observer-examiner must be convinced that the candidate will get value from his/her examination skills.

Another benefit will come out of this exercise. For those who have not yet mastered a logical sequence, others will contribute to improve this deficiency. Also, if you only practice on your own in front of a mirror, you may use medical jargon without noticing while explaining to the non-existent patient what you are going to do. Real patients do not know what percussion and auscultation are. Feedback given by colleagues will correct these minor, but important, errors.

Miscellaneous

The way each medical school runs its own OSCE will vary and every potential candidate must find out the details that should be available to examinees. Being unaware of these arrangements may lead to unnecessary loss of marks. Below is a checklist of 'must-know' information so that the final preparations can factor this information in and reduce tension caused by the unknown:

- How long is each station? Usually five minutes, but it can be seven to ten, depending on the number of stations.
- If a bell ring system is used, make sure you understand what the bell ring means.
- Are the candidates provided with an OSCE book in which instructions for each station are given and answers at unmanned stations written?
- Some schools provide a map to show where the stations are placed. If not in one exam hall, arrows will be placed on the floor to indicate the flow and direction of movement from station to station.
- If printed, self-adhesive labels are provided with candidates' names and IDs, these should always be checked to see that they are correct.
- Each station has a sign stating the OSCE station number. However, if in doubt, this should be double-checked.
- Most schools place a rest station at an interval of approximately 5–6 stations. If an OSCE book is provided, this can be an opportunity to read the instructions for the further 4–5 stations.
- Present yourself in a clean white coat, suitably trimmed hair, smart clothes and polished shoes. Female medical candidates should avoid fashion accessories and not wear shoes with more than an approximate one-inch heel and well polished. Appear ready to be the professional that you are being examined for.
- Remember to take your stethoscope, a tape measure, a tendon hammer if needed and a small torch with new batteries.

Conclusion

It is impossible to be all conclusive. Today, so much has been written about OSCE that it is worthwhile investing in one good textbook on the subject. Several suggestions are given and some are highly recommended; see below. In these books are many examples of stations and how to make the most of your skills, and a website constructed by students for students.

Reading

1. Burton NL, Birdi K, 2006. *Clinical skills for OSCEs*, second edition. Informa Healthcare, UK. May be ordered online, but consult www.tandf.co.uk/medicine
2. Byrne G, Hill J, Dornan T, O'Neill P, 2007. *Core clinical skills for OSCEs in surgery*. Churchill Livingston, Elsevier. May be ordered online, www.elsevier.com
3. Dornan T, O'Neill P, 2006. *Core clinical skills for OSCEs in medicine*. Churchill Livingston, Elsevier. May be ordered online, www.elsevier.com
4. Bhangu, 2008. *Crash course: OSCEs in medicine and surgery*. Churchill Livingston, Elsevier. May be ordered online, www.elsevier.com
5. Hurley, 2005. *OSCE Clinical Skills Handbook*. Elsevier. May be ordered online, www.elsevier.com   http://www.oscehome.com/

Summary

- Get a list of the previous stations.
- Have the list of tasks mastered.
- Read the local OSCE rules.
- Practice for mastery.
- Understand the marking system.
- Check out what is in the skills lab store.

Chapter 27

Student Portfolios

Nadia Al Attas

Objectives

After reading this chapter, you will be able to answer the questions:
- What is a student portfolio?
- What educational principles do student portfolios incorporate?
- What are the benefits of the portfolio as an assessment tool?
- What does educational research conclude regarding the effects of portfolios on learning?

Introduction

The assessment of student performance is an essential part of educational programs necessary to evaluate progress of knowledge and acquisition of skills for both summative and formative purposes. Assessment is important in determining *summative* decisions such as educational promotion or passing to the next academic level, and also has a *formative* value for assessing students' current standings and identifying strengths and areas for improvement.[1]

Students experience many internal and external stressors that influence how they perform on exams. Making decisions of competence, especially in medical education, requires a comprehensive and multi-step approach to assessing progress in knowledge, skills and professional behavior which cannot always be achieved by any single assessment method.[2]

Additionally, despite the awareness that assessment tools can and should advance learning (i.e. formative value), often this aspect is missed or overlooked.[3]

Student portfolios have been introduced and promoted internationally in health professional education over the past three decades as a tool capable of bridging obvious gaps in assessment programs.[4-7]

So what do student portfolios add to an already long list of assessment methods? Should all curricula incorporate portfolios in student assessment programs?

This chapter will briefly explore what is meant by a student portfolio, identify its educational and assessment value, and finally report on what current research has concluded on implementing this assessment method.

What is a student portfolio?

Unlike other forms of assessment, portfolios are *student-developed* documents that incorporate reflection on their educational performance as well as self-selected evidence of learning progress that is collected from multiple sources.[7] A portfolio is both a learning tool and an assessment method used to promote the achievement of knowledge, skills and professional behavior, and is unique in its ability to document educational performance trends over time (longitudinal assessment).[8] It is a flexible instrument that can be tailored to serve the identified needs of any program such as clinical knowledge and patient care issues,[9] personal and professional development,[10] or a combination of outcome competencies the students are expected to obtain.[11] Recent years have seen the shift from paper-based portfolios to electronic or web-based formats.[4, 12] Faculties have a responsibility to structure the portfolio program by determining objectives, content requirements and assessment guidelines on the basis of needs and available resources.[13] For example, assessment programs that use MCQs, OSCEs and clinical exam formats to adequately measure knowledge and skills acquisition may consider incorporating portfolios to address gaps in assessing personal and professional development skills such as critical reflection, management, leadership and teamwork. With the recent trend towards competency-based education, the robustness of portfolios has provided a valuable method to reliably assess competencies that are difficult to measure by more traditional assessment methods.[7, 8, 11]

Portfolio programs have been implemented for undergraduate students,[10,14] postgraduate trainees[15] and the teaching faculty.[16, 17] Mentors guide the reflective process, help students identify learning goals and provide feedback on reflection and progress.[18] In some settings, portfolios have replaced the final summative assessment methods to inform decisions on whether students pass or fail their medical training.[11, 19]

What educational principles do student portfolios incorporate?

Assessment strategies need to be well aligned with educational principles of medical curricula[8] in order to enhance the learning process, promote active self-directed learning and incorporate critical reflection as an important aspect of student development.

- *Assessment should enhance student learning processes:*
  It is well established that assessment drives learning as students are known to focus efforts on what is expected to be assessed.[1] In order to promote learning, portfolio assessment should incorporate both summative and formative components.[14] The development of clear assessment guidelines with the integration of mentors and the use of constructive feedback is used to enhance the learning value of portfolios.[11]

- *Assessment should promote active self-directed learning:*
  Current thinking in medical education focuses on principles of active knowledge construction,[20] learning through collaboration and a process of sharing and discussing,[20, 21] as well as receiving appropriate guidance and constructive feedback.[22]

  Portfolios have been shown to promote active, meaningful and self-directed learning[5,11] in addition to allowing student creativity and self-expression.[23] Students engage in collaborative learning with mentors and are able to use guidance and feedback to identify their own needs and devise necessary action plans.[18]

- *Assessment should incorporate critical reflection as an important aspect of learning:*
  Learning to reflect on personal performance is a skill that initially requires sufficient guidance and feedback to stimulate the development of reflective practice in students. Once this is established, learning from experiences can support professional development.[14] In order to graduate reflective practitioners, a process is needed where students are "rewarded for identifying gaps in their abilities and developing effective ways to correct those gaps".[11, p. 494] Portfolios can foster reflective practice through mentor support in an open, non-judgmental setting where students are guided on what and how they should reflect.[6]

What are the benefits of the portfolio as an assessment tool?

- A holistic assessment approach able to assess educational competencies and a broad spectrum of knowledge, skills and professional behavior including critical reflection.[5, 18]
- A flexible tool that can assess different educational levels using different formats and objectives while allowing for student creativity.[18]
- A longitudinal assessment method able to assess performance trends over time, providing an overall appreciation of performance rather than a single "snapshot" view.[1, 24]
- An assessment method with opportunities to reflect on experiences and benefit from mentor feedback.[11]
- A method that incorporates triangulation of data by gathering educational evidence from multiple sources to establish that a student has achieved or shown progress in the portfolio objectives,[11] and to improve assessor judgments on decisions of student competence.[18 ,24]

What does educational research conclude regarding effects of portfolios on learning?

A recent systematic review identified that most portfolio programs in medical schools are conducted during the clinical phase, are compulsory, include general guidelines, combine student reflection and gathering of evidence, include formative and summative assessments and are shared with mentors or peers.[4]

Most reports on the effects of portfolios on learning are positive, but mainly rely on *self-perceived* satisfaction and educational gains, which may be seen as a limitation of the current available evidence.[4,10,14]

- *Perceived benefits of portfolios include:*[4,6,9–11]
  - improving skills in critical reflection, decision-making and communication;
  - supporting students emotionally in coping with new and difficult situations;
  - providing opportunities for open discussion and learning through a process of constructive feedback; and
  - providing mentors a better understanding of student needs and helping to modify teaching approaches based on this new understanding.

The literature also reports on drawbacks of the portfolio assessment method that may limit its successful implementation and value as a learning tool. These drawbacks are centered on the need for more resources and further consideration of time constraints, other commitments and motivational incentives.[4,6] Based on experience, the literature provides the following advice:

- Prior to implementation, portfolio programs require planning in the following areas:
  - Identify objectives, content requirements, assessment guidelines and measurable outcomes.[1,4,11,13,14]
  - Identify and train mentors on the portfolio and assessment process.[1,4,6]
  - Orient and train students on portfolio development and assessment processes.[1,4]
  - Allocate sufficient resources to support mentor and student needs.[4]

During the implementation phase, the following issues should be considered:

- Allocate adequate time for students to complete the portfolio. Students have found the portfolio process time-consuming and detracting from their training.[4,6]
- Support students and mentors through the process and provide administrative and IT support.[4,6]
- Provide mentors with incentives to maintain a commitment to the portfolio process despite other clinical or teaching duties.[11]
- Evaluate the effectiveness of the portfolio process as a learning and assessment tool.[25]

Conclusion

Student portfolios are robust assessment tools that support self-directed learning and reflective practice. They have the advantage of allowing flexibility in design, providing a longitudinal view of achievement and combining formative and summative assessment components. Incorporating portfolios in an assessment program should be based on the need to support specific educational objectives or competencies. Portfolios should contribute to an existing assessment program and not just add an additional workload for students and staff. Preparing for student portfolios requires extensive planning, training and resource allocation as well as the establishment of a support system during implementation and continuous evaluation of the process and outcomes. There is growing evidence in the literature to support the educational benefits of student portfolios, but their value will ultimately depend on the individual program's needs, structure, support and resources.

References

1. Epstein RM. Assessment in medical education. *N Engl J Med* 2007; 356: 387–396.
2. van der Vleuten CPM, Schuwirth LWT. Assessing professional competence: from methods to programmes. *Med Educ* 2005; 39: 309–317.
3. Rushton A. Formative assessment: a key to deep learning? *Med Teach* 2005; 27(6): 509–513.
4. Buckley S, Coleman J, Davidson I et al. The educational effects of portfolios on undergraduate student learning: a Best Evidence Medical Education (BEME) systematic review. BEME Guidance No. 11. *Med Teach* 2009; 31: 282–298.
5. McCready T. Portfolios and the assessment of competence in nursing: a literature review. *Int J Nurs Stud* 2007; 44(1): 143–151.
6. Dreissen E, van Tartwijk J, van der Vleuten CPM, Wall V. Portfolios in medical education: Why do they meet with mixed success? A systematic review. *Med Educ* 2007; 41: 1224–1233.
7. Davis MH, Friedman BDM, Harden RM et al. Portfolio assessment in medical students' final examinations. *Med Teach* 2001; 23: 357–366.
8. Hawkins RE, Holmboe ES. *Practical Guide to the Evaluation of Clinical Competence.* Philadelphia: Mosby-Elsevier, 2008.
9. Driessen EW, van Tartwijk J, Vermunt JD, van der Vleuten CPM. Use of portfolios in early undergraduate medical training. *Med Teacher* 2003; 25(1): 18–23.
10. Gordon J. Assessing students' personal and professional development using portfolios and interviews. *Med Educ* 2003; 37: 335–340.
11. Dannefer EF, Henson LC. The portfolio approach to competency-based assessment at the Cleveland Clinic Lerner College of Medicine. *Acad Med* 2007; 82: 493–502.
12. Driessen EW, Muijtjens AM, van Tartwijk J, van der Vleuten CPM. Web- or paper-based portfolios: is there a difference? *Med Educ* 2007; 41(11): 1067–1073.
13. Wade RC, Yarbourgh DB. Portfolios: a tool for reflective thinking in teacher education? *Teach Teacher Educ* 1996; 12(1): 63–79.
14. Driessen EW, van Tartwijk J, Overeem K, Vermunt JD, van der Vleuten CPM. Conditions for successful reflective use of portfolios in undergraduate medical education. *Med Educ* 2005; 39: 1230–1235.
15. Lee AG, Carter KD. Managing the new mandate in resident education: a blueprint for translating a national mandate into local compliance. *Opthalmology* 2004; 111(10): 1807–1812.
16. Speer AJ, Alnicki DM. Assessing the quality of teaching. *Am J Med* 1999; 106(4): 381–384.

17. McColgan K, Blackwood B. A systematic review protocol on the use of teaching portfolios for educators in further and higher education. *J Adv Nurs* 2009; 65(12): 2500–2507.

18. Wilkinson TJ, Challis M, Hobma SO, Parboosingh FT, Sibbald RG, Wakeford, R. The use of portfolios for assessment of the competence and performance of doctors in practice. *Med Educ* 2002; 36: 918–924.

19. Fishleder AJ, Henson LC, Hull, AL. Cleveland Clinic Lerner College of Medicine: an innovative approach to medical education and the training of physician investigators. *Acad Med* 2007; 82(4): 390–396.

20. Hmelo-Silver C. Problem-based learning: what and how do students learn? *Educ Psychol Rev* 2004; 16(3): 235–266.

21. Ormrod JE. *Human Learning* (5th edition). Ohio: Prentice Education, 2008.

22. Ericsson KA. Deliberate practice and the acquisition and maintenance of expert performance in medicine and related domains. *Acad Med* 2004; 79(10): S70–S81.

23. Dent JA, Harden RM. *A Practical Guide for Medical Teachers* (2nd edition). London: Elsevier, 2005.

24. Freidman Ben David M, Davis MH, Harden RM, Howie PW, Ker J, Pippard MJ. AMEE Medical Education Guide 24. Portfolios as a method of student assessment. *Med Teach* 2001; 23(6): 535–551.

25. Tiwari A, Tang C. From process to outcome: the effect of portfolio assessment on student learning. *Nurse Educ Today* 2003; 23(4): 269–277.

Chapter 28

Formative Assessments

Clarke Hazlett

Objectives

The goal of this chapter is to assist you in developing skill in how to teach yourself and in using formative assessments to determine whether your present strategies for learning are appropriate (or whether other learning tactics need to be also adopted). These skills enhance the likelihood that you will successfully complete your medical education. The related, detailed learning objectives follow at the end of the chapter.

The challenge

The "Iditarod" is one of the most challenging races on earth. Each participant has a team of sledge dogs to help race across nearly 2000 kilometers of northern wilderness, referred to as the Iditarod Trail. In the winter of 1925, this trail served as a life-saving route for the diphtheria-stricken town of Nome, Alaska. Serum could only be brought into Nome by sledge dogs. Today, an annual race commemorates the heroic efforts of those who rushed to supply Nome with the life-saving medicine.

The Iditarod crosses mountains, rivers, forests, tundra and the windswept coastline of the Bering Sea. Racers use different tactics in order to succeed. These include various training schedules, special menus for their dogs, and skipping essential rest periods. The trail is marked with stakes. However, long distances between the stakes, frequent blinding snow conditions and the build-up of fatigue during the several days that it takes to complete the race, all contribute to some going off-course. Given the many hardships, some do not finish the race. Those who do are given a heroes' welcome. Whether finishing first or last, each racer accomplishes a feat that few dare to attempt.

A medical undergraduate program has some similarities to the Iditarod. Not unlike the Iditarod's topography, a medical program has varied and challenging components – i.e., basic medical and social and clinical sciences that require extensive knowledge as well as sound behavioral and clinical skills. A medical program requires more time to complete than most other university programs, paralleling the unusual length of the Iditarod race. Medical students also use varying strategies in order to succeed: allocating differential times and importance to lectures, library research, ward experience, study groups and individual study time; working long hours; and skipping sleep. Few can successfully tackle either a medical program or the Iditarod; however, for those who successfully finish, special recognition awaits.

Given the race conditions, the stakes that mark the Iditarod trail are often insufficient guideposts. Medical programs also provide markers in the form of program, course and case-base objectives. However, the degree of clarity and complexity of these objectives sometimes can make them difficult to follow, not unlike conditions in a blinding snowstorm. Fortunately, many medical programs recognize that an additional resource can help students remain on course. These augmented markers are referred to as *formative assessments*.

> Similar to the Iditarod (one of the most daunting races on earth), undergraduate medical education is sufficiently challenging that few can tackle, and even fewer complete successfully. However, formative assessments are specifically designed to help you meet the challenges.

The resource

A medical program that specifically delineates what is expected of its students and how the student can successfully meet these requirements is regarded as having clearly *mapped* outcomes. In describing formative assessments, MAPPED is used as an acronym for introducing six key reasons why and how you can use formative assessments to help you successfully complete your medical program:

> **M**onitor your own progress
> **A**nalyze your learning strategies
> **P**ractice taking a variety of tests
> **P**roduce data that improves teaching
> **E**nhance your learning
> **D**evelop your lifelong learning skills

Purpose

Monitor your own progress

Tests designed to determine whether one should pass, be promoted, obtain a degree or qualify for professional licensure are so-called *summative* assessments.[1] The information from a summative test is primarily designed for others (teachers, professional bodies and society), so that they can make decisions about a candidate's qualifications.

"Formative" assessments have an entirely different purpose. They are designed to provide students with assistance before a summative test is taken. Formative assessments are a means for you, as a student, to independently determine, at any time throughout your training, "how am I doing?" The goal is for you to check whether you are making adequate progress (and thus continue with your present learning strategies) or, if not, to make some adjustments.[2]

Formative assessments provide feedback after you have taken the assessment. The feedback needs to be quickly available and to provide an appropriate amount of information.[3]

Stimulus-response theory explains why timely feedback optimizes learning.[4] Feedback is a form of reward for making a response (an answer) to a stimulus (a question). People can become addicted to a stimulus if positive rewards are provided. For example, slot machine gambling can be addictive because of its capability to intermittently provide varying amounts of reward (winnings). Similarly, learning is addictive (i.e. enjoyed and effective) if helpful feedback is provided in a timely manner.

To be most beneficial, feedback needs to be appropriately designed.[3] Feedback has limited usefulness if it only indicates that your answer was, or was not, correct. This simple form of feedback can help you to remember the answer to the same question; but usually you are not being adequately helped if later questions incorporate some variations – for example, a summative item may address similar signs and symptoms but the disease stage or age of patient is modified.

Therefore, appropriate feedback will provide information for you to meaningfully reflect on your answer.[5] For example, if your answer is incorrect, an explanation would be provided as to why it is not correct and would often be followed with an indication of a new direction for you to consider. Depending on the test's format, the feedback may suggest further reading materials, relevant case notes or patients to clerk. Frustration develops if an inordinate amount of time researching every incorrect answer is required. Thus, some feedback will be more prescriptive. Regardless, provided you have partial knowledge, the feedback will help you solve the problem after reflecting on your previous incorrect response.

To illustrate, a question from the IDEAL Consortium's formative item bank[6] is cited. It is an extended matching item, developed by a medical student, Angie Au of the Chinese University of Hong Kong. The question assesses diagnostic skill in relation to pediatrics suffering from dehydration and is available as an on-line, formative item that is scored by the computer, with an option of feedback.[7]

Options

A. Diabetes insipidus
B. Diabetic ketoacidosis
C. Food poisoning
D. Gastro-oesophageal reflux
E. Hypoglycaemic attack

F. Norwalk-gastroenteritis
G. Pyloric stenosis
H. Salmonella-gastroenteritis
I. Sepsis
J. Vaso-vagal attack

Question
Based on the above options, what is the most likely diagnosis for the following child?

Scenario
A 16-month-old boy had a history of intermittent fever for 10 days. His maximum body temperature was up to 38.6°C. His mother indicated that his fever was associated with an increased frequency in diaper changing. For two days, he ate poorly and appeared lethargic. He developed labored breathing the day prior to hospital admission. On examination, he was found to be irritable and tachycardic. Physical examination revealed dry mucosa, reduced skin turgor, prolonged capillary refill and mottled skin. Blood culture was normal. Arterial blood gas results were: pH 7.05; pCO2 2.0 kPa; base excess −26.3.

The feedback provided varies depending on the answer given by the candidate. If an answer does not include option A, B, I, the feedback is as follows:

> Dehydration can be caused by, or is a consequence of, various conditions. For example, it can result from conditions causing vomiting and diarrhea, such as gastroenteritis or food poisoning or from conditions causing excessive urination, such as poorly controlled diabetes mellitus, diabetic ketoacidosis, diabetic insipidus or from conditions causing an increase in evaporation from the body's surface such as burns or from conditions leading to third space loss, such as septicaemic shock or hypoalbuminaemia. Dehydration can also result from poor feeding or poor absorption such as cystic fibrosis or sprue. On the other hand, it can lead to heat exhaustion, when the body can no longer adequately dissipate heat because of extreme environmental conditions or increased endogenous heat production. Among all the conditions, dehydration, secondary to diarrheal illness, is the most common.
>
> Given the child's clinical presentation, you should be aware, that the differential diagnosis includes sepsis, diabetes insipidus and diabetic ketoacidosis. Before re-answering the question, review the material on dehydration in pediatrics.

However, if a candidate's answer is either option A or I, then the feedback is as follows:

> Given the child's clinical presentation, differential diagnosis includes three possibilities. However, a normal blood culture is indicative that metabolic acidosis, due to sepsis, is less likely and diabetes insipidus per se, cannot explain the blood gas derangements. Consider these points when you re-answer the question.

Finally, if the candidate chooses option B as the answer, then the feedback is confirmatory:

> **Correct.** The case fits a classical presentation for diabetes ketoacidosis, as evidenced by polyuria (usually associated with polydipsia), signs of dehydration, metabolic acidosis and Kussmaul breathing (that the mother regarded as labored breathing). Fever indicates that the child might have concomitant infection,

or more often, an underlying infection that predisposes development of diabetic ketoacidosis in type I diabetes mellitus.

To enable a candidate to readily follow up on the particular feedback she/he got, relevant literature is cited.

Diabetic reaction (emedicine): Scott H Plantz, Michael E Zevitz; Francisco Talavera, et al.
Dehydration (emedicine): Dan L Ellsbury & Caroline S George,
Heat exhaustion and heat stroke (emedicine): Amy Kunihiro & James Foster

---

The most useful form of feedback does not specify the correct answer, but rather provides information for you to discover or deduce the correct answer.

Analyze your learning strategies

Given the type of feedback illustrated above, you have the means for independently determining how well you are mastering a particular case. Use this technique to reflect on your chosen strategies for learning the content being covered in your courses. Some issues to consider are as follows:

- Are you able to answer questions for which the answers can be memorized, but are weaker in applying the information for different circumstances?
- Are you having more difficulty answering knowledge-based questions or with executing clinical skills?
- Was the assessed material adequately addressed or taught in the course?
- How well you are doing in comparison to others in your group?

For example, what should you do if you are very capable in remembering specific clinical facts and findings, but are less able to develop generalizations so that the information can be used with different patients (age/gender), conditions (acute/chronic) or environments (inpatient/ outpatient)? If so, allocate more time for discussions with your tutorial group, raise more queries with your clinical teachers and reflect in your private study time how clinical conditions or outcomes will or will not change if the underlying mechanism, stage of disease, place of practice or type of patient was different.

Medical schools vary in the weight allocated to assessing memorized information and problem-solving ability, and to the relative importance of clinical knowledge and skills.[8] Regardless, all schools recognize that the amount of relevant information and skills far exceeds the time they can allocate to administering assessments. Thus, your teachers will try to determine:

- whether you have an adequate base of information, as estimated by a sample of assessed scientific and clinical facts;

- whether you can think laterally by applying sampled factual information to different clinical situations; and
- whether your clinical skills are rooted in your baseline knowledge and rational decision making.

Few medical students are deficient in allocating enough time and effort to enable them to succeed. However, many more have difficulty determining the optimal way to utilize their relatively limited time for learning all the materials being taught.

> Given information you acquire from taking formative assessments, you can make better decisions about how much time to spend in memorizing scientific and clinical factual information, developing problem-solving skills and acquiring appropriate clinical skills.

Practice taking a variety of test formats

Formative assessments can be administered in many formats – i.e. multiple choice and short answer questions, essays, OSCEs, projects and orals. Orals can be in the form of case discussions among students (in study groups or PBL tutorials) or between students and a clinical supervisor (during ward rounds). Each format has some limitations and strengths.[9] Ensure you participate in all forms of formative assessments in order to compensate for the inherent weakness of answering only one type. Overall, your summative assessments will incorporate many formats because your teachers know that use of only one or two types is far too limited for correctly determining whether you are entitled to pass or graduate.[10]

For example, consider the above multiple questions in pediatrics. Although it is illustrated as an on-line, formative assessment, a clinical supervisor could orally ask a similar question while you are rotating through a pediatric ward, and also provide you with appropriate feedback.

> Actively participate in ward discussions as well as take on-line, hard copy or any other form of formative assessments that your medical school provides.

Produce data for improving teaching

After reflecting on the feedback provided in the formative assessment, you might think that the assessed information, or skill, was not adequately addressed within the medical program. Confirm this by checking how well you did in comparison to others who took the same formative assessment. If others are having similar difficulties, your concerns might be valid. Discuss this with your instructors, as they will want to know, *not* for purposes of assigning grades, but rather to help in tailoring their further instruction and guidance.[11]

If, however, you are among a small group who are performing less than expected on a formative assessment, then consider whether you have been spending too much or too little time in the library, on the wards, with your tutorial group or in studying independently. For example, if you have been unable to do well in a formative OSCE, you may have been allocating insufficient time on the wards (e.g., clerking patients, discussing case notes with your ward supervisors or talking to patients' relatives). You may need to book extra time in the clinical skills laboratory and practice deficient clinical skills on mannequins or classmates.

> What you need will be diagnosed from the type of knowledge or skill that you did not answer correctly in the formative exercises. Where to focus your remedial efforts will be indicated in the corresponding feedback.

Enhance your learning

Research has shown that students who participate in formative assessments will outperform those who do not by 21 to 41 percentile points.[12] This is a statistically significant and educationally meaningful benefit.

Your school may provide fewer formative assessments than you would like to have. What you might view as a shortfall should not be an educational liability. You need also to participate in formative assessments other than those set by the teaching faculty.

Research has also established that students who cooperatively work together in groups will outperform those who study independently. This beneficial effect is independent of gender, social class, culture, ethnicity, geographical region or content of material studied.[13] Thus you need to complement your medical school's formative assessments with group work in which each member takes responsibility for raising questions that lead to improved learning.

It is important to recognize that there are two types of questions that can be asked, i.e. *"closed-ended"* and *"open-ended."*[14] Although both forms aid learning, open-ended questions are more effective aids.

Closed-ended questions require answers that are clearly right or wrong. These questions can be easily answered if you memorized the related factual information. In contrast, **open-ended** questions require reasoning and justifiable logic in order to be correct. The latter are more easily answered if you practice analyzing and synthesizing new information in order to derive principles and generalizations.

For example, again consider the above example item dealing with a dehydrated pediatric patient. An example of a closed-ended question might be "What are the common causes of dehydration in pediatrics?" In contrast, an open-ended question would query not only the diagnosis, but related issues such as "Why would a diagnosis of sepsis and diabetes insipidus be less likely?"

You will find that it is relatively easy to formulate and answer closed-ended questions. However, you also need to learn how to ask and answer open-ended questions in your study groups. First, summative tests will include both closed- and open-ended questions. Thus you need to practice answering both forms. Secondly, open-ended questions lead to discussions that create an understanding of when and how certain clinical factual information will (or would not) be relevant for different patients, disease stages and/or practice environments.

As a guide for learning how to pose an open-ended question, begin with a phrase such as:

"Could this happen if . . .?"	"Can you apply this method to . . .?"
"How was this similar to . . .?"	"Can you explain what must have happened when . . .?"
"How would you deal with . . .?"	"How would you have handled . . .?"
"How important was . . .?"	"What questions would you ask of . . .?"

> Participate in cooperative study groups in which each member is responsible for asking as well as answering open-ended questions.

Develop your lifelong learning skills

It has been estimated that the amount of medical knowledge doubles every three to five years. Thus your medical program provides only a basis for starting a medical career. Unless you are able to continue learning after leaving medical school and without the benefit of dedicated instructors, it is inevitable that you will not be up-to-date clinically, you will increase your risk of malpractice litigation and, most importantly, your patients will not receive optimal care.

Thus, while medical school, it is essential to develop lifelong learning skills, i.e. "learning how to learn." Development of your self-learning skills is an educational goal held by all medical schools. It is a skill that summative tests will try to assess as you progress through your medical program. The key prerequisite for those who can teach themselves is an ability to self-monitor. Self-monitoring is the highest form of formative assessment.[15]

> An essential component in the skill of lifelong learning is the ability to monitor one's own level of competency – the essence of all formative assessments.

Conclusion

Strategically, you should avail yourself of most formative assessments that present while you are in medical school. By doing so, you will, similar to a successful racer in the Iditarod, avoid going off-course. You will successfully finish a task that few others dare to attempt. Rewards waiting at the end of your medical program will justify the time you spend in using these formative assessments as guideposts.

Detailed objectives

- To develop lifelong learning skills while in medical school, i.e. develop the skill of how to teach yourself.
- To remember that formative assessments are designed to provide timely, useful feedback for you, and not for others to decide whether you should pass or obtain a degree.
- To use feedback from marked formative assessments by reflecting on your learning strategies, adopting alternative tactics if your progress at that time is inadequate.
- To remember useful strategies for learning (besides course attendance, library research and individual study time) including participating in study groups; asking and answering questions with your peers, teachers and patients; observing and working on wards.
- To become a strategically informed medical student by taking many formative assessments.
- To appreciate that time taken to answer formative assessments will help you successfully complete your medical program.

References

1. Miller AH, Imrie BW, Cox K. *Student Assessment in Higher Education: a handbook for assessing performance.* London: Kogan Page, 1998, pp. 33, 34.
2. Ibid., pp. 32, 33.
3. Nicol DJ, Macfarlane-Dick D. Formative assessment and self-regulated learning: A model and seven principles of good feedback practice. *Studies in Higher Education,* 2006, 31(2), 199–218.
4. Custers EJFM, Boshuizen HPA. The psychology of learning. In: Norman GR, van der Vleutin CPM, Newble DT (eds). *International Handbook of Research in Medical Education, Part One.* Dordrecht: Kluwer Academic, 2002, pp. 163–203.
5. Schon DA. *Educating the Reflective Practitioner.* San Francisco: Jossey-Bass, 1987.
6. http://www.hkwebmed.org
7. Hazlett CB, Yip S, Nicholls J, Au W, Tan J. *IDEAL-HK™: Students' Guide.* Hong Kong: Don Bosco, 2008.
8. Curry L. Individual differences in cognitive style, learning style and instructional preference in medical education. In: Norman GR, van der Vleutin CPM, Newble DT (eds). *International Handbook of Research in Medical Education, Part One.* Dordrecht: Kluwer Academic, 2002, pp. 263–276.
9. Schuwirth LW, van der Vleuten CPM. Different written assessment methods: what can be said about their strengths and weaknesses. *Medical Education,* 2004, 38, 974–979.
10. Epstein RM. Assessment in medical education. *New England Journal of Medicine,* 2007, 356(4), 387–396.
11. Gibbs G, Simpson C. Conditions under which assessment supports students' learning. *Learning and Teaching in Higher Education,* 2004, 1, 3–31.
12. Black P, Wiliam D. Inside the black box: raising standards through classroom assessment. *Phi Delta Kappan,* 1998, 80(2), 139–149.

13. Johnson DW & Johnson RT. *Learning Together and Alone: Cooperative, Competitive and Individualistic Learning*. (5th Ed): Allyn and Bacon, 1999.

14. Dillon J. Questioning. In: Hargie DW (ed). *The Handbook of Communication Skills*. New York: Routledge, 1997, pp. 103–133.

15. Eva KW, Regehr G. Self-assessment in the health professions: a reformation and research agenda. *Academic Medicine*, 2005, 80 Supplement, S46–S54.

Chapter 29

The Student's Role in Evaluation: Rationale and Benefits

Francis Michael Seefeldt

Objectives

- To posit the grounded validity of students as evaluative data sources.
- To link the promotion of effective critical thinking in students with effective evaluative contribution in academe.
- To address major concerns of those opposed to the use of student evaluation in medical and other health professional education.
- To support evaluation in the context of higher level objectives in education.

No one – neither the department heads, nor the curriculum or executive committees – experiences as much of the curriculum and related educational activities, formal or informal, as does the student. From the first day of matriculation to that of final commencement, bestowal of the certificate and the oath-giving ceremony, the student sees it all. Whether in lecture auditoria, small-group classrooms or laboratories, whether in clinics or wards, the student experiences it all and struggles through it all. The student experiences virtually every full-time faculty member and many part-time and adjunct faculty members. Wide varieties of residents, nurses and unit coordinators are encountered in clerkships and clinical electives. Thus, despite occasional anti-student chimes from certain retrogressive faculty members (often the very ones doing the worst job teaching), the student is the most valid, most well grounded and experientially the most familiar data source we can include when evaluating the educational program and its contributing educationists and practitioners. The student also arguably has the most investment in the success of the program, not only branded with it as she/he will always be, but also as the direct product of its ministrations, good or bad. And after four or five years in medical school, after all that accumulating experience as a student, this data source knows whereof it speaks.

We should also recall, further, that in virtually every country on the globe selection for medical school often draws the highest levels of students, the *crème de la crème* of that nation's future generation. High performance, determination, ambition, commitment, quality educational background – all these attributes may well be as representative of the prototypical medical student body as of that of any other field. This is not to say that other fields, from art to engineering, do not get worthy students, but taken as a whole no discipline sports as broad an array of scholarly ability as medicine. Not only have medical students scored highest in national exams, but in countries using the US model they have already completed a baccalaureate degree, usually of particular rigor, and usually with science majors. Neither medical students nor pre-med students are credibly characterized as slackers, and the match results for residency placement toward which each student tensely strives are, themselves, as arduous a milestone as any stepping stone in academe.

Students not only see the whole program but they also constitute the most reliably accomplishing of the various pools of a nation's young talent. So, why not capitalize on their proven commitment, their demonstrated quality, their accumulated program experience and perceptual advantage? Why not tap the talent that leads to such selection and performance and the maturity that grows out of it to help inform us about our educational program? It would seem to any reasonably progressive educator that the onus of explanation for failure to do so should rest squarely on the shoulders of those arguing against using student data in program or faculty evaluation. I see little to support such negativity, particularly in this day of consumer-consciousness and student-centered educational philosophy.

In revolutionizing Japanese industry, W. Edwards Deming put forward the concept of Total Quality Management (TQM). He advocated measures to fulfill quality assurance aims through enlisting viewpoints from all along the organizational hierarchy and divisions of operation. He recognized that consumer satisfaction builds on a dependable product; that a dependable product requires alert quality maintenance; and that that maintenance flourishes on a perspective more closely attuned to day-to-day operations than is possible from upper management's remote vantage point. He recognized that TQM functions most effectively when the entire collective body, at all cohort levels from top to bottom, is engaged in a kind of critical vigilance. And the incorporation of the ideas of those closest to the productive action secures one of the most essential data sources for success in this vigilance. A vital alternative to the antiquated top-down industrial-age factory model, this less hierarchic, more inclusive, participatory, post-industrial model, gains even more plausibility in educational circles confronted by accreditation-related entities with their vigorous advocacy of sustained quality assurance through continuous renewal. Continuous renewal depends on continuous, meaningful self-scrutiny, and effective self-scrutiny depends on a well triangulated database. Both the professionalism of competent auto-criticism and the full incorporation of often overlooked stakeholder groups are key to practical, effective and meaningful continuous renewal.

So the question arises, not whether student data should be employed in any health profession's commitment to quality in its educational programs, but why that data source is not given more predominance in programmatic and personnel decision-making in many places; for we know that progressive program and faculty evaluation is not universally embedded in all medical school operations.

Utilization of student data is a frequent omission; and even where it is not omitted it is often susceptible to, if not outright subjected to, unbridled skepticism, if not outright disparagement and hostility. But, whether trusting students' experiential perspective, or respecting their tested class ability, or acting on regard for the theory and practice of quality assurance, the importance of the medical student as data source seems undeniable. Hence, their utilization for evaluative purposes is ineluctable in any respected educational program; they must play a key role in effective educational program and personnel evaluation.

So why the resistance in certain quarters? Because it does exist, whether definitively across an institution or defiantly in certain nooks within it. How can it be explained? Does it have validity? While these questions may elicit many earnest attempts at explanation, consideration of them may be parsed into five areas: faculty defensiveness, perceptions of interference with research priorities, concerns for scientific rigor, limitations due to process or resource feasibility, and time-honored tradition.

The last two are most easily dismissed: feasibility, though always an issue, is less of a concern with medical education units, which are typically administratively well staffed by comparison with other disciplines, many of which manage to conduct evaluation with far humbler resources. The arguments for faculty-elitist tradition hold almost nowhere in contemporary education that considers itself in the least progressive.

But perhaps the most serious of these contentions is the concern about scientific rigor. Data are not solicited under "controlled" experimental conditions. Nor is isolation of variables possible, as factors such as impact of exams, ease of grading and so forth are alleged by some to impact student ratings. But we must remember, on the first point, that we are not attempting to generalize to large populations, so consideration of threats to external validity is functionally moot. And, as far as extrinsic factors affect student ratings, decades of research simply do not support the alarmist levels to which some naysayers raise this argument. In fact, most studies indicate that student perception of faculty is fairly well settled within the first weeks of a class. Those who claim "opinionnaires" are not sufficiently rigorous would have to eliminate all studies using survey forms in their methodology, which is simply absurd. Our modern society uses such strategies in virtually every walk of life – marketing, political strategizing, sociological studies, product performance, etc.

Some faculty members also resist evaluating teaching generally, and students are only the scapegoats. These often wish to be left alone for their research and publication promotional interests only, and not be bothered by accountability to the institution for their teaching. This is a narrow and even arrogant argument, which fails to notice that the first duty of an educational institution is just that – education. Research institutes are the proper venue for their claim, but colleges have a broader mission: research matters of course, with service, but only as part of "the three-legged stool." And what institution, with or without full educational evaluation activity, puts ratings for teaching ahead of vigorous publication records, fund- and grant-raising, or high performance money-generating clinical service?

In well-regarded institutions of higher learning, the centrality of critical thinking to scholarly reputation is nonpareil. While this is most clearly manifest in research activity, it should apply to educational processes too. Modern learning theories promoting student-centered methods, adult learning principles, situated learning, problem-based learning, etc., almost universally aspire to "higher levels" of learning, shifting away from more traditional rote and patterned learning activities to multi-mode, analytical, creative and evaluative learning functions. Fluency in critical thinking is important to the actively engaged student, to the flexibility and future utility of his/her learning, and, ultimately, to the future of the respective professions they enter, depending for their progress, as they inevitably do, on forthcoming generations.

Many recent innovations in health professions have emerged in response to this fervor: problem-based learning, increased early use of clinical paper cases, standardized patients, earlier patient exposure, better contextualization through vertical integration of basic and clinical sciences, development of higher quality manikins, and assessment using high-order items or comparative essays, to note a few. It is clear that the aspiration to provide higher level learning episodes promoting critical thinking permeates medical education today. The student as critical thinker represents the outcome-apogee of these new directions. And, if we assume success in this intention, does not the employment of evaluative data from such critical-learning students only further sharpen that capacity within those students, particularly when they clearly see it applied to decision-making in the academic setting? Such realization on their part can only reinforce the twin charges to heighten critical-thinking ability and to apply it in everyday performance. Not only is the program the beneficiary with improved student commitment and informed utilization of their data, but the consequences reverberate to the ultimate benefit of the academic community as a whole.

In an additional related social concern, since physicians are not only drawn from the intellectual heights of a society's manpower but are also, virtually by definition, faced with life-and-death decisions, they are natural candidates for decisions-based leadership roles in the future. Whether applied in intraprofessional or extramural venues, critical thinking and effective decision-making, as well as openness to input from all valid data sources in the process, are essential components of effective leadership. The experience of participating in critical program and faculty evaluation as students is not only practical and informative to institutional decision-making, as argued above, but it also offers students a consonant higher-learning process toward their demanding future, in addition to daily medical responsibility: eventual critical-thinking life skills, judicious professionalism, and responsive leadership. After all, it is not for naught that "Evaluation" is the highest level on Bloom's Taxonomy of Cognitive Development.

Chapter 30

Receiving Feedback

Zubair Amin

Objectives

On completing this chapter, you will be able to:
- Develop a positive attitude towards feedback as an essential element in education.
- Accept that the purpose of feedback is to improve your learning and behavior.
- Recognize the key elements and process of receiving feedback.

Introduction

Feedback is one of the most fundamental mechanisms governing the human body and its functions. It is essential for the survival of all living beings. Feedback allows information about performances or output to be relayed back to a central control system in order to make necessary adjustments in inputs or processes. These adjustments could be either positive or negative. For example, an increase in oxygen demand at the tissue level sets off a chain of motions in the central control system. This leads to an increase in cardiac output to meet the increase in oxygen demand. Similarly, information resulting from low blood glucose feeds back to the central control system, which leads to a decrease in insulin and an increase in glucagon production in the body.

In education, feedback provides information about your performance to the central control system: your psyche. In more formal terms, feedback denotes a structured communication technique in which teachers or observers provide meaningful information about knowledge, performance and behavior of students in a way that is intended to result in a positive change in the recipient's learning or behavior. In addition, feedback may be used to reinforce prior learning and to correct mistakes.

As a specific communication technique in education, you should expect to receive feedback. The essential elements of a proper feedback are:

- Observed behavior or performance, e.g. an answer provided by you during the class;

- The effects – positive or negative; and
- How this information can be utilized in future. Thus, feedback in education tends to be specific and focuses on elements of behavior that can be changed.[1]

Essential elements of feedback
Dealing with a positive behavior:

1. Description of the behavior
2. The positive effects
3. How this can be utilized in the future

Dealing with a negative behavior:

1. Description of behavior
2. The negative effects
3. How this can be avoided in the future

There is a clear distinction between feedback and the more familiar praise and criticism. Praise and criticism are not synonymous with feedback. They are not intended to bring about meaningful changes in students' behavior or learning, but rather tend to be generic, non-specific statements without any direction provided. In addition, praise and criticism tend to be directed towards the person rather than the specific aspects of behavior. They are not as effective as feedback in bringing about intended change.

Feedback is an essential element of learning

Feedback is a critical element of learning and has a very significant influence on achievements. Feedback is one of the most powerful educational interventions.[2,3] For example, a meta-analysis of twelve meta-analyses from general education literature shows that feedback has the largest influence on achievement, with an effect size of 0.79.[2] Effect size is a name given to a family of indices that measure the magnitude of a treatment effect, especially in meta-analyses.

A close relationship exists between learning, assessment and feedback. From a traditional point of view, assessment is seen primarily as a test to determine whether learning has taken place in a given situation. In other words, the principle governing education focuses on "assessment of learning." However, assessment can also be a powerful learning tool. This is particularly true in medical education where the focus should be on "assessment *for* learning" as well. To achieve this noble objective, data collected during assessment needs to be conveyed to the students in a systematic and usable manner. Feedback is the essential link that connects assessment and learning (Figure 30.1).

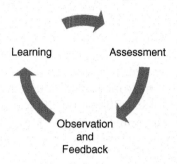

FIGURE 30.1

Nature of feedback

In the most simplistic schema of classification, feedback can be directed towards either positive or negative aspects of behavior or learning. Feedback on positive aspects is intended to reinforce a particular behavior or knowledge so that the behavior or knowledge becomes permanent. Feedback on negative aspects is intended to correct a specific behavior or faults in knowledge. As a result, undesirable behavior may become extinct or a faulty knowledge may get corrected.

Feedback may include any observable knowledge, behavior or skills. In the domain of knowledge, you might ask for feedback on content (i.e. understanding of a concept) or processes (e.g. reasoning process, analysis of facts). In the behavioral domain, you might ask for feedback on your empathy, demeanor, or other specific aspects of your quality. Similarly, in skills, you should take initiative to get feedback on your history-taking, communication, bedside physical examination and other aspects of patient management. You might also ask for global feedback on your performance.

It is important to appreciate that feedback is necessary even when your response is correct and behavior is appropriate. You may provide a correct answer to your teacher's question without fully appreciating the underlying knowledge structure or reasoning process. Even worse, a right answer could be given for an entirely wrong reason! Feedback and a subsequent discussion surrounding the right answer ensure that the accurate information becomes a permanent element of your knowledge. Reinforcement from an authoritative figure, such as your teacher, would ensure that information is retained as a part of long-term memory.

Feedback may take place in group situations. For example, group feedback may be given after a problem-based learning session or a communication skills training workshop. Group feedback is often favored by the students because it does not target any specific person. You should also ask for an examination review or a feedback session after an exam. However, you have to be very clear about the purpose of such review sessions, which is to highlight important concepts, correct wrong answers and address specific knowledge deficiencies. The purpose is not to criticize the questions or question setters!

When should you ask for feedback?

Fortunately, you have many opportunities to receive feedback. Any teaching and learning activity can be a potential source of feedback. For example, an answer to a question could be an important trigger point for feedback. Many assessment instruments used in contemporary medical education have an in-built mechanism for provision of feedback. For example, mini-Clinical Evaluation Exercise (mini-CEX) typically reserves a certain time for feedback. Similarly, Objective Structured Clinical Examination or OSCE might include feedback on your performance, either in real-time or at a later date. Finally, you should ask for feedback from your patients and colleagues whenever you interact with them. In particular, feedback from your patients can be very meaningful as this involves an authentic interaction.

Ask for feedback during the following:

- Question and answer sessions during the lectures
- Problem-based learning sessions
- Ward rounds
- During an interaction with your patients and fellow colleagues
- After written examinations
- Daily activities (e.g. attitude and behavior in class)
- Performance assessment, such as OSCE and mini-CEX

Feedback is rare

Despite its well-known association with positive learning, feedback is rarely practiced in medical education. Much valuable information about knowledge, behavior and performance that should have been to the students remains underutilized. Students and trainees are rarely observed directly by their teachers. In one study, researchers noted that structured observation of clinical skills was carried out for only 7–23 percent of students in medical schools.[4]

The reasons for not giving feedback are many. From teachers' perspective, the most common reason could be the ubiquitous problem of "not having time." Moreover, many medical teachers are unaware of the beneficial effects of feedback on learning. They might believe feedback would undermine the delicate harmony between teachers and students. Finally, they might unfamiliar with proper feedback techniques.

Students are also reluctant to ask for feedback. Finding an opportune moment is always difficult. Identifying the right person for providing feedback could pose a challenge to the students. Finally, students, like teachers, might be unaware of the positive impact of feedback.

In addition to problems specific to teachers and students, there are structural problems in the healthcare system that might hinder meaningful feedback. Medical education tends to be highly fragmented with little or no long-term follow-up of students by a dedicated mentor or teacher. Without opportunities for such follow-up, teachers might not have credible data on students' performance. The end result tends to be cursory comments rather than honest, meaningful feedback.

Reasons for not asking for feedback

- You are uncertain about the value of the feedback –
  - Feedback is one of the most important educational interventions. Feedback improves students' learning and corrects inappropriate behavior or knowledge.
- You are unsure about the purpose of the feedback –
  - The purpose of feedback is to improve your learning. It is not intended to criticize or make adverse comments about your performance.
- You worry feedback will be negative –
  - Feedback is a well-balanced view on your knowledge and performance. It should contain both positive and, if necessary, negative aspects of your knowledge and performance.
- You believe feedback will be personal –
  - On the contrary, feedback targets observable behavior. The person is not the target of feedback.
- You do not know whom to ask for feedback –
  - Teachers are the traditional source of feedback. However, you should expand the list of feedback providers and include fellow students, nurses, patients, and other members of health-care teams.
- Your past experience with feedback was not helpful –
  - You might have received unhelpful or even harmful feedback. Try a new person, a new approach, or a new domain. For example, if you have already asked for feedback on your knowledge in the past, try asking for feedback on your clinical skills this time.
- You are not sure how to ask for feedback –
  - Try to be specific. Instead of stating "Would you kindly give me a feedback?" ask "Would you kindly give me a feedback on my history-taking skills?"
- You are not sure when to ask for feedback –
  - This very much depends on the context. In a typical module, it might be useful to ask for feedback while the module is still in progress. During bedside clinical teaching, ask your tutor to provide immediate feedback after you have finished your assigned task.

Getting the most out of feedback

Feedback alone does not cause change; it is the goals that people set in response to feedback. (Locke et al., 1990)

Feedback helps you to identify your strengths and weaknesses and directs you towards personal and professional development in the future. It is essential that you set a goal towards achieving a specific target with a defined timeline. Once a goal is set, develop some specific action plans. It is also advisable that you share your goal with your feedback provider and arrange a specific meeting to discuss whether you have achieved the goal. Without specific targets and action plans, learning remains undirected and you might miss out on a golden opportunity to improve your education.

Help teachers to provide feedback

It might seem counter-intuitive, but teachers also need help from students to provide honest, meaningful feedback. First and foremost, it is important that both parties are clear about the goal of the feedback. Clarity about the purpose will avoid confusion and misunderstanding. Second, be proactive in soliciting feedback from your teachers. Seek feedback after an assignment is over or after a presentation. With time, this will become a routine for both teachers and students. Third, provide feedback to the teachers. It might not be apparent, but teachers love to receive feedback from their students. Feedback from students is highly appreciated and one of the greatest sources of joy and motivation for teachers. Write a note of thanks to your teachers highlighting the value of the feedback received by you.

Helping your teachers to provide meaningful feedback

- Encourage and expect feedback from the teachers.
- Seek both positive and negative feedback.
- Set aside dedicated time for feedback. This is a part of learning.
- Ask specific questions, e.g. "How can I benefit from this information? How can I improve myself?"
- Do not take feedback personally. The purpose of feedback is to improve your learning.
- Set a clear action plan from the feedback, e.g. "I will incorporate this behavior in future."
- Provide feedback to your teachers, e.g. "You have helped me understand the benefits of asking psychosocial history. Now I routinely elicit psychosocial history from my patients."

Important learning points

- Feedback is one of the most effective educational interventions.
- The intention of feedback is to bring about positive change in learning.
- Feedback tends to focus on specific, observable behaviors that are amenable to change.
- Set a specific goal and action plan to implement the change required according to the feedback given.
- Provide feedback to your teachers.

References

1. Amin Z, Khoo HE. Providing effective feedback. In: *Basics in Medical Education*, 2nd edition. Singapore: World Scientific Publishing Company, 2008, pp. 135–141.
2. Hattie J, Timperley H. The power of feedback. *Review of Educational Research*. 2007; 77(1): 81–112. Web address: http://rer.sagepub.com/cgi/content/full/77/1/81#B62-0770081. Last accessed March 2009.
3. Veloski J, Boex JR, Grasberger MJ, Evans A, Wolfson DB. Systematic review of the literature on assessment, feedback and physicians' clinical performance: BEME Guide No 7. *Medical Teacher*. 2006; 28(2): 117–128.
4. Kassebaum DG, Eaglen RH. Shortcomings in the evaluation of students' clinical skills and behaviors in medical school. *Academic Medicine*. 1999; 74: 841–849.

VIII
STUDENT'S SUPPORT

Chapter 31

Involving Patients in Medical Education: Ethical Guidelines for Clinical Teachers and Medical Students [1]

Merrilyn Walton

Objectives

- To educate medical students about clinical experience involving patients and to learn medicine "at bedside."
- To teach medical students how to deal with "ethical dilemmas" in a clinical situation.
- To know what they should do as medical students, and their professional responsibilities to each other.
- To know the responsibilities of clinical teachers to medical students.

Introduction

To be a good doctor requires practical clinical experience involving patients. One of the most valuable components of a medical program is the opportunity for students to learn medicine "at the bedside." This involves students observing the full range of emotional and physical symptoms that are experienced by patients.

It is important for students to remember that the opportunity to interview and examine patients is a privilege granted by each individual patient. Patients should not become engaged in any personal or physical interaction without their express permission. A patient has the right to withdraw this privilege at any time and for any reason.

Particular care must be taken when involving patients in teaching activities because, from the patient's perspective, student learning is not directly necessary for their care and treatment. Nevertheless, most patients welcome the opportunity to contribute to the education of students and junior doctors.

Explicit guidelines for clinical teachers and medical students provide protection for everyone. They are designed to protect patients, to promote high ethical standards and to avoid misunderstandings.

Bedside teaching

Clinical teachers must ensure that patients understand that medical students are *not*_qualified doctors. When introduced to patients or their families, they should always be described as 'medical students'. Please do not describe students as 'junior doctors', 'student doctors', 'young doctors', 'assistants' or 'colleagues'. Students must advise patients of their correct status, even if that means correcting what their clinical teacher has said. Students must explain that they are medical students studying to become doctors.

Patient consent

Clinical teachers must advise patients that their cooperation in educational activities is entirely voluntary. Clinical teachers and medical students must obtain verbal consent from patients before the students interview or examine them. Patients should be told that the examination is mainly for educational purposes. An appropriate use of words would be: "Would you mind if these students ask you about your illness and/or examine you, so that they can learn more about your condition?" Please take care to ensure that patients understand that their participation is voluntary, and that a decision not to participate will not compromise their care.

While verbal consent is sufficient for most educational activities, students should be aware that the law requires patients to be fully informed in advance about their care and treatment. Much of healthcare requires written consent. If a student is unsure about the type of consent required, he/she should check with a clinical supervisor.

When education is an integral part of clinical care

If a student is presented with a learning opportunity that involves assisting, observing or examining a patient during the patient's treatment or therapy, then specific, verbal consent is not necessary, as long as the patient is aware that students may be involved in their care and treatment. For example, when a patient is in theater and the surgeon directs the student to assist in or perform a relevant examination, then separate consent is not necessary provided that the activity is directly related to the patient's management.

Supervisors must obtain consent for students to conduct a physical examination and for other students to be present during the examination. An appropriate choice of words would be: "Would you mind if (student X) examines you while we observe?"

Students requesting supervision

There will be times when students require supervision but are not able to be supervised due to ward activities or patient care load. Notwithstanding these conflicting interests, it is important that students ask for supervision when they think they need it. If the supervision is not immediately available, then a time should be scheduled with the appropriate person (doctor or nurse) so they can supervise the student during the procedure.

Students are obliged to do the following prior to performing a procedure on a patient:

- read about the procedure and how it is done;
- observe another person performing the procedure;
- practice the procedure on a model or surrogate patient; and
- arrange for a supervisor to be present when the student is performing the procedure for the first time.

A patient must give prior written consent to any invasive, intimate physical examination, such as a rectal or vaginal examination under general anesthetic, when it is for primarily educational purposes separate from treatment. The prior written consent must indicate the nature of the examination intended, and must be recorded in the medical notes. Patients who are unconscious or incapacitated for other reasons must only be involved in such examinations with the explicit written agreement of their responsible clinician and after appropriate consent from a parent (if a child) or appropriate relative or appointed guardian (if an adult).

Clinical teachers and students must obtain explicit verbal consent from patients for procedures such as taking blood, suturing or giving injections. If the procedure is one that is normally written in the notes, then consent must also be recorded. Procedures that do not require supervision are to be performed only if the supervisor or staff member has satisfied him or herself that the student is competent to perform the procedure.

Patient confidentiality

Medical students must respect the confidentiality of all information to which they have access, whether or not it is related to the patient's condition or treatment.

Clinical teachers and medical students must respect patient confidentiality when discussing a patient in any way. Students must never provide information that would identify a patient unless there is a specific reason. Students must obtain a patient's written authorization to record identifying information that they intend to use for educational purposes. An "educational purpose" is when the activity is undertaken separately from the care and treatment of a patient, and the explicit intention of the activity, contact or communication is educational.

Medical students must not discuss cases in public places such as elevators, corridors, coffee shops and waiting rooms, where a third party could overhear their conversation. This is the case even if patients' names are not used.

A patient must be informed if medical students, in the patient's best interests, are obliged to divulge confidential information to a responsible clinician about the patient's care and treatment. An example would be a patient who expressed an intention of self-harm.

Medical records

Medical students must identify themselves and their status in medical records. They must take care to record only information they believe to be factual and accurate or representing accurately the words of the patient or the patient's relatives.

Ethical dilemmas

Several studies highlight the problem of the "hidden curriculum" in medical education. Students report that the most difficult situations to resolve involve teachers who appear to show unethical behavior towards patients[2–6]

Hicks et al.[2] surveyed 108 clinical students, one year from graduation, at a medical school in Toronto. Forty-seven percent of students reported that they had, at times, been placed in a clinical situation in which they felt pressured to act unethically. Sixty-one percent said they had witnessed a clinical teacher acting unethically very frequently and occasionally. The same study reported that ethical problems reported by the students were seldom discussed or resolved with the clinical teachers.

All students and doctors in training potentially face similar ethical dilemmas. There may be rare occasions where clinical supervisors direct medical students to participate in patient management that is perceived by the student to be unethical or misleading to the patient. Many students are not confident enough to raise the inappropriateness of such involvement with their supervisors, and are unsure of how to respond.

This role confusion can lead to student stress and can have a negative impact on morale and the developing professionalism of the students.

What students should do

Students should be aware of their legal and ethical obligations to put patients' interests first.[7] This may include refusal to comply with an inappropriate instruction or direction.

The best way to resolve conflict (or at least gain a different perspective) is for the student to speak directly with the person concerned in private. The patient concerned should not be part of this discussion.

The student should explain the problem(s) and why they are unable to comply with the instruction or direction. If the clinician or responsible staff member ignores the issues raised, and continues to instruct the medical student to proceed, he/she should use discretion to proceed or withdraw from the situation. If the decision is to continue, patient consent must be confirmed. If the patient does not consent, the student must not proceed.

If a patient is unconscious or anesthetized, the student should explain why they cannot proceed. It may be necessary to point out the requirement of the Faculty of Medicine to comply with these guidelines. It may also be appropriate to discuss the situation with another person in the faculty or clinical school.

If a medical student is uncertain about the appropriateness of any behavior by another person involved in patient care, he/she should discuss the matter with a senior colleague of choice, usually the Associate Dean.

Any student who feels that he/she has been subjected to unfair treatment because of a refusal to do something that he/she deemed to be wrong, should seek advice from senior colleagues.

Students' responsibilities to each other

Every member of a profession has a responsibility for the standards of the profession as a whole. If a student has reason to believe that a fellow student is impaired, he/she has a professional responsibility to report the matter to a faculty member. This duty to report overrides any obligations regarding confidentiality between students. Encourage the 'impaired' student to self-report, but if they refuse, ask them to nominate the person whom they would prefer to receive the information about them. If the impaired student cannot nominate such a person, the concerned student needs to report the matter to the Associate Dean.

Students may find the following use of words helpful in discussing reporting with the fellow student: "I need to report (the matter of concern). I am happy to negotiate with whom I should inform and how much I will reveal, but I am not willing to keep this problem concealed."

Clinical teachers' responsibilities to students

Students are sometimes unsure about raising ethical issues with their clinical teachers because they fear they may be discriminated against if they are perceived to be "trouble makers" or "soft."

This is unfortunate, since ethical issues are interesting and challenging and they raise important learning opportunities. Students should be encouraged to raise ethical issues throughout the term with teachers and not just when a specific issue arises. They should also be encouraged to speak directly with the teacher involved during an ethical dilemma. Because students are new to the hospital environment, they may be mistaken in assuming that their position is being compromised. A simple explanation about the reasons for managing a patient in a particular way may be sufficient for the student to gain a new understanding.

Teachers should be receptive to ethical dilemmas or problems that students raise and seek to explain the ethics involved or change the circumstances so that students are not ethically compromised and patients are respected. If there is a particular practice that is routine in the hospital environment but raises ethical issues for medical students, the matter should be discussed with the Associate Dean of the clinical school, because he/she is in a position to resolve the issue at a systems level.

Problems in the workplace

Like all workplaces, hospitals and other health facilities are legally required to protect their staff (including students) from harassment. A study[1] involving students in an Australian university medical school showed that female students encountered an unacceptable amount of sexual harassment in medical training from fellow students, patients, faculty and doctors that they worked with. Two hundred and ninety-three out of 310 students returned questionnaires. The results showed that the type of behavior most reported concerned inappropriate comments by fellow students. Complaints against patients ranked second, with concerns about "unwelcome attention" and "unwanted physical contact." Faculty members and doctors were mainly criticized for "inappropriate comments." Research shows that medical students in other countries have similar problems.

What is sexual harassment?
Generally, this is sexually related behavior that:

- a person does not want, or
- offends, humiliates or intimidates,

in circumstances that a reasonable person should have expected would offend, humiliate or intimidate.

What to do
- You can privately ask the person to stop the behavior.
- You can seek the assistance of a clinical tutor.
- You can seek the assistance of a faculty member.
- You can seek the assistance of the Associate Dean.
- The hospital will have protocols and an identified officer to provide advice and guidance on how to deal with a problem of harassment.

References
1. These guidelines are adapted and expanded from: "Policy on the rights of patients in medical education." *BMJ* 2001; 322: 685–686.
2. Hicks LK, Lin Y, Robertson DW, Robinson DL, Woodrow SI. Understanding the clinical dilemmas that shape medical students' ethical development: Questionnaire survey and focus group study. *BMJ* 2001; 322: 709–710.
3. Swenson SL, Rothstein JA. Navigating the wards: teaching medical students to use their moral compass. *Acad Med* 1996; 71: 591–594.
4. St Onge J. Medical education must make room for student-specific ethics dilemmas. *Can Med Assoc J* 1997; 156: 1175–1177.
5. Bisonette R, O'Shea RM, Horwitz M, Route CF. A data-generated basis for medical ethics education: Categorisating issues experienced by students during clinical trials. *Acad Med* 1995; 70: 1035–1037.

6. Feudtner C, Christakis DA, Christakis NA. Do clinical students suffer ethical erosion? Students' perceptions of their ethical and personal development. *Acad Med* 1994; 69: 670–679.
7. White GE. Sexual harassment during medical training: the perceptions of medical students at a university medical school in Australia. *Med Educ* 2000; 34: 980–986.

Chapter 32

Stress and Stress Management

Henk T. Van der Molen and Abdullah Mohammed Al Zahem

Objectives

- To define the concept of stress and to be able to present a theoretical stress model.
- To describe different sources, symptoms and consequences of stress in medical students.
- To describe the different ways of dealing with stress; how can stress be prevented and how can it be managed?

When I (the first author) was 18 years old, I left my parents' home in the north of the Netherlands to study psychology at a university in another city. My first preference was to study medicine, but I didn't pass the lottery system for admission to this popular program. Therefore, I decided to choose my second option, psychology, because I was not only interested in the hard core of the human body but also in the 'softer' psychological aspects. However, my questions were: would psychology be interesting, would it fulfill my wish to help other people and what would be my job prospects on completion of the program?

The move to another city meant that I had to stand on my own two feet for the first time in my life. I rented a small student apartment that was 12 square meters and on the sixth floor of a block of flats. The apartment was big enough for a single bed, a tiny desk, a small table and a small bookshelf. I shared a communal kitchen with other students and had to watch that they didn't steal my cheese from the fridge!

I had been used to my dear mother's cooking, but now I had to learn how to cook potatoes and vegetables and how to bake meatballs. Not that easy. Furthermore, I had to live on a rather limited amount of money, which I received on a monthly basis, about 50 percent as a scholarship from the government and about 50 percent from my parents.

Only a few acquaintances from the same high school as myself chose to study psychology. A female friend who started to study medicine in the same city decided to move to the capital of the Netherlands because her boyfriend was living there. I felt quite sad about that because I was really close to her. Therefore, I had to make new friends and decided to become a member of the *student union. However, I did not click with fellow members of this union, so I felt quite lonely at times at the beginning of my academic career.*

During the weekends I was happy to go home to see my old friends. I took my laundry with me so that my mother could drop it in the washing machine. At the end of the weekend, I would return by train with a bag filled with clean clothes.

In the meantime, I enthusiastically began my academic studies. I liked the courses on clinical psychology, social psychology and the practicals on communication skills. But compared to high school, where I had 34 lessons of 50 minutes per week, the university program offered only a limited number of 10 hours of lectures per week and a couple of small working groups. For the rest of the time, I was supposed to have enough discipline for self-study and to prepare for the examinations at the end of each semester.

This personal example illustrates how the beginning of academic study may be accompanied by various sources of stress. In this case, the following factors were causing some stress. First, the *choice to study* psychology. This was in fact my second choice. Would I remain motivated throughout the whole program that in those days was of six years duration? Second, my *living situation* changed dramatically. From having lived in a rather big house, I now found accommodation in a very small room. Third, I had to deal with *limited finances* for my living and study costs. Fourth, I had to learn *how to care and cook for myself*. Fifth, there was the issue of *losing touch with old companions*, and therefore the need to *create new friendships*. Lastly, for study itself, I needed good *self-discipline* to excel and pass examinations.

All these different factors led to a certain level of stress. For most students, the start of the first year after leaving their home and family causes more stress than the start of the next year when they have become acquainted with their new living environment, new friends and new teachers. In the course of their study, other stressors may arise, such as writing a thesis or – as in the study of medicine – the first interactions with real patients and exposure to human pathology. Let us hasten to say that some stress in itself is not problematic; it is a part of life for everyone, including medical students.

Definition of the concept of stress

The word 'stress' is quite common in daily language. When people say that they are 'stressed', it means that they have difficulties in coping with the demands of the environment. Psychologists have tried to give a more specific definition of this concept. Lovallo[1] makes a distinction between two components of stress. The first one is the *physical component* that has to do with bodily symptoms such as an increased heartbeat or increased secretion of sweat when people are confronted with a difficult situation. The second is the *psychological component* that involves the way people perceive circumstances in their lives.

Sarafino[2] describes three ways in which these components can be examined. The first approach focuses on the environment. In this approach stress is considered as a *stimulus*. In the example above the small apartment and the loss of old friends were physically and psychologically challenging. Such factors are called *stressors*. The second approach considers stress as a *response*. An example of this approach is when students use the word 'stress' to refer to their state of mind when they are nervous before an exam. Responses can be physiological (getting cold hands, shivering) or psychological (like when people say: "I feel very nervous"). Together, the psychological and physiological response is called *strain*. The third approach considers stress as a *process* that includes stressors and strains, but adds an important dimension: the *relationship* between the person and the environment.[3] "This process involves continuous interactions and adjustments – called *transactions* – with the person and environment each affecting and being affected by the other."[2] In our definition, we follow Sarafino[2] who defines stress as: *"the circumstances in which transactions lead a person to perceive a discrepancy between the physical or psychological demands of a situation and the resources of his/her biological, psychological, or social systems."*[1-4]

Theoretical model

Below, we present a model for the relationship between demands of the study in medicine, stress and (physical and psychological) health in medical students. This model is based on a general model within the general framework of work stress.[5] The development of stress responses in medical students can be explained on the one hand by characteristics of their study environment, and on the other hand by their personal characteristics. Environmental factors are, for example: one's living situation, financial situation, and the degree to which the medical program is well structured. Personal characteristics that can play a part in the development of stress are: sex, age, level of education, intelligence, personality structure and motivation. These individual characteristics determine the coping capacity of the student. Within the causes of stress there are three main dimensions: (1) the educational and other environmental demands for the study of medicine; (2) the opportunities for the student to control their own study behavior during the curriculum; and (3) the amount of social support during their study. When there is no balance between the demands of the study and the coping capacity of the student, this may lead to a situation of stress. (see Figure 32.1)

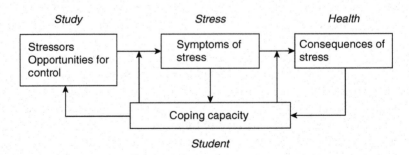

FIGURE 32.1   Theoretical stress model[6]

In the first box to the left of this figure, we see the concepts *stressors* and *opportunities for control*. In fact these concepts are competing with each other. When a student lacks the opportunity for controlling the influence of stressors, it may be that the student develops physical and psychological *symptoms of stress*. When the opportunities for control compete with stressors, no symptoms of stress will emerge. When the symptoms of stress last for an extended period of time, they may have negative *consequences* on the health of the student. These consequences of stress may negatively influence the *coping capacity* of the student, and when this coping capacity is reduced, this in itself may function as a new stressor for the student. This may lead to a reduction in the opportunities for control. Altogether, the figure shows that there is a *vicious circle* that is difficult to break through.

In the next sections, we will discuss what specific stressors play a part for medical students, which symptoms these stressors may lead to, and the consequences which may impact on the physical and psychological health of students.

Stressors: Sources of stress in medical students

Reviews of the literature[7, 8] show a high prevalence of stress among medical students. A study[9] among third- and fourth-year medical students from two Californian universities showed that the prevalence of stress was 51%. Among those who reported stress in this study, 38% reported severe stress or distress. In a recent review[10] concerning literature about stress among dental students, written by the present authors, the following group of stressors has been identified:

- living situation factors
- personal factors
- factors related to the medical curriculum and educational environment
- clinical factors

The fourth group of factors (clinical factors) is an extension of the third group (factors related to the medical curriculum and educational environment), and is related to the phase of the curriculum in which students have to deal with real patients, for example during their internships. Although we have not been able to do an extensive review of the literature concerning stress in medical students, we assume that the same groups of stressors are important for this specific group as well.

Living situation factors

As in the example of the first author at the beginning of this chapter, when he became a student of psychology, a common stressor for all students (including medical students) is to find suitable accommodation when they start a new program at the university. This may cause some temporary stress, but once they have found a room or apartment they may get used to it, and even prefer to live independently from their parents. In the latter case, the accommodation is no longer a stressor. However, when the room is small or the student has to live with other students in a noisy dormitory and where privacy is compromised, they may experience stress for a longer period of time. Another factor is whether the accommodation offers enough recreational facilities such as a bar or sport facilities. When their parents live in close proximity to where the university is located, students may postpone their decision to live independently and stay at home for the first years of their study. However, the relationship with their parents can then be a stressor; for example, when the parents have marital problems or when they do put some pressure on the student to go and live independently.

Personal factors

There are many personal factors that may act as a stressor for the medical student. The first factor is their *intelligence* or *cognitive ability*. Courses in a medical curriculum are about physics, chemistry, biology etc., and to understand the content of these courses the students need a certain minimal knowledge; otherwise they will never achieve good examination results.

The second factor is their *personality structure*. Personality psychologists have found that people differ from each other on five personality dimensions: the so called "Big Five."[11,12] Most "Big Five" personality tests contain measures for: (1) Extroversion; (2) Agreeableness; (3) Conscientiousness; (4) Emotional stability; and (5) Autonomy (for more detail about the nature of dimensions, see Table 32.1).

Research among Norwegian medical students[13] showed, for example, that the personality traits of neuroticism (which is the opposite of emotional stability) and

TABLE 32.1   Examples of items from the *Five Factor Personality Inventory (FFPI)*; (+) = a positively phrased item, (–) = a negatively phrased pole item.

Factors	Items
Extroversion	Likes to chat (+) Keeps at a distance from others (–)
Agreeableness	Respects others' feelings (+) Imposes his/her will on others (–)
Conscientiousness	Likes to follow a regular schedule (+) Acts without planning (–)
Emotional stability	Can take his/her mind off his/her problems (+) Invents problems for himself/herself (–)
Autonomy/Openness	Can easily link facts together (+) Follows the crowd (–)

conscientiousness were independent predictors of stress in later years of the curriculum. Another personality factor is *self-efficacy;*[14] this is comparable to the personality dimension *self-confidence*. Students' self-efficacy is dependent on their achievements. So, when a student fails the first two examinations in the first year of the curriculum, this may lead to a low self-efficacy, and when another student passes these exams that may result in a higher self-efficacy. Once a student has developed low expectations for his/her next achievements, either in the theoretical or in the more practical aspects of the course, this may act as a stressor, because a negative thought pattern might prevail. "However well I prepare for the examination, I am still afraid that I will not succeed" is a concrete example of such a thought pattern.

Other personal factors that may act as stressors are: *financial problems, lack of leisure time, lack of new friends* and *problems with time management* (compare the example at the beginning of this chapter).

Factors related to the medical curriculum and the educational environment

Different aspects of the medical curriculum and the educational environment may also be a stressor. The first aspect of the educational environment that is very important is the extent to which the educational program is well structured. If students understand what is expected from them during the blocks or semesters of the program, there is little reason to become stressed. However, when the structure is not very clear and they are left to their own devices, they may then develop stress.

A second aspect is the difficulty of the subject matter. Courses that are generally considered as difficult by the students will easily become a stressor for each student. Of course, students differ in their capacities and preferences. Achmed may be better in biology than in chemistry, whereas Leila prefers mathematics courses above communication skills. For Achmed, the examination in chemistry may act as a stressor, whereas he is looking forward to proving his abilities in the biology exam. Leila is not stressed in her preparation for the maths examination, but it makes her quite nervous when she looks ahead to the first practical exercise with a simulated patient in the diagnostic interview.

A third aspect is the approachability of staff members. If students are allowed to ask questions about difficult subject matter and the teachers are willing to take time to give further explanation, that will be helpful and the students will become less stressed. However, when there is an attitude among the staff that questions from students take too much time and that they have to be able to find out themselves, students may become uncertain and develop stress.

A fourth aspect of the educational environment is the workload that goes together with the academic program. It will be clear that the students' personal experience of the workload is dependent on their intellectual capacity and their prior knowledge. For the smarter students who easily filter the headlines from a voluminous academic textbook and have to study for their exam in physiology, this textbook may not act as a stressor, but for the less gifted it can be a huge stressor. Sometimes there is an academic overload for all the students, for example in the case of the professor who has little idea about how much subject matter students are able to deal with.

Examinations and preparation for examinations are the fifth general stressor for the students. Students may develop anxiety about exams when they have failed one or more. They may also become anxious as to the reactions of their parents when they do not succeed in passing an examination. Furthermore, once they have failed one or more examinations, they may become anxious that they will lag behind or even that they will not pass the transition from one year to the next.

A sixth important aspect is the degree to which the students receive social support from their parents, other family members and their peer students. Students who are reassured by their parents after failing an exam will develop less stress than students who receive a lot of negative feedback from their parents after failing.

Clinical factors

A six-year longitudinal, nationwide and comparative study among medical students in Norway[15] showed that satisfaction with life decreased during medical school for the students. Medical students were as satisfied as other students in the first year of study, but reported less satisfaction in their graduation year. This finding was in line with the findings of a longitudinal study of depression among medical students.[16] Which stressors may play a part to explain these findings?

The first stressor is the *real patient contact* and the *responsibility for comprehensive patient care*. Acquiring sufficient academic medical knowledge during the first years of the curriculum may be stressful, but dealing with complex medical complaints and psychological problems of the real patient is probably even more stressful.

A second stressor is the *feedback of the supervisor* on the attitude and professional behavior of the new physician. If the students make inadequate diagnoses or prescribe the wrong treatments, they will be criticized by their supervisor. When this happens several times, they may be anxious over receiving feedback.

A third stressor can be *differences in opinion between supervising staff members concerning diagnosis or treatment*. The medical profession is often confronted with ambiguous situations in which there is no clear solution.

A fourth stressor is that medical students are sometimes *overloaded with work during their internships*, which can also lead to a shortage of time to do the job properly. A final stressor lies in the *general atmosphere* that is created by other clinical faculty. If this atmosphere is positive and rewarding, it will probably not act as a stressor, but if it has become negative, it will.

Symptoms of stress

Stress may become manifest in many different symptoms. A distinction can be made between physical, psychological and behavioral symptoms of stress.[5]

Physical symptoms

In a situation of stress the human body is activated in many regards. People may breathe more quickly, which sometimes leads to hyperventilation. They may blush and their hands may sweat. There may be an increase in heartbeat and hormones, producing more adrenaline and cortisol. All these changes are caused by the activation of the autonomous nervous system.

Table 32.2 gives an overview of the responses of the different organs on stress.

People differ in their physical responses to the same stressors. Table 32.3 presents an overview of different psychological symptoms of stress.[5,9] The most common symptoms are anxiety, worry, nervousness and tension. Chronic stress may even lead to depression, emotional exhaustion and burnout. Depression goes together with symptoms such as fatigue and sleeplessness, indecision, unhappiness, guilt, irritability and hostility.

Consequences of stress

The physical and psychological symptoms of stress can be followed by different behavioral symptoms. Table 32.4 gives an overview on the consequences of chronic stress on the behavior of medical students. They may put less effort into their study and may even begin to develop bad habits such as drug and alcohol abuse. They may also resort to tranquillizers as a way of dealing with stress. As for social interaction, because they feel ashamed of their low academic achievements they may display cynical behavior and avoid their friends.

TABLE 32.2 Responses of different organs on stress.[5]

Organ	Stress response
Heart	Increased heartbeat Decreased variability in the frequency of the heartbeat
Veins	Increased high blood pressure in the vein system Increased low blood pressure in the vein system
Breathing	Increased frequency of breathing Decreased depth of breathing
Skin/Secretion glands	Increased sweating
Muscles	Increased muscle tension
Hormones	Increased production of adrenaline and secretion in the blood Increased production of cortisol and secretion in the blood
Stomach	Upset, painful

TABLE 32.3   Psychological symptoms of stress.

Anxiety, worry, nervousness	Fatigue, sleeplessness
Tension, being upset	Indecision
Depression	Unhappiness
Lack of confidence	Guilt
Distress	Irritability
Emotional exhaustion	Hostility
Burnout	

Finally, chronic stress may have negative consequences on physical and psychological health. Stress increases the vulnerability for infectious diseases such as catching a cold or a fever, and may also lead to complaints of the muscular system, i.e. headaches, neck pain and pain in the wrists.[17] When psychological symptoms last for a longer period of time, the student may be diagnosed as suffering from anxiety disorder, depression, alcoholism or substance abuse. In that case, the future physician needs medical and/or psychological help for him or herself.

Stress management: How to deal with stress?

In this final section, we will try to answer the question on how to deal with stress. Before discussing different approaches that are found in literature, we have to emphasize that some stress, in an interesting and intriguing study such as medicine, is unavoidable. Life is not always fun and that is maybe even more true in the life of a medical student, and later on as a physician. However, as we discussed before, chronic stress may lead to somatic and psychological diseases. The first question is: how can we prevent this? Prevention is better than healing. The second question is: what to do when students have not been able to prevent stress-related complaints? When we answer this question, we will take into account both the perspective of the student, and that of the management having the responsibility for the medical curriculum.

TABLE 32.4   Behavioral stress symptoms.[5,10]

Putting less effort into study	Sudden changes in productivity
Showing restless behavior	Excessive use of alcohol or drugs
Panic reactions	Avoidance of social contacts
Excessive use of tranquillizers	Excessive complaining
Cynical behavior	Showing hostility

Prevention of the development of stress-related complaints

Based on literature,[15,16] we give some general advice. As we have seen before, personal characteristics such as intelligence and personality play a role in the development of stress. However, it is not easy to change these rather stable dispositions. Although personality characteristics may be changed by psychotherapy to some extent, most students take them for granted. Your own behavior and habits are more under the direct control of your will. Therefore, below we focus on your study and social behavior.

Time management

Try to study on a regular basis. If you procrastinate on your self-study time and there is an exam in two weeks' time, for example, life will be very stressful in that period. However, studying on a regular basis enhances the probability that you will remember the subject matter better than when you have to rush through voluminous textbooks. It is better to spend 5 days x 2 hours per day in self-study, than 2 days x 5 hours per day. In general, you need a study plan that is based on a calculation of how much time you need to finish all the preparatory work for the examinations. Of course, personal differences play a role here, because some students are quicker than others in acquiring relevant knowledge.

Make adequate time for a social and personal life.[15] When your student life only consists of attending lectures, doing practicals, studying literature and working at the hospital, you may eventually develop burnout.

Try to find one or more peers from your academic year that you can share your concerns with.

As you might give advice to other patients suffering from work stress: do some sport or physical activity. This clears your head and creates new energy.

Pay attention to your diet. If you arrive at a stage in which you realize your intake is actually related to a reduction in your stress levels, then try to set limits for yourself. If you do not succeed, then it might be time to ask for professional help, for example from a student counselor.

Stress management

Several investigators[18,19] recommend that the management responsible for the medical curriculum should pay attention to the fact that stress has such a high prevalence among medical students. Below we present a number of measures that can be taken to help medical students deal with the stressful aspects of their academic program and life:

1. General advice for managing stress reduction is to *create a student-friendly atmosphere* in which students' concerns are treated seriously.
2. Offer sufficient *counseling services* to discuss study progress and any personal problems. Students should have access to qualified staff who can offer professional help.

3. Organize *effective support* for students by offering *workshops on stress management* or *assertive training*. A concrete example hereof is the *Student-led stress management program for first-year medical students* at Oklahoma State University (USA).[19] This program has been offered to students for the past 16 years and they can participate on a voluntary basis. It involves small groups (6–8 students) in which first-year medical students meet with second-year student co-leaders at noon on the same day of the week, and two psychologists (faculty members) serve as program coordinators. At the beginning of the fall semester, each group meets weekly for one hour per week. The program has seven sessions.

Table 32.5 gives an overview of the activities during the seven sessions.

Evaluations showed that there was a very high participation rate of 94% over the last 16 years and that the results were positive. Most components were considered to be useful. The authors argue that, among other factors, the use of second-year medical students as group leaders is fundamental for the success of the program, because they are close to the experience of the first-year students.

Summary

The prevalence of stress among medical students is high. In this chapter we have presented a definition and a theoretical model of the concept of stress. Stress was defined as: "*the circumstances in which* **transactions** *lead a person to* **perceive a discrepancy** *between the physical or psychological* **demands** *of a situation and the re-* **sources** *of his or her biological, psychological or social systems.*" The main elements in the theoretical model are: stressors and opportunities for control, stress symptoms, coping capacity, and consequences for physical and psychological health. An overview was given of different stressors. These have been categorized into four groups: (1) living situation factors (2), personal factors, (3) factors related to the medical curriculum and educational environment, and (4) clinical factors. An overview was presented of different physical and psychological symptoms of stress. Chronic stress may lead to physical and psychological illness. Therefore, it is important for medical curricula to pay attention to the prevention and cure of these illnesses by offering a student-friendly learning environment and adequate counseling services, and by offering modules such as stress management and assertiveness training programs for those students who need it.

TABLE 32.5 Overview of the sessions in the student-led stress management program.

Session 1	Icebreaker exercises to get acquainted. Group contract to keep personal information confidential and to treat each other with respect. No studying during group meetings.
Between session 1 and 2	Lecture on the effects of stress on health and instruction on relaxation methods during a lab session.
Session 2	Follow-up of the lecture. Discussion of study and test-taking skills.
Session 3	Role of peer support in maintaining health. Focus on empathic listening. Humorous video with good and bad responses to a fellow student who is disappointed by a failing exam grade.
Session 4	Reframing thoughts. Students practice identifying their thoughts about stressful events and adopting a new perspective that results in a decreased level of stress.
Session 5	Medical student wellbeing and personal relationships. Groups' review "A Primer on Medical Student Well-Being," prepared by the American Medical Student Association.
Session 6	Conflict resolution skills. Video examples and discussion.
Session 7	Oral and written evaluation.

References

1. Lovallo WR. *Stress and health: Biological and psychological interactions.* Thousand Oaks, CA: Sage; 1997.
2. Sarafino EP. *Health Psychology. Biopsychosocial interactions*, 5th edition. Hoboken, NJ: John Wiley & Sons; 2006.
3. Lazarus, RS, Folkman S. *Stress, appraisal, and coping.* New York: Springer; 1984.
4. Trumbull R, Appley MH. A conceptual model for examination of stress dynamics. In: Appley MH and Trumbull R (Eds.). *Dynamics of stress: Physiological, psychological, and social perspectives* (pp. 21–45). New York: Plenum; 1986.
5. Kompier MAJ, Houtman ILD. Stressreacties [Stress responses]. In: Smulders PGW, Op de Weegh J. (Eds.). *Arbeid en Gezondheid. Risicofactoren* [Work and Health. Risk factors]. Utrecht: Open Universiteit/Lemma; 1995.
6. Kompier MAJ, Marcelissen FHG. *Handboek Werkstress: een systematische aanpak voor de bedrijfspraktijk*, 3ᵉ druk. [Handbook on Work Stress: a systematic approach, 3rd edition]. Amsterdam: Nederlands Instituut voor Arbeidsomstandigheden; 1990.
7. Shapiro S, Shapiro D, Schwartz G. Stress management in medical education: a review of the literature. *Acad Med* 2000; 75: 748–759.

8. Kiessling C, Schubert B, Scheffner D, Burger W. First year medical students' perception of stress and support: a comparison between reformed and traditional track curricula. *Med Educ* 2004; 38: 504–509.

9. Bughi SA, Sumcad J, Bughi S. Effect of brief behavioral intervention program in managing stress in medical students from two southern California universities. *Med Educ* 2006; 40: 11–17.

10. Al Zahem AM, Van der Molen HT, Alaujan AH, Schmidt HG, Zamakhshary MH. Stress amongst dental students: A systematic review. *Eur J Dent Educ* 2011; 15: 8–18.

11. Hendriks AAJ. The construction of the Five-Factor Personality Inventory (FFPI). PhD Dissertation: Rijksuniversiteit Groningen, The Netherlands; 1997.

12. Hendriks AAJ, Hofstee WKB, De Raad B. The Five-Factor Personality Inventory. Manual. Lisse: Swets Test Publishers; 1999.

13. Tyssen R, Dolatowski FC, Rovik JO, Thorkildsen RF, Ekeberg O, Hem E, Gude T, Gronvold NT, Vaglum P. Personality traits and types predict medical school stress: A six-year longitudinal and nationwide study. *Med Educ* 2007; 41: 781–787.

14. Bandura A. *Self-efficacy: The exercise of control.* New York: Freeman; 1997.

15. Kjeldstadli K, Tyssen R, Finset A, Hem E, Gude T, Gronvold NT, Ekeberg O, Vaglum P. Life satisfaction and resilience in medical school – a six-year longitudinal, nationwide and comparative study. *BMC Med Educ* 2006; 6: 48.

16. Rosal MC, Ockene IS, Ockene JK, Barrett SV, Ma Y, Hebert JR. A longitudinal study of students' depression at one medical school. *Acad Med* 1997; 72: 542–546.

17. Hendrix WH, Schultz SA, Steel RP. Job stress and life stress: their causes and consequences. *J Soc Beh and Pers* 1987; 2: 291–302.

18. Shah C, Trivedi RS, Diwan J, Dixit R, Anand AK. Common stressors and coping of stress by medical students. *J Clin and Diagnostic Res* 2009; 6(3): 1621–1626.

19. Redwood SK, Pollak MH. Student-led stress management program for first-year medical students. *Teach Learn Med* 2007; 19(1): 42–46.

Chapter 33

Career Choices and Opportunities after Medical School

Rogayah Jaafar and Zulkifli Ahmad

Objectives

By the end of this chapter, you will be able to answer:
- Is there a place in medical school for you as a medical student to nurture your career development?
- The number of medical specialty aptitude tests and instruments that may offer an accurate assessment of your career options.
- How to develop your interest in a specific clinical discipline as a career choice during your medical school.
- How important is the period of medical school for you to form a decision concerning your future career?

Introduction

Alice asked the cat, "Would you tell me please, which way I ought to walk from here?"
"That depends a good deal on where you want to get to," said the cat.
"I do not much care where," said Alice.
"Then it doesn't matter which way you go," said the cat.

The above quote, taken from the *Adventures of Alice in Wonderland,* reflects the varied ways medical students view their career options and choices after medical school. While some medical students do consider this aspect rather seriously while in medical school, most medical students just go with the flow and delay their decision on a career choice until after they have graduated and have had a chance to work in a number of clinical postings and thereafter.[1,2]

Therefore, the question to ask is: Is there a place in medical school for you as a medical student to be nurtured in your career development? The social milieu offered by medical schools, clinical teaching hospitals and other teaching settings does influence career choice and future specialty training options for medical students, albeit in a limited way. This fact has been confirmed by a number of studies on the topic. Markert reviewed 12 studies of changes in medical student specialty preferences, and found agreement between early and late choices on average only 39% of the time.[3] In a Malaysian study (of Malaysian doctors) on timing and stability in choices of medical specialty, it was discovered that while 48.5% of the doctors had made an earlier career choice as medical students, only 15.2% of them actually made their eventual specialty choices by the end of medical school.[4] This is especially true with regard to psychiatry (42.9%) and, to a lesser extent, surgery (25.7%). By the end of their internship, another 17.7% of the graduates had made their decision while the remaining 67.1% made their final decision only when they were medical officers.[5] Zeldow et al. noted that specialty choices that seemed to be most powerfully influenced by the clinical clerkship experience during medical school were pediatrics, psychiatry and surgery.[6] Other studies have claimed that interest in surgery and psychiatry was already present prior to entering medical school.[7, 8]

The choice of a career in the medical field is a complex, personal decision, influenced by a multitude of factors. In the developing world, factors may differ from those operating in the developed countries. Most developing countries continue to experience a shortage of doctors in certain specialties.[9] There are shortages in 'service' specialties such as anesthesiology, radiology and pathology. Deficiencies are also felt in rural areas, which involve primary healthcare and preventive medicine. Medical schools also have difficulties in recruiting medical graduates to basic medical sciences (non-clinical) departments.

Many medical schools have embarked on an innovative medical curriculum to foster and nurture medical students into becoming doctors who are sensitive to the country's health manpower needs and who are able to prioritize health issues. Emphasis is placed on producing future doctors who not only possess the technical skills of healing but also have the mind and soul to empathize, promote well-being and focus on and understand the whole patient and community, rather than just the disease.[10] As such, problem-based learning, early clinical exposure and communication skills training and community-based education have become the mainstream of medical education around the world. Early clinical skills training and student-centered learning activities have replaced much of the teacher-centered lectures and demonstrations of the older educational system. As students, you should take these educational approaches into consideration when you start thinking about opportunities to serve and work with your healthcare system, especially in rural communities and in primary healthcare, regardless of which specialty you choose to pursue after medical school.[11]

The period in medical school is an important phase during which many of you will begin to form a decision concerning your future career. Depending on your gender and marital status, your career choices may differ. Surgery and orthopedic surgery tend to attract male students, while female students have been shown to choose less rigorous disciplines such as family medicine, public health and anesthesiology.[12-14] However, female specialty preferences may have changed in the last few years and may still be in the process of transition. The choice of obstetrics and gynecology (O&G), for example, may point to your social and religious ideals that female patients should be managed by female doctors, especially if you are a female student. However, do remember that this idealistic obligation will need to be fulfilled alongside your own responsibilities of marriage and family.

One thing is for sure: there is evidence that personality changes are occurring among female medical students. Female students have become more action-oriented, autonomous and aggressive and just as ambitious as your male colleagues.[15] This is particularly true if they are female mentors in the more vigorous clinical specialties whom students look up to and try to emulate in terms of their professional work and family commitments.

Fixed working hours are found to be an important factor affecting career choices for female doctors.[16] So if you are a female with an interest in the surgical specialties such as orthopedic surgery and O&G during medical school, there is a strong possibility that you may reconsider that option later on in your career pathway. This decision may also reflect on whether you will consider marriage after completion of study, commitment to your partner's career or decisions about child care. Combining a full-time medical career with domestic responsibilities and taking care of a partner and children may pose greater and more serious considerations for you than for your male counterparts. Most male doctors, but few female doctors, can expect their spouses to take responsibility for child care. Since professional medicine imposes exhaustive work schedules on practitioners in most medical specialties, the combination of domestic responsibilities and professional career demands is a major challenge, especially if you are a female doctor.[17,18] Thus, serious attention to time management and the ability to balance responsibilities on both the work and home fronts are fundamental in considering your future career options, especially in the more demanding specialties such as O&G and surgery.

Both male and female medical students, as well as young doctors, generally choose clinical-based specialties rather than the more administrative and preventive specialties such as family medicine and public health. In line with clinically oriented career choices and academic careers in general, teaching hospitals are prime choices for a vocational setting. Other relevant sites for medical vocations are private medical centers/hospitals, private practice, health office, administration of a hospital and the armed forces.[19,20]

When starting to form a career interest in medical school, you may want to examine your own personal inclination towards certain specialties. You may have already developed a preference for counseling and listening to other people's problems prior to medical school that may lead you to a choice of psychiatry. You may be very good with your hands, enjoy working with instruments and able to manage dramatic situations, which may direct you to an interest in surgery, orthopedics and trauma or emergency medicine. If you are hard-working and have empathy for children, then pediatrics may be your choice; otherwise, general medicine could be an option. If you have an interest in sleeping and putting people to sleep, then anesthesiology may just be the right career choice for you. A love for criminology and dealing with the dead could lead you to pathology. Respect for motherhood and empathy for women's wellbeing could make you choose O&G.

The flowchart (Figure 33.1) provides a hilarious but scientifically supported framework on a career pathway for medical students and young doctors in relation to personality-matched specialty options.[21] While it is not exhaustive and does not cover the whole spectrum of specialty choices, it does provide a basis to get medical students to start thinking about their future career direction, albeit in a tongue-in-cheek fashion. Of course this approach to selecting a career option must be taken with a large pinch of salt.

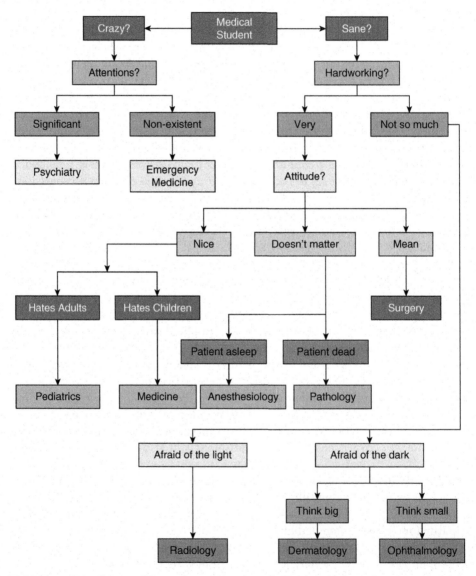

FIGURE 33.1 Career choices for medical students (a hilarious framework by Vagus, 2006)

On a more serious note, you may want to explore the Medical Specialty Aptitude Test, offered by the University of Virginia Health System website.[22] It consists of an on-line survey of 130 questions that can accurately rank your total personality score to a list of possible specialty options in medicine. This aptitude test offers an accurate assessment of your career options, based on your perceived personality traits.

Also described is a study on mapping career preferences for medical students that uses the hexagon of Holland's general typology of careers and Prediger's derived orthogonal dimensions.[23] Holland's general career typology comprises six categories, namely: realistic, investigative, artistic, social, enterprising and conventional (RIASEC),[24] while Prediger's orthogonal model comprises Things–People and Ideas–Data axial dimensions.[25] Petrides and McManus found that there are close parallels between these two elements and the structure found in medical careers. Medical specialties typical of Holland's six RIASEC categories are Surgery and its related fields (Realistic), General Medicine and its related fields (Investigative), Psychiatry and its related fields (Artistic), Public Health and its related fields (Social), Administrative Medicine and its related fields (Enterprising) and finally Laboratory Medicine and its related fields (Conventional).[26] These career choices can be represented graphically as shown in Figure 33.2.

You can actually plot your medical career choices in relation to six proto-typical dimensions on a general career model. They reflect realistic, investigative, artistic, social, enterprising and conventional (RIASEC) specialties of medicine, along with the Things–People and Data–Ideas axial dimensions of those chosen disciplines.

The following statements illustrate the link between these specialties and the RIASEC personality dimensions:

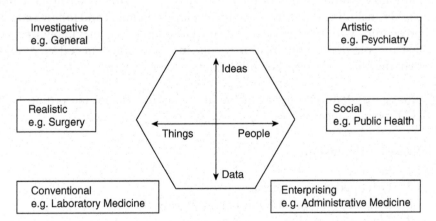

FIGURE 33.2   The hexagon of Holland's RIASEC typology along with the Things–People and Ideas–Data dimensions proposed by Prediger[24]

- *Surgery etc. – Realistic*
  Surgeons can be seen as the engineers of medicine, solving problems at high levels of mechanical and technical proficiency with an emphasis on practical skills, craftsmanship, and immediate and effective results.
- *Internal medicine etc. – Investigative*
  The core of internal medicine is diagnosis, which is achieved by carrying out appropriate investigations. Physicians typify the model of the scientist-practitioner, investigating signs and symptoms and relating them to the underlying pathophysiology of the patient.
- *Psychiatry etc. – Artistic*
  Psychiatrists and general practitioners have a more artistic approach to medicine – seeing, interpreting and responding imaginatively to a range of medical, social, ethical and other problems. The emphasis in many ways is on the uniqueness of the patient, the ideas that they are expressing and the psycho-social theories and concepts which are necessary for interpreting the individual.
- *Public Health etc. – Social*
  Although most medicine is concerned with individual patients, the remit of Public Health is primarily social in the sense of applying medicine to society as a whole, treating the 'body politic.' Public Health manages social and community health by the appropriate analysis of data.
- *Administrative medicine etc. – Enterprising*
  The management of hospitals and healthcare requires the creative skills of the business executive, the lawyer and the personnel director to achieve a smooth-running system. People, both patients and caregivers, are at the heart of any health care system, and therefore administrative medicine is at the people-end of the dimension.
- *Laboratory medicine etc. – Conventional*
  The running of efficient systems in hematology, histopathology or chemical pathology requires many of the attributes shared with an accountant and a banker, including the willingness to develop, implement and follow standard procedures within a complete system. The emphasis is inevitably upon the instruments that do the measurements and upon the data collected, rather than the ideas or people behind the data and technology.

Common specialty choices available after medical school (according to the RIASEC Topology) include:

1. **Realistic dimension**
   1.1   Surgery
   1.2. Orthopedics and trauma
   1.3. Ear, nose and throat (Otorhinolaryngology)
   1.4. Medical researcher

1.5. Anesthesiology
1.6. Ophthalmology

2. Investigative dimension
2.1. General medicine
2.2. Pediatrics
2.3. Infectious diseases
2.4. Respiratory medicine
2.6. Obstetrics and gynecology

3. Artistic dimension
3.1. Psychiatry
3.2. General practice
3.3. Family medicine
3.4 Dermatology

4. Social dimension
4.1. Public Health
4.2. Community medicine
4.3 Geriatric medicine
4.4. Genitourinary medicine
4.5. Oncology

5. Enterprising dimension
5.1. Administrative medicine
5.2. Pharmaceutical medicine
5.3. Industrial medicine
5.4. Forensic medicine

6. Conventional dimension
6.1. Laboratory medicine (hematology, microbiology, etc.)
6.2. Basic Medical Sciences (anatomy, physiology, etc.)
6.3. Pathology
6.4. Radiology
6.5. Radiotherapy

In starting to develop an interest in career choices at medical school, you may wish to consider the following strategies:

1. Begin by playing an active role in all your basic sciences programs and clinical postings during your clerkship years.
2. Keep an open mind to the various career and specialty options available after graduation.

3. Choose appropriate basic science teachers, consultants and clinicians as role models and mentors in basic sciences/clinical postings that you will be undertaking.
4. Find out about your Ministry of Health manpower requirements as well as specialty needs and the labor market.
5. Start to develop an interest in a clinical discipline or posting of your choice.
6. Explore career options in basic sciences and laboratory services.
7. Discuss career options with your peers, seniors, academic advisors, clinical consultants, career counselors and your family.
8. Remember that you will probably modify or change your career choice as you move into internship and also as a future medical officer.
9. Keep in mind that a final career decision is a complex, personal choice, influenced by a multitude of factors.
10. Do not worry too much about the need to finalize your career decision at the end of medical school – just enjoy the ride!!

Numerous factors such as your ease and confidence level in handling patients, your marital status and financial aspirations may influence your career choices in medical school during your internship training and postgraduate practice. You may thus wish to consider the following aspects in your decision to select your career options after graduation:

- The ability to have direct contact with patients
- Marriage and family considerations
- Work experience in your specialty
- The possibility of pursuing specialty training locally
- The offer of a good salary and financial incentives
- Fixed hours of work e.g. office hours
- Opportunities for teaching
- Opportunities for research
- Higher social status.

Apart from your own personal and individual interests as well as inclination, your career choices may be determined on the basis of your selection of location and site of your practice. Therefore, you may want to consider the following location or site of practice in the context of your career pursuit:

1. Clinical consultant in a general hospital
2. Clinical lecturer in a teaching hospital
3. Specialist in a private medical center or hospital
4. General practitioner in a private clinic
5. Non-clinical lecturer in a medical school
6. Service consultant in a general hospital

7. Health officer/Public health practitioner
8. Administrator in a hospital
9. Doctor/specialist in the armed forces
10. Pharmaceutical representative
11. Medical researcher in a public medical institution
12. Medical researcher in the private sector

Conclusion

Medical school is an exciting starting point for you, as medical students, to start to formulate ideas about the specialties and practicing sites you would like to pursue for your future vocation. You and your medical teachers should seek updates and be kept regularly informed by the Ministry of Health on manpower and labor requirements in various medical specialties. This would enable your active participation in career guidance, counseling and mentoring at all levels in medical school. You would then be able to make realistic choices on careers, based not only on your personal interests, but also on the current health needs of the population of your country in general and the manpower requirements of your national healthcare system.

Take-home messages

1. The choice of a career in the medical field is a complex, personal decision, influenced by a multitude of factors.
2. The period in medical school is an important phase during which many of you will begin to form a decision concerning your future career.
3. There are a number of medical specialty aptitude tests and instruments that may offer an accurate assessment of your career options, based on your perceived personality traits.
4. You will be exposed to an interesting social milieu and varied working experiences during your medical school program.
5. There will be both positive and negative role models among your basic medical sciences and clinical teachers.
6. The social milieu and mentorship opportunities in your medical school will spur your career aspirations.
7. Many of you will start to develop an interest in a specific clinical discipline as a career choice during medical school.
8. There are specific strategies during your medical program that can help you to sharpen your selection of career options.

(Continued)

9. Preferred site and location of practice will influence your career decision.
10. In most instances, you will probably need to review, affirm or modify your career choices as you enter internship and also later on as a practicing medical officer.

References

1. Tardiff K, Cella D, Seiferth C. Selection and change of specialties by medical school graduates. *J Med Educ* 1986; 61: 48–49.
2. Zulkifli Ahmad, Rogayah Jaafar. Career preferences of medical students of Universiti Sains Malaysia. *Malaysian J Med Sci* 1996; 3(1); 58–61.
3. Markert RJ. Change in specialty choice during medical school. *J Fam Pract* 1983; 17: 295–300.
4. Babbott D, Balwin DC, Jolly P et al. The stability of early specialty preferences among US medical school graduates in 1983. *JAMA* 1988; 259: 1970–1975.
5. Rogayah J, Zulkifli A. The timing and stability of choice of medical specialty among Malaysian doctors. *Med J Malaysia* 2001; 56; 324–329.
6. Zeldow PB, Preston RC, Daugherty SR. The decision to enter a medical specialty, timing and stability. *Med Educ* 1992; 26: 327–332.
7. Geertsma RH, Grinos DR. Specialty choice in medicine. *J Med Educ* 1972; 47: 509–517.
8. Deva MP. Career choices of Malaysian medical students. *Med J Mal* 1981; 36: 188–192.
9. *Annual Report 1991.* Ministry of Health, Malaysia, 1991.
10. Wayne K, Davis et al. (Eds). *Moving Medical Education from the Hospital to the Community.* Report of the 7th Cambridge Conference in Medical Education, 1995.
11. Victor Neufeld, Richard Pickering, Janice Simpson (Eds). *Priority Health Problems in the Education of Health Professionals.* Network Publications, 1997.
12. Rogayah Jaafar. Editorial: Social accountability of medical schools: Between reality and fantasy. *Mal J Med Sci* July 1997: 5–8.
13. Zulkifli A, Rogayah J. Career preferences of male and female medical students in Malaysia. *Med J Mal* 1997; 52: 1–6.
14. Shahabuddin SH. Career choices of final year female medical students at Universiti Kebangsaan Malaysia (UKM). *Med J Mal* 1986; 41: 327–330.
15. William AP, Domnick-Pierre K, Vayda E. Women in medicine: practice patterns and attitudes. *Can Med Assoc J* 1990; 143: 194–201.
16. Wakeford RE, Warren VJ. Women doctor's career choice and commitment to medicine: Implications for general practice. *J Rol Coll GP* 1989; 39: 91–95.
17. Ulstad VK. How women are changing medicine. *J Am Women c* 1993; 48: 75–78.
18. Frey H. Representation of women in medical specialties with particular reference to Sweden. *J Am Med Womens Association* 1980; 14: 428–433.
19. Nortzer N, Brown S. The feminization of the medical profession in Israel. *Med Educ* 1995; 29: 377–381.

20. A Zulkifli, J Rogayah. Specialty choices of male and female doctors in Malaysia. *Med J Malaysia* 1998; 53(4): 327–333.
21. *Career Choices for Medical Students.* 9th March 2006. Malaysian Medical Resources website: http://medicine.com.my/wp/
22. *Medical Specialty Aptitude Test 2004.* University of Virginia Health System website: http://www.med-edu.virginia.edu/specialties/QuestionList/cfm
23. Pretrides KV, McManus IC. Mapping medical careers: Questionnaire assessment of career preferences in medical school applicants and final year students. BMC *Med Educ* 2004; 4: 1–17.
24. Prediger DJ. Dimensions underlying Holland's hexagon: Missing link JL between interests and occupations? *J Vocational Behaviour* 1982; 21: 259–287.
25. Holland JL. *Making Vocational Choices: A theory of careers.* New York: Prentice Hills, 1973.
26. Prediger DJ. Locating occupations on Holland's hexagon: Beyond RIASEC. *J Vocational Behavior* 1992; 40: 111–128.

Chapter 34

Preparing for Practice

Chris Roberts and Mohamed Al Moamary

Objectives

- To prepare students for their medical practice.
- To learn the domains of practice required by an intern and how they are measured.
- To teach medical students how to acquire sound clinical reasoning skills developed in the clinical environment.

Introduction

Claims are often made that medical schools are not preparing students well enough for entering the workforce. Problems for interns include a perceived lack of self-reflection and improvement, poor organizational skills, underdeveloped professionalism, and lack of medical knowledge.[1] Directors of clinical training or their equivalent in hospitals have been the most vocal in this regard. Universities do have a role in considering the needs of the workforce and must ensure that their graduate outcomes reflect the knowledge, clinical skills and professional behavior expected of a junior doctor commencing in the intern year.

International context

Internationally, there is considerable variation in the quality of both undergraduate medicine programs and vocational training. In developed nations, there appears to be little difference in how modern curricula prepare students for practice. Graduates from the graduate-entry, problem-based programs are at least as well prepared for their intern year as graduates from traditional and undergraduate problem-based programs.[2] However, there is evidence to suggest that graduate-entry students are more self-confident and less anxious than those from undergraduate schools.[3]

In several developing countries, the situation is similar to that described by Flexner a century ago in North America, where medical education had become a commercial enterprise with proprietary schools of variable quality, lectures delivered in crowded classrooms, and often no laboratory instruction or patient contact, leading to severe inadequacies in the quality of physician training.[4] This is partly the result of decreasing public spending on higher education over the last two decades, such that some countries have seen rapid growth in the number of private medical schools. There is an imbalance whereby, in some countries, the shortage of qualified faculty and insufficient clinical exposure are expected to give new graduates not enough opportunity to achieve pre-set competencies or provide satisfactory preparation for practice. At the same time, other countries have seen more investment in higher education.[5,6] Moreover, constraints in the availability of postgraduate training slots will mean new graduates will have to compete strongly in the selection process for those places that are available. Therefore, it is the responsibility of the governing bodies in these countries to ensure the quality of medical education by strengthening the accreditation process, investing in health profession education and enhancing the teaching abilities of their faculty.

Most developing countries implement a traditional, unstructured, 12-month medical internship. Internationally, there have been innovations in medical internship. For example, in the United States, specific standards have been set to assess the trainees during the first postgraduate year (PGY1) on a variety of expected competencies that include: patient care, medical knowledge, practice-based learning and improvement, interpersonal skills, communication, and professionalism.[7] In Canada, where universities are responsible for providing postgraduate training for PGY1, which has replaced the internship period, the Canadian Medical Education Directions for Specialists (CanMEDS) framework[8] is competency-based and aims to graduate a doctor who is a medical expert, communicator, collaborator, manager, health advocate, scholar and professional. There have been similar initiatives in Australia and the UK.[9,10] In countries applying traditional internship, a Framework for Medical Intern's Competencies (FMIC) is an example, proposed by Saudi Arabia, that covers the domains of clinical management, medical practice, professionalism and communication.[6] One challenge for all of these frameworks is the relationship between the curriculum framework itself, the quality of education and training in the various clinical rotations, and the meaningfulness of any associated assessment in determining fitness to practice.

Measuring preparedness for practice

The Preparation for Hospital Practice Questionnaire scale (PHPQ)[11] gives some insight into how the domains of practice required by an intern might be measured. The PHPQ is a valid and reliable 41-item questionnaire which contains eight subscales designed to assess key areas of medical hospital practice (see Box 34.1).

How can medical educators ensure that their curricula give graduates strength in all these areas, and develop curricular innovation where there are gaps? Some schools have taken the approach of having a generic preparation for the internship

---

Box 34.1   The Preparation for Hospital Practice Questionnaire scale

- interpersonal skills
- confidence and coping
- collaboration (team approach to care)
- self-directed learning (evaluation of performance, identification of learning needs)
- patient management and practical skills
- understanding science (as the basis of disease and therapeutics)
- prevention (preparedness to incorporate health promotion and disease prevention with hospital practice)
- holistic care (appreciation of the impact of multiple variables on patients' health and disease)

---

block in the final year. Others have taken to building customized courses with an emphasis on specific components, e.g. basic science refreshers, developing professionalism skills such as teaching or leadership, or providing specific career-related preparation, for example surgical skills. The hospital and community sectors also have their responsibilities in ensuring that new graduates are prepared for practice. There are many examples of hospital-based induction and orientation programs, often with ongoing, continuing professional development, with some even offering protected time for education and training.

Teaching and learning of professionalism

This covers the domains of interpersonal skills, confidence and coping, collaboration and self-directed learning. Coates et al.[12] found that a mentoring scheme, where senior students were matched with mentors in their intended specialty in time to plan a well-rounded, elective schedule, helped students prepare adequately for residency selection. An important consideration for new doctors is dealing with stress. Leeder[13] notes that moving from medical school to the workplace is an important transition. Medical schools can only do so much and hospitals and community settings need to provide the appropriate training and support for interns. This is particularly important in an increasingly globalized world where students may work in a setting very different from the one in which they were trained. International Medical Graduates are an important cohort of newly qualified doctors. Medical schools can provide some preparation by taking a global health perspective in their curriculum,[14] and encouraging students to undertake some of their education in another country.

It is now recognized that there is a significant impact on students' learning through the 'informal curriculum.' This is the term used to describe the often unintentional lessons learned by students from everyday encounters in healthcare settings.[15, 16] Here medical students engage in complex, interpersonal dynamics with patients and their families, teachers and other healthcare staff. Concerns have been raised that the assimilation of this rich experience into evolving clinical practice has been neglected because of a prevailing focus on the formal curriculum,[16] which is the "stated, intended and formally offered and endorsed curriculum." Critical to this assimilation are professional role models, some of whom can be supportive and constructive, but sadly in some cases uncaring and destructive. Professionalism in medicine has many facets, but all doctors must take responsibility for their role-modeling behavior and reflect on its effects on others. Medical students must try and seek out positive role models and not always expect to be sought out. It is particularly important for newly qualified doctors to have good role models.

Facilitating clinical competence and performance

This covers patient management and practical skills. Much of the literature assumes a generalist type of internship in internal medicine or primary care. Specifically, surgical internships have focused on practical skills; for example, dedicated skills courses may help to prepare senior medical students for surgical internships.[17,18] However, many medical students are undecided about their future medical career even at this stage.

The old adage that assessment drives learning means that medical school assessment strategies are important in shaping how students prepare in their senior years for practice. There has been international recognition that work-based assessment strategies may have a significant role in providing authentic clinical situations where students can be observed during a relatively short encounter. There are many reasons why medical educators have challenged traditional competency-based assessments on the grounds of subjectivity with regard to marking and lack of similarity to everyday practice. For example, the Long Case and the Objective Structured Clinical Examination (OSCE) assess a student at the level of 'shows how' in Miller's pyramid,[19] rather than at the level of 'does;' i.e., they are assessing competence rather than performance. There is a gap between competence and performance,[20] and while testing for competence may be appropriate for junior clerkships, senior clerkships should include an element of work-based assessment in preparation for working as an intern.

The tools all have in common the notion that in order to assess the capability of the student in some domain, e.g. clinical performance, there needs to be multiple ratings on multiple occasions by multiple raters. Particular examples already used in both student and postgraduate settings include the Mini Clinical Evaluation Exercise (Mini-Cex)[21] and multi-source feedback.[22] There is now good evidence of their validity, reliability, feasibility and acceptability to students and staff.

In suggesting that newly graduated doctors lack medical knowledge, the issue is often more of the application of that knowledge and the demonstration of sound clinical reasoning skills. Thus, typically, a clinical supervisor might suggest that a new intern was not able to give a short and focused summary of history, examination, differential diagnosis and proposed management plan following a patient encounter. To give an example of how students' clinical reasoning skills might be developed in the clinical environment, there are various brief educational strategies designed to encourage them to present their case summary to the clinical tutor in a succinct and reasoned way. One example is SNAPPS[23] (an acronym for S – summarize the case, N – narrow the differential, A – analyze the differential, P – probe the preceptor, P – plan management, S – select an issue for self directed learning), which is a brief intervention developed to support the clinical reasoning of medical students. In a SNAPPS session, students would recognize their learning needs in relation to clinical cases that they have seen, be encouraged by their tutor to justify their differential diagnosis or management plan, and then go and look up the things they did not know to encapsulate their clinical knowledge. This repeated and deliberate practice would be expected to lead to a better demonstration of their clinical knowledge, particularly in critical care situations after graduation.

How much basic science is enough?
A solid foundation in the basic mechanisms of basic sciences is essential for sound clinical reasoning. Internationally, regulatory bodies have attempted to cut down the number of facts that medical students need to learn, with an emphasis on promoting an understanding of key mechanisms. Traditional schools that emphasis a Flexnerian[24] pre-clinical/clinical divide may find their students do well on written knowledge tests, but are still unable to integrate their basic science with the history, examination and differential diagnosis at the bedside. Some medical schools try to ensure they maintain a vertical theme of case-based learning. Alternative approaches to integrating science with clinical competence include refresher courses, for example in anatomy.[25]

Community-engaged education
An appreciation for holistic care is problematic where the student spends his/her senior years in a number of short subspecialty attachments. Increasingly, it has been recognized that it is important for students to follow the pathway of care from the community through the acute episode and back into the community. This is a way of understanding how the complexity of medical care is organized, and socializes medical students into the realities of the clinical environment. Longer term, integrated attachments, where students may cover three or more discipline areas, for example medicine, surgery, and primary and community care, in one block of 24 weeks instead of three separate blocks of eight weeks, are thought to promote such holistic attitudes in students. Krupat et al.[26] describe an example which embodies some of these approaches. Longitudinal clinical clerkships were created in which learners spent their entire clerkship in a single setting. A 'longitudinal pedagogy' was adopted to allow for long-term relationships with patients

and families, sustained relationships with faculty members that promote mentorship and feedback, opportunities to work and learn in teams and to process experience through reflection, writing and group support, and opportunities to become meaningfully involved in the work of the community.

Public health

Modern healthcare professionals are faced with a plethora of public health challenges. There have been international concerns over the skills of newly graduated doctors and the need to appropriately train public health workforces. Accordingly, there have been several calls for curriculum innovation in this field. Medical students' attitudes toward epidemiology suggest that although they may find this topic dry, boring and difficult to understand, they appear to appreciate its relevance to clinical practice as they pass further through their medical degree course.[27] That said, evidence from studies of the skills of evidence-based medicine (EBM) demonstrates that newly qualified doctors are lacking in such skills. Several schools are encouraged to look at how they deliver EBM teaching to ensure a commitment to integrated best evidence at the point of care.

There is a relative paucity of information as to how medical schools go about arranging their health promotion teaching.[28] There have been some innovative curriculum developments around issues of social accountability, largely in rural and community-engaged settings, so far. Universities need to be socially accountable, defined by the World Health Organisation (WHO) as the obligation to direct their education, research and service activities towards addressing the priority health concerns of the community, region and/or nation they have a mandate to serve.[29] In practice, medical schools can ensure that their learning outcomes encompass regional and national priorities. It is apparent from reviewing global priorities, for example in cardiovascular health and diabetes, that significant impact may be made in attending to lifestyle interventions in smoking, obesity and diet. However, many medical educators would see a more important aspect of public health, not mentioned in the PHPQ scale in Figure 34.1, as that of patient safety. It is unfortunate that a small number of newly qualified doctors will make errors in judgment, resulting in a significant adverse event for the patient. Many medical schools are considering how they can build patient safety into their curricula. One example of the guidance available is the WHO patient safety curriculum,[30] which has many useful resources that medical educators can adapt for local issues and concerns.

Conclusion

Medical schools have a duty to prepare students for practice in the clinical workforce. This does not exclusively refer to the intern year, but more to laying down a foundation for lifelong learning, a commitment to providing safe, effective and compassionate care, and an ability to look after one's self in demanding working conditions. Internationally, there is a need to strengthen quality assurance of medical education, adopt curriculum frameworks for pre-vocational training tied to robust assessment, foster frameworks for the governance of pre-vocational training, and for medical school curricula to refine their learning outcomes so that they align with those of the intern year. There is a need for ongoing curricular reform to ensure monitoring of the often repeated gaps in interns: self-reflection, poor organizational skills, underdeveloped professionalism, and lack of medical knowledge. Areas which seem to have a good basis of evidence include the teaching and learning of professionalism, particularly around positive role modeling, work-based assessment, vertical integration of science, clinical competence through case-based clinical reasoning, longitudinal integrated placements both in metropolitan and rural areas, systematic teaching of clinical skills, and the integration of patient safety. Areas for which there is a theoretical case but less evidence include moving public health to a socially accountable model, focusing on national and regional concerns. How much science seems a vexatious debate, and the anatomy question[25] will probably never go away as a rule of thumb for seniors to measure the quality and preparedness of their juniors.

References

1. Lyss-Lerman P, Teherani A, Aagaard E, Loeser H, Cooke M, Harper GM. What Training is Needed in the Fourth Year of Medical School? Views of Residency Program Directors. *Acad Med.* 2009; 84(7): 823–829. 10.1097/ACM.0b013e3181a82426.

2. Dean SJ, Barratt AL, Hendry GD, Lyon PM. Preparedness for Hospital Practice among Graduates of a Problem-based, Graduate-entry Medical Program. *Med J Aust.* 2003, Feb 17; 178(4): 163–166.

3. Evans DE, Roberts CM. Preparation for Practice: How can Medical Schools Better Prepare PRHOs? *Med Teach.* 2006, Sep; 28(6): 549–552.

4. Flexner A. Medical Education in the United States and Canada: A Report to the Carnegie Foundation for the Advancement of Teaching. New York, NY: *Carnegie Foundation for the Advancement of Teaching*, 1910.

5. Bray M, Borevskaya N. Financing Education in Transitional Societies: Lessons from Russia and China. *Comp Educ.* 2001; 37(3): 345–365.

6. Al-Moamary MS, Mamede S, Schmidt HG. Innovations in Medical Internship: Benchmarking and Application within the King Saud bin Abdulaziz University for Health Sciences. *Educ Health (Abingdon).* 2010, Apr; 23(1): 367.

7. Goroll AH, Sirio C, Duffy FD, LeBlond RF, Alguire P, Blackwell TA et al. A New Model for Accreditation of Residency Programs in Internal Medicine. *Ann Intern Med.* 2004, June 1;140(11): 902–909.

8. Frank JR, Danoff D. The CanMEDS Initiative: Implementing an Outcomes-based Framework of Physician Competencies. *Med Teach.* 2007; 29(7): 642–647.

9. Graham IS, Gleason AJ, Keogh GW, Paltridge D, Rogers IR, Walton M et al. Australian Curriculum Framework for Junior Doctors. *Med J Aust.* 2007, Apr 2; 186(7 Suppl): S14–S19.

10. Beard J, Strachan A, Davies H, Patterson F, Stark P, Ball S et al. Developing an Education and Assessment Framework for the Foundation Programme. *Med Educ.* 2005; 39(8): 841–851.

11. Hill J, Rolfe IE, Pearson SA, Heathcote A. Do Junior Doctors Feel they are Prepared for Hospital Practice? A Study of Graduates from Traditional and Non-traditional Medical Schools. *Med Educ.* 1998, Jan; 32(1): 19–24.

12. Coates WC, Crooks K, Slavin SJ, Guiton G, Wilkerson L. Medical School Curricular Reform: Fourth-year Colleges Improve Access to Career Mentoring and Overall Satisfaction. *Acad Med.* 2008; 83(8): 754–760. 10.1097/ACM.0b013e31817eb7dc.

13. Leeder S. Preparing interns for practice in the 21st century. *Med J Aus.* 2007; 186: S6–S8.

14. Drain PK, Primack A, Hunt DD, Fawzi WW, Holmes KK, Gardner P. Global Health in Medical Education: A Call for More Training and Opportunities. *Acad Med.* 2007; 82(3): 226–230. 10.1097/ACM.0b013e3180305cf9.

15. Stern DT. In Search of the Informal Curriculum: When and Where Professional Values are Taught. *Acad Med.* 1998, Oct; 73(10 Suppl): S28–S30.

16. Hafferty FW. Beyond Curriculum Reform: Confronting Medicine's Hidden Curriculum. *Acad Med.* 1998, Apr; 73(4): 403–407.

17. Zeng W, Woodhouse J, Brunt LM. Do Preclinical Background and Clerkship Experiences Impact Skills Performance in an Accelerated Internship Preparation Course for Senior Medical Students? *Surgery.* 2010; 148(4): 768–777.

18. Brunt LM, Halpin VJ, Klingensmith ME, Tiemann D, Matthews BD, Spitler JA et al. Accelerated Skills Preparation and Assessment for Senior Medical Students Entering Surgical Internship. *J Am Coll Surg.* 2008; 206(5): 897–904.

19. Miller GE. The Assessment of Clinical Skills/Competence/Performance. *Acad Med.* 1990; 65(9): S63–S67.

20. Rethans JJ, Norcini JJ, Barón-Maldonado M, Blackmore D, Jolly BC, LaDuca T et al. The Relationship between Competence and Performance: Implications for Assessing Practice Performance. *Med Educ.* 2002; 36(10): 901–909.

21. Norcini JJ. Work Based Assessment. *BMJ.* 2003, April 5; 326(7392): 753–755.

22. Davies H, Archer J. Multi Source Feedback: Development and Practical Aspects. *Teach.* 2005; 2(2): 77–81.

23. Wolpaw TM, Wolpaw DR, Papp KK. SNAPPS: A Learner-centered Model for Outpatient Education. *Acad Med.* 2003; 78(9): 893–898.

24. Cooke M, Irby DM, Sullivan W, Ludmerer KM. American Medical Education 100 Years after the Flexner Report. *N Engl J Med.* 2006; 355(13): 1339–1344.

25. Bergman EM, Prince KJAH, Drukker J, van der Vleuten CPM, Scherpbier AJJA. How Much Anatomy is Enough? *Anat Sci Educ.* 2008; 1(4): 184–188.

26. Krupat E, Pelletier S, Alexander EK, Hirsh D, Ogur B, Schwartzstein R. Can Changes in the Principal Clinical Year Prevent the Erosion of Students' Patient-centered Beliefs? *Acad Med.* 2009, May; 84(5): 582–586.

27. Moffat M, Sinclair HK, Cleland JA, Smith WC, Taylor RJ. Epidemiology Teaching: Student and Tutor Perceptions. *Med Teach.* 2004, Dec; 26(8): 691–695.

28. Wylie A, Thompson S. Establishing Health Promotion in the Modern Medical Curriculum: A Case Study. *Med Teach.* 2007, Oct; 29(8): 766–771.

29. Boelen C, Woollard B. Social Accountability and Accreditation: A New Frontier for Educational Institutions. *Med Educ.* 2009; 43(9): 887–894.

30. Walton M, Woodward H, Van Staalduinen S, Lemer C, Greaves F, Noble D et al. The WHO Patient Safety Curriculum Guide for Medical Schools. *Qual Saf Health Care.* 2010, Dec 1; 19(6): 542–546.

Chapter 35

Developing a Career as a Medical Educator

Julie Browne and Jamie Read

Objectives

- The objective of this chapter is to introduce medical students and junior doctors to medical education as a possible career choice.
- The authors outline ways in which medical students can become involved in their own education and that of others. They describe the Academy of Medical Educators' *Professional Standards* which sets out a curriculum for the study and practice of medical education, and discuss the steps medical students and junior doctors can take to improve their skills and knowledge of medical education.

"In this life, we want nothing but Facts, sir; nothing but Facts!" The speaker, and the schoolmaster, and the third grown person present, all backed a little, and swept with their eyes the inclined plane of little vessels then and there arranged in order, ready to have imperial gallons of facts poured into them until they were full to the brim.

Charles Dickens, *Hard Times* (p 47)[1]

How is medical education changing?

The traditional view of medical teaching is that it involves a teacher transmitting knowledge into the heads of the students.[2] The clinical teacher is seen as the source of knowledge, information, skills and values and is the role model whom the students are expected to follow obediently.

In recent decades, this 'transmission' approach to education has been challenged because it ignores the place of both the student and the patient in medical learning. It has been criticized, particularly because medicine is changing so quickly that even if a medical student were capable of learning everything that is known about the practice of medicine today, much of that knowledge would be obsolete within a short time. To respond to this challenge, a more active, collaborative, student-centered approach has been advanced by educational theorists.

Such an approach, designed to encourage students to take more responsibility for their own learning and to continue to learn throughout their working lives, is now in widespread use in medical schools across the world.[3,4]

We hope that reading through this book will have given you a better insight into how these modern perspectives on medical teaching and learning are influencing your education as a doctor. Each chapter will have shown you how, using a variety of techniques and methods, your tutors and lecturers are trying, not just to teach you facts, but to inspire you to learn more for yourself, to become an active participant not just in your own learning but also in the education of others, and to develop professional attitudes, skills and habits that will be of lifelong use to you as a medical practitioner, benefiting the patients with whom you will come into contact with throughout your career.

Do students teach as well as learn?

It is easy as a student to forget how much influence you can have on the learning of others in your daily life.

To learn effectively in medicine, you need to interact with a wide variety of people. As you are learning from them, they will also learn from you. Consider the following extracts from the diary of Saira, a medical student:

> I haven't really enjoyed my obstetrics placement very much so far. The clinics are so busy, everyone seems terribly overworked and I felt as if I was in the way. I finally got up the courage to talk to one of the residents about how I could make more of a contribution and he said he'd bring it up with the other staff on the ward.
>
> The ethics assignment was really thought provoking. Maria and I spent ages over lunch discussing the various scenarios.
>
> Dr Hegazy's hematology lectures are useful, but there's always far too much to take in. Hana and I have decided to compare notes afterwards to see what we missed. Then we can ask Dr Hegazy about it at the tutorial.
>
> I had to ask Dr Ahmed what he'd written on the feedback form because I couldn't read his writing. He was very nice about it and said he'd use the online forms in future.
>
> The renal unit was quite quiet today, so I asked if I could sit and talk to some of the dialysis patients for my case study. The patients taught me loads about how kidney disease affects their daily lives and they said they had enjoyed talking to a medical student.
>
> One of the children didn't want to have his stitches covered with a dressing, so I let him stick some surgical tape on me to show it didn't hurt!

Saira may not be entirely aware of it, but in all of these examples she is actually teaching as she is learning. She is having a constructive effect on the people around her. She is asking polite and relevant questions, encouraging and helping others to learn, giving feedback and influencing the way teaching and learning happens in her medical school. By taking responsibility for her own learning and that of others, Saira is already modeling some of the key roles she will have to fulfill during her career as a doctor.

One of the key things to remember as a student is that learning and teaching do not always take the form of a lecture or structured teaching with patients at the bedside. All experience within the clinical setting is both an opportunity to teach and learn, and often you will be quite unaware that this is even happening!

Teaching as a doctor will also be a vital part of the care that you provide to patients. As a doctor you are often going to know more than your patients about the diseases and conditions that they have. Being able to teach patients about their conditions, how they are managed and the preventative measures that they can take to improve their health, is going to be an important part of being a doctor, and therefore, acquiring these skills will be vital during your time at medical school. Teaching can be especially valuable in helping to cement your own knowledge. Students often find that once they have taught a topic they are able both to remember and to apply it more easily, improving their own skills and knowledge as a doctor as well as benefiting those that they have taught.

How can students get more formally involved in teaching?

Students are taught, of course, but they also teach and contribute to the education going on around them by getting involved in learning. Deliberate practice as a medical educator starts at medical school, so make the most of learning and teaching opportunities.[5] There are often opportunities to become more involved in groups and organizations that are involved in teaching others, especially medical students in years below you at medical school.

Many medical schools offer all sorts of formal and informal opportunities to get involved in teaching; for example:

- Get involved in the life of your medical school. Many medical students feel that they need to study all the time, but learning and teaching are not always solitary or static activities. Your medical school may have journal clubs, study groups, and special interest societies such as an anatomy or surgery group, a student parliament or medical society and a whole range of other opportunities for learning and teaching. Some medical schools have staff–student liaison groups where students are encouraged to comment on and contribute to the curriculum. If your medical school does not offer these types of opportunities, why not start a group of your own, either formally or informally?
- Peer support. Talk to your fellow students about the course, what improvements could be made, what is particularly challenging and what you feel is going well. Help other students where you can. Teaching is about being a good colleague and encouraging those who are having difficulties.

- Small-group learning offers excellent opportunities to practice your teaching skills and to see how others do it too. Next time you are in a small group, think about what is going on within the group. Some participants have characteristics that make their contributions particularly helpful. What are these, and what qualities do you, yourself, bring to a successful group?
- Presentations. Many students find presentations hard, but the more you do them the better you will become. Take opportunities to practice your presentation skills. Observe how other people make presentations and think about what they are doing particularly well and what could be improved. Remember that presentation skills are exceptionally useful in all areas of medicine and that getting good at presenting early on will make your life much easier.
- Posters and abstracts. You may be lucky enough to attend a medical school which offers you opportunities to showcase your work in more formal settings. Writing posters and abstracts is part of the role of the medical academic. Why not seek out opportunities to publish your work more widely?
- Start writing! Many medical students keep portfolios, but they also produce blogs and diaries, and some even contribute to journals, websites and magazines such as *Student BMJ* or *Medical Student Newspaper*. Preparing an original piece of writing is an excellent way of learning new material, but it can also have a valuable teaching function for those who read it.

Lots of ideas for how you can improve your learning and teaching skills are described in this book. Look through it and think about what you can do to make yourself a better teacher.

How can medical students and junior doctors become medical teachers?

In the following case study, medical student Jamie Read describes how his interest in the education he is receiving has blossomed into an interest in being an educator himself.

Case study:

Jamie Read is a final-year medical student studying at the Peninsula Medical School in the UK. His involvement in medical education started through becoming involved in student representation with his Student Parliament. This role involved teaching both his peers and members of medical school staff about important issues, and also gave an insight into the inner workings of medical education. From here, Jamie began working for the UK General Medical Council, assessing other medical schools to check that the graduates that they produce are both competent and confident to be doctors. This involvement later introduced Jamie to the Academy of Medical Educators and a presentation at a national conference about the importance of medical education to medical students and ensuring that the student voice is always considered in the development of medical schools.

Jamie says: These experiences that I have had as a student have been provided through my interest in medical education. This is an ever-expanding international speciality in medicine that allows you not only to further your own education but also the education of others. The skills that such involvement produces are invaluable and also transferable to many areas of being a good doctor. Medical education is also an exceptionally friendly area of medicine and I have found everyone involved to be very supportive, which has greatly assisted my development as a medical student as well as a medical educator. I would definitely recommend exploring this area of medicine and examining how you could become involved within your own medical school.

If you get actively involved in your medical education you may, like Jamie, find that your interest in learning, coupled with your enjoyment in teaching, stimulates you into thinking about making medical education a major part of your career as a doctor.

The next step in developing a career as a medical teacher is to make some deliberate moves into education. Teaching has often been seen as just another of those things that doctors do as part of their overall professional duties, but we hope we have shown that medical education has in recent years become a real career choice for doctors. With study, practice and experience, all practitioners can improve their skills in teaching to the benefit of both students and patients. As a result of this new understanding of the importance of developing skills in medical education,[6] opportunities are emerging for doctors who wish to make teaching a significant part of their careers – and you can even make a start while still at medical school. For example, some medical schools offer special study modules and even the opportunity to undertake intercalated degrees in medical education. Junior doctors may get opportunities to do rotations in medical education and some may work towards certificates, diplomas and even higher degrees in medical education. In the UK, the National Institute for Health Research supports academic clinical fellows and clinical lecturers who want to develop their research skills in medical education. There is a wide variety of short training courses and conferences offering professional development in areas such as simulation, assessment and appraisal. Specialty boards and professional organizations are now offering 'train the trainers' courses for those who are delivering continuing professional education, and in some specialties these courses are mandatory. There is a multitude of interest groups and learned societies for those who want to know more about teaching in medicine and who wish to develop a special interest in a particular area of medical education, such as simulation or assessment, and all welcome interested students to become involved from an early stage.

What is an excellent medical teacher?

The Academy of Medical Educators' *Professional Standards*

For the first time, a set of clear professional standards exists for those involved in the education of medical students and doctors, applicable to all medical educators, whatever the level or subject area they teach and wherever they are based.[7] The Academy of Medical Educators (AoME) was established in 2006 as a professional standard-setting body for medical educators, and, to this end, it has been working since its inception on developing a set of standards against which anyone involved in teaching medical students and doctors can measure their progress and plot their career development.

The *Professional Standards* are a tool designed to help medical educators to work towards excellence. They are necessary because medical teaching is not like other types of teaching in higher or professional education, as a consequence of the central place that patient care occupies not only in teaching and learning but also in assessment and feedback, and in quality assurance.

The Academy's *Standards* were developed through a long process of consultation in which over a hundred groups, individuals and organizations were asked for their views and feedback. As a result, they represent a real consensus on the essential skills, knowledge and attitudes a medical educator needs to have and are subdivided into a set of core values plus 5 domains:

- Domain 1 – *Design and planning of learning activities*
- Domain 2 – *Teaching and supporting learners*
- Domain 3 – *Assessment and feedback to learners*
- Domain 4 – *Educational research and evidence-based practice*
- Domain 5 – *Educational management and leadership*

All practicing medical educators are expected to have a commitment to the core values. Each of the five other domains is sub-divided into three levels and most medical educators will be able to demonstrate a range of attainments at various levels in some or all of these. A few exceptional individuals will have achievements at the very highest levels. The *Professional Standards* enable medical educators to map their professional progression at all stages of their career.

Why are the *Professional Standards* relevant to medical students?

If you read the *Standards*, you may be surprised to see that you are already working towards or have even reached level 1 standard for some items, especially if you have been actively involved in teaching at medical school. Even if you do not feel you are at this stage, but would like to start working towards level 1, you might still consider joining the Academy as an Associate Member, and in fact, many medical students have already done so.

The *Standards* are relevant to medical students who want to follow a career in medical education beyond the minimum requirements for professional practice, because they can act as a blueprint for your career as a teacher.

Summary

All doctors are expected to teach – they teach each other, they teach students and other healthcare professionals, and above all, they teach their patients. Learning to teach starts at medical school; because to be a good medical student is to be an active participant in the education that is going on all around you. Not all medical education is formal or even recognized for what it is, but anyone who is involved in teaching and assessment has a responsibility to reflect on his or her skills, to take time and opportunities to improve them and to seek feedback to improve quality. All medical students have unparalleled opportunities for learning and teaching if they make the most of them.

Some medical students find teaching so rewarding that they decide to take it further, but it is sometimes difficult to know what is expected of a good medical educator. To this end, the Academy of Medical Educators' *Professional Standards* can act as a guide to career development in the field.

References

1. Dickens, C. *Hard Times.* Harmondsworth: Penguin Books, 1980.
2. Bleakley A, Bligh J. Students Learning from Patients: Let's Get Real in Medical Education. *Adv Health Sci Educ* 2008; 13(1): 89–107.
3. Spencer J, Jordan R. Learner Centred Approaches in Medical Education. *BMJ* 1999: 318: 1280–1283.
4. Dacre J, Fox RA. How should we be teaching our Undergraduates? *Ann Rheum Dis* 2000; 59: 662–667.
5. Rodrigues J, Sengupta A, Ramoutar D, Maxwell S. Are UK Junior Doctors being taught to teach? *Med Educ* 2010; 44(3): 324.
6. GMC. *Tomorrow's Doctors.* London: General Medical Council, 2009.
7. Academy of Medical Educators. *Professional Standards 2012.* London: Academy of Medical Educators, 2012. Available for download from www.medicaleducators.org

IX

INTERNATIONAL STUDENT EDUCATION

Chapter 36

The International Federation of Medical Students' Associations (IFMSA)

"Think Globally, Act Locally"

Nayef Dajim and Robert J. Duvivier

Objectives

The aspiration of the organization is to serve medical students, in the Kingdom of Saudi Arabia in particular, by achieving the following goals:

- To represent the Kingdom of Saudi Arabia in the International Federation of Medical Students' Associations meetings and activities as well as taking part in other health or youth-related activities on the international level.
- To obtain growth and development of Saudi medical students' knowledge, attitude and practice on the personal, professional and social level within the cultural and traditional morals and to strengthen the bonds between students all over the kingdom.
- To emphasize cooperation and bonds between the students themselves, and to strengthen the ties between the students and the academic and administrative officers within the medical schools of the kingdom to create a suitable educational atmosphere.
- To empower the medical students to use their knowledge and capacities for the benefit of society through programmed activities and events.
- To allow medical students in Saudi Arabia to join the world debate on global health-related topics and to formulate policies from such discussions.
- To promote and facilitate professional and scientific exchanges, projects and extracurricular training for medical students, thereby sensitizing them to other cultures and societies and subsequently to their health problems.

- To link medical students in Saudi Arabia with the international medical community in order to increase the learning opportunities available to students and to allow them to communicate their knowledge and share their experiences with other medical institutions in the interest of the common goal.
- To develop leadership between the medical students as future community leaders; to give them a chance to responsibly express, exchange and even implement their best thoughts and ideas.

Introduction

The International Federation of Medical Students' Associations (IFMSA) is an independent, non-governmental and non-political medical student organization. Currently, IFMSA has 98 National Member Organizations (NMOs) from 91 countries on six continents and represents more than one million medical students worldwide. The IFMSA was founded in May 1951 and is run for and by medical students on a non-profit basis. It is officially recognized as a Non Governmental Organization (NGO) within the United Nations and recognized by the World Health Organization (WHO) as the international forum for medical students. It exists to serve medical students all over the world. IFMSA was established in the Netherlands as a charity organization.

In order to make its approach more organized, IFMSA created six standing committees as follows:

- Standing Committee on Medical Education (SCOME)
- Standing Committee on Public Health (SCOPH)
- Standing Committee on Reproductive Health and AIDS (SCORA)
- Standing Committee on Human Rights and Peace (SCORP)
- Standing Committee on Professional Exchanges (SCOPE)
- Standing Committee on Research Exchanges (SCORE)

Twice a year, more than 800 students from 91 countries hold two General Assemblies; the March Meeting (MM) and the August Meeting (AM), each lasting more than two weeks. These medical students from different backgrounds and schools participate with the aim of gaining experience and acting to make a change in medicine.

In these meetings, medical students run lectures, workshops, small working groups and training sessions. Moreover, they exchange ideas and projects that can be implemented in their own countries and start transnational positive approaches.

IFMSA – Saudi Arabia

The International Federation of Medical Students' Associations – Saudi Arabia (IFMSA-SA) is the first students' organization on the national level. It was founded at the beginning of 2007 and successfully obtained international official membership in the International Federation of Medical Students' Associations (IFMSA) in the UK in August 2007 as the Saudi national affiliate of this global well-known federation.

Mission

To create and sustain an environment whereby medical students become empowered and culturally sensitized to practically generate exchange and implement their outstanding ideas and thoughts regarding various health-related issues.

To provide comprehensive programing and opportunities on the national, regional and international scales for medical students to build their capacities, develop their schools, benefit their societies and interact positively with their counterparts around the globe.

Vision

Medical students are a powerful source of hope for the future and our vision is to use our medical training to benefit all members of society and with commitment to share our knowledge and skills internationally.

IFMSA's involvement in medical education

Medical education should be a concern of every medical student as it shapes not only the quality of future doctors but also the quality of future healthcare. IFMSA has a dedicated working group of enthusiastic medical students who aim to implement an optimal learning environment for all medical students around the world, known as the **Standing Committee on Medical Education (SCOME)**.

SCOME was one of IFMSA's first standing committees from the beginning of its foundation in 1951. It acts as a discussion forum for students interested in different aspects of medical education, and aims to achieve excellence in medical education throughout the world.

IFMSA in general and SCOME in particular work on two levels: *locally* and *nationally*.

Locally

The most promising strategy for change is a local approach. Even if students do not have official representation within the faculty decision-making bodies, they could convince deans, professors and other stakeholders to develop their education. It may not be possible to change the whole curriculum at once; however, small changes in each of the different subjects will slowly but steadily improve the curriculum as a whole.

To enable local IFMSA officers to facilitate improvements in their own institutions or country, the main activities within SCOME are training sessions. Training covers all fields within medical education, such as assessments, evaluation, and problem-based learning.

Tasks of SCOME

- Provide training on relevant topics.
- Facilitate discussions between students and faculty.
- Participate in evaluation of medical education.
- Collect local students' opinions and review and consider them for applicability or implementation.
- Set up related projects such as seminars, courses, conferences and workshops.
- Represent students in faculty/university boards and committees.

One example of IFMSA's activities is the SCOME-Wikipedia. This project aims to share ideas, to describe, and to discuss latest developments in the field of medical education worldwide. Medical students are invited to contribute on relevant topics, such as the educational system, admission criteria for studying medicine or the different faculties in their country.

For more information log-on to http://wiki.ifmsa.org/scome

Internationally

IFMSA cooperates with organizations in the field of medical education in order to represent students' voices on an international level. These initiatives often find their way back to the national and local level.

Currently, IFMSA is represented on the executive board by the Association for Medical Education in Europe (AMEE) and in the council of the World Federation of Medical Education (WFME).

AMEE promotes scholarship in medical education and hosts the largest educational research conference in the world to share developments in the field of health professionals' education.

WFME is the global organization concerned with medical education and training of medical doctors as well as undergraduate students. WFME serves as an umbrella organization for six regional organizations for medical education. IFMSA works actively together with the regional associations for medical education in the future development of medical training.

Standing committee on medical education in Saudi Arabia

Realizing the importance of this standing committee to address many curricular gaps as well as all student-related concerns, SCOME-SA is dedicated to make safe those doctors who are able to make a change in medicine. SCOME-SA has continued and developed the same tasks as SCOME.

SCOME-SA has initiated its approach at the national level by starting with nine faculties of medicine. In each faculty we have a Local Officer on Medical Education (LOME) who conducts projects, ideas and suggestions to and from his/her faculty.

Within a span of one year, SCOME-SA has achieved many projects that have left a positive impact on the process of medical education nationally and internationally. This was made possible through teamwork and organizing targets according to action plans.

Some of the projects currently running at local, national or international levels are:

- **PASS (all levels)**
  PASS stands for "Professional and Academic Support for Students." It is the first international project for SCOME-SA with a broad comprehensive approach that aims to fill defects in the curricula by running full-day courses on a weekly basis. It carries very important medical educational themes (e.g. Psychomotor, effective and knowledge). It is purely conducted by medical students for medical students. There is also an annual calendar of all courses running in the kingdom. Also, we act in parallel with the international day's events. Topics, for example, are: Art of Antibiotics, World Diabetes Day, TB day, Basics of Radiology, SPSS, and ECG.
- **Hi Tech Dr Club (all levels)**
  Information technology is changing tremendously every day, and a big chunk of that concerns medicine. We believe that medical students have to be highly skilled in all aspects related to medicine in terms of technology. Through this project we aim to standardize the current medical students' (future doctors') awareness of these changes and to keep pace with its importance in medicine. Ultimately, we expect these students to participate in medicine significantly in the future.
- **Abroad Prep Club (APC, local level)**
  As time passes, the chance for medical students to apply abroad is getting difficult and challenging. Moreover, it requires students to fulfill a number of obligations and requisites to succeed in getting acceptance. BPC aims to help prepare students to have the international exams before they graduate: USMLE[1], PLAB[2], AMC[3], TOEFL. These exams will help students to review their basic sciences level and work on their weaknesses to make them better doctors in the future.
- **Interns Future Day (national level)**
  This is a one-day course, where students in their final year and interns go through different themes important for them to address before they graduate

---

[1] United States Medical Licensing Examination.
[2] Professional and Linguistic Assessment Board, UK.
[3] Australian Medical Council.

or even apply for residency – for example, how to prepare a CV, passing interviews, specialties tutorials.

- **Reading Club (local level)**
  This club aims to widen students' horizons by encouraging them to look at things differently and subsequently reflect on their mental ability to regard medicine in a different and effective manner, and to invent or improve current practice or science.

Other standing committees in IFMSA – Saudi Arabia

Standing Committee on Public Health (SCOPH)

SCOPH-SA is the first national committee to serve all medical students across the kingdom, providing a strong dynamic base where they can begin their active role in the community.

Active medical students used to face great difficulties when starting a new project and their work was hardly ever appreciated. SCOPH-SA's greatest aim is to facilitate the work of future doctors.

Standing Committee on Human Rights and Peace (SCORP)

SCORP and IFMSA have arranged a number of successful workshops and international projects that give medical students the opportunity to work alongside non-governmental organizations towards the improvement of specific situations.

SCORP offers global peace and defines human rights by acting locally in our community with various activities:

- Fundraising
- Workshops
- Exhibitions
- Lectures
- Campaigns

SCORP aims to:

- Educate people and encourage their human nature to turn our world into a peaceful place for all of us.
- Make the difference in our community that leads to a peaceful place on earth.
- Act together to make the world one peaceful community.
- As medical students and health professionals, achieve good health in our area as part of a healthy planet.
- Erase the word "violation" from our dictionary, and replace it by the word "protection."

Standing Committee on Global Opportunities (SCOGO)

In addition to exchange programs (professional and research), SCOGO's main concern is to open the eyes of medical students in Saudi Arabia towards a better horizon. Students are given the chance to participate in any opportunity that would improve their personality in all aspects, whether improving their medical, professional or social skills, and to keep abreast with the world.

SCOGO also helps students to get in touch with other medical students from all over the world to exchange and share their own experiences.

Also, it is our duty to show the world that medical students in Saudi Arabia are competent and can succeed anywhere they are placed, if given the chance.

Index